BONE

Volume 5: Fracture Repair
and Regeneration

BONE

Volume 5: Fracture Repair and Regeneration

Brian K. Hall
Department of Biology
Dalhousie University
Halifax, Nova Scotia
Canada

CRC Press
Boca Raton Ann Arbor London

Library of Congress Cataloging-in-Publication Data
(Revised for volume 5)

Bone.

   Includes bibliographical references and index.
   Contents: v. 1. The osteoblast and osteocyte — v. 2. The osteoclast —
   v. 3. Bone matrix and bone specific products — v. 4. Bone metabolism and
   mineralization — v. 5. Fracture repair and regeneration.
   1. Bones. I. Hall, Brian Keith, 1941–
[DNLM: 1. Bone and Bones.   WE 200/B7113]
QP88.2.B58   1991   599′.01852   89-20391
ISBN 0-93692-324-5 (v. 1)
ISBN 0-8493-8822-8 (v. 2)
ISBN 0-8493-8823-6 (v. 3)
ISBN 0-8493-8824-4 (v. 4)
ISBN 0-8493-8825-2 (v. 5)

Developed by Telford Press

This book represents information obtained from authentic and highly regarded
sources. Reprinted material is quoted with permission, and sources are indicated. A
wide variety of references are listed. Every reasonable effort has been made to give
reliable data and information, but the author and the publisher cannot assume
responsibility for the validity of all materials or for the consequences of their use.

Preface

This is the fifth of seven volumes devoted to bone. The impetus for initiating this series was to fill the need for an up-to-date, comprehensive, and authoritative treatment of all aspects of bone. Cartilage has been covered in the three volume series, *Cartilage* (Hall, 1983), and in *Cartilage: Molecular Aspects* (Hall and Newman, 1991), published by CRC Press in 1991.

The seven volumes in this series are organized thematically, each volume integrating structure, function, biochemistry, metabolism, and the molecular and clinical aspects of a particular aspect of the biology of bone. The chapters are written by authors actively engaged in basic, applied, and/or clinical research upon bone, ensuring that each chapter is both authoritative and up-to-date.

Bone-forming cells were covered in *Volume 1: The Osteoblast and Osteocyte.* The second volume, *The Osteoclast,* dealt with bone-resorbing cells, both multicellular osteoclasts that resorb the mineral and organic phases of bone, and mononuclear cells that resorb only the latter. The third volume, *Bone Matrix and Bone Specific Products,* extended coverage from bone-forming and -resorbing cells to the synthesis of bone specific products and their deposition into the extracellular matrix. Volume 4, *Bone Metabolism and Mineralization,* summarized the current status of knowledge on bone metabolism and mineralization of the bone matrix. Volume 5, *Fracture Repair and Regeneration,* treats the dual processes of repair of complete fractures of bones and the potential for regeneration of lost skeletal units, from regeneration of microfractures to the replacement of complete skeletal elements.

This volume begins with a comprehensive analysis of the metabolism of the fracture callus. This chapter provides a link between the metabolic studies on normal bone described in Volumes 1, 2, and 4 and the remaining chapters on repair and regeneration in Volume 5. Activation of the pentose-phosphate shunt, NADPH, pentose sugars, and the vitamin K cycle are crucial for formation and mineralization of the fracture callus. The potential role of vitamins B6 and K in activating delayed healing are discussed.

The second chapter discusses the stress dependence of tissues of synovial joints, a dependence that is manifest both in maintenance of normal joint homeostasis and in the processes needed to regain homeostasis during repair. Both basic studies on mechanical stimuli as signals to cell receptors and the clinical application of principles of stress dependence are discussed.

The theme of stress dependence in fracture repair is continued in Chapter 3 in the context of macromolecular synthesis. Biochemical and tissue heterogeneity follow mechanical instability at a fracture site. Why non-unions do not progress beyond the stage of fibrous repair is discussed in this context.

The potential use of cultured cells to augment repair and/or regeneration is discussed in Chaper 4. Such "cell therapy" requires the knowledge of metabolism and macromolecular synthesis discussed in Chapters 1 and 3 and will be an important adjunct to the use of implants as discussed in Chapter 5. The important issues of the integration of grafted cells and mechanical stability of the resulting repaired skeletal site are discussed in these two chapters.

Chapter 6 provides an evaluation of the use of bone inductive molecules to initiate and/or enhance repair and regeneration. Clearly, we are approaching the time when an integration of knowledge of implant vehicle (Chapter 5), cells (Chapter 4), and molecules (Chapter 6) will enable us to engineer precise physical-cellular-molecular systems for bone repair.

With Chapter 7 we move into three chapters devoted explicitly to bone regeneration. Limb lengthening is the topic of Chapter 7, a chapter that includes a discussion of growth plate morphology, distraction, and how growth plates respond to trauma. Whether the mammalian growth plate can be stimulated to regenerate is discussed in Chapter 8, and digital regeneration is discussed in Chapter 9.

The final chapter provides a discussion of bone formation in soft tissues. The rationale for including this topic is that knowledge of how cells can be stimulated to form ectopic or heterotopic bone aids the search for mechanisms to stimulate bone repair and regeneration within the skeleton.

In summary, Volume 5 provides a forward-looking review of prospects for the repair and regeneration of bone. The treatment of metabolic, mechanical, macromolecular, inductive, and therapeutic factors provides a compendium of the approaches most likely to increase the prospects for bone repair and regeneration.

Brian K. Hall
Halifax, 1991

The Editor

Brian K. Hall, Ph.D., D.Sc., is Izaak Walton Killam Research Professor in the Department of Biology, Faculty of Science, Dalhousie University, Halifax, N. S., Canada. He also holds an appointment as Professor of Physiotherapy, Faculty of Health Professions, Dalhousie University.

Professor Hall received his B.Sc. (Hons.) degree in 1965, his Ph.D. in Zoology in 1969, and a D.Sc. in Biological Sciences in 1978 from the University of New England, Armidale, N.S.W., Australia. He was appointed a Teaching Fellow in the Department of Zoology, UNE in 1965, Assistant Professor in the Department of Biology, Dalhousie University in 1968, Associate Professor in 1972, Professor in 1975, and Killam Research Professor in 1990. He served as Chair of the Biology Department, Dalhousie University from 1978 to 1985.

Professor Hall is a Fellow of the Royal Society of Canada and a member of the American Society of Zoologists, International Society for Differentiation, British Society for Developmental Biology, International Society for Developmental Biology, Society of Vertebrate Palaeontology, The Bone and Tooth Society, and the British Connective Tissue Society. He is an editor of *Anatomy and Embryology*, editorial board member of the *Journal of Craniofacial Genetics and Developmental Biology*, international advisory board member of the *Croatian Medical Journal*, past associate editor of the *Canadian Journal of Zoology*, and a past member of the advisory editorial board of *Bone*.

Professor Hall has worked on the development and differentiation of cartilage and bone for 25 years. He has presented invited lectures at international meetings and symposia and guest lectures at universities and institutes. He is the author or coauthor of 5 books, 130 papers in referenced scientific journals, and many chapters in edited works or conference proceedings. He edited a 3-volume series on cartilage (1983) and is coeditor of *Cartilage: Molecular Aspects* published by CRC Press in 1991. The current focus of his research is on the development and evolution of neural crest-derived craniofacial cartilage and bone.

Contents

1

Metabolism of the Fracture Callus

JANE DUNHAM
Division of Cellular Biology
The Mathilda and Terence Kennedy Institute of Rheumatology
London, United Kingdom

Introduction

The metabolism of the fracture callus is studied with the ultimate aim of attaining the knowledge necessary to influence the healing process to advantage. This might mean accelerating or modifying the metabolism in order to prevent non-union or delayed union of the fractured bone, or the associated disorders of muscle wasting, fibrosis, and joint stiffness. Knowledge of the metabolism of calcified tissue in general is extremely limited when compared to that of other tissues. The reasons for this are twofold. First, the physical nature of bone, particularly of adult bone, has created technical difficulties in studying this tissue. This has previously meant either isolating the cells from the dense matrix, or modifying the matrix itself. Second, the fracture callus is composed of a heterogeneous population of cell types which is constantly changing.

For metabolic studies the cells of the callus should ideally be studied *in situ* and their biochemical characteristics related to the morphology of the fracture callus. In this way it is hoped that both the temporal and spatial pattern of fracture healing may be defined.

Techniques Available for Studying the Metabolism of the Fracture Callus

Biochemical Techniques

Adult mineralized tissue generally does not lend itself to biochemical analysis; consequently, most work has been restricted to fetal or neonatal tissue, or isolated cell preparations. Tissue or organ culture, most commonly of calvariae and limb long bones of fetal and neonatal mice and rats, was first initiated by Fell and Robison (1929), Fell and Canti (1932), and modified by Raisz (1965). Isolated bone cell techniques, again mainly from fetal calvariae, were developed on the premise that they could reveal more biochemical information on bone formation and resorption than the cells *in vivo* (Wong, 1980). This situation allows short term biochemical characterization of bone cells but has the disadvantage of being a non-physiologic environment, which may either lack or possess different factors from those found *in vivo*. The isolation of cells relies either on mechanical separation or the enzymatic digestion of periosteum or extracellular matrix. However, there may still be problems with heterogeneity since cells could well be at different stages of development. The problem of cell damage is particularly evident with osteoclasts which are easily damaged by crude collagenase (Silbermann and Maor, 1984). Methods have been developed for looking at the energy metabolism of mineralized tissue, but for this the cells have been removed from the region of the epiphyseal plate (Shapiro, 1984).

Fracture Callus

Although the fracture callus in the early stages of healing consists predominantly of soft tissue, biochemical analysis has been hampered by access to a sufficient weight of tissue composed of a homogeneous population of cells. As the fracture heals and woven bone fills the fracture gap, technical problems associated with handling adult bone are encountered. Even with sensitive microchemical techniques it is difficult to isolate a homogeneous population of cells containing the necessary 10^4 to 10^6 cells required for biochemical analysis. However, Kulhman and Bakowski (1975) have reported such microchemical techniques possible in rabbit fracture callus.

Histochemical Techniques

The main approach to studies on the metabolism of the fracture callus has hitherto been histochemical. However, the light microscopical identification of enzymes has been fraught with problems. First, there have been the technical difficulties inherent in sectioning mineralized tissue, and second, a problem common to all tissues, one of loss or diffusion of enzymes, cofactors, and activators from their original sites and the susceptibility of enzymes to histochemical procedures in general. Decalcification of bone has been a widespread procedure and is still often a prerequisite for certain histochemical demonstrations of enzymes (Sheehan and Hrapchack, 1980). The use of decalcifying agents at low pH often interferes with substrates and enzymes and may produce invalid results even in the case of nucleic acids or polysaccharides. The more favorable EDTA also has severe limitations, for example, interfering with both the alkaline and acid phosphatase reactions (Anderson, 1984). The decalcifying process is also a lengthy one when considering the retention of enzyme activity. Fixation, dehydration, and embedding are common histochemical procedures, and for histological appraisal, mineralized tissue prepared in this fashion may be excellent. However, for the demonstration of enzyme activity the techniques can significantly alter the nature of the tissue. For example, the use of alcohol, either as a fixative or in embedding, causes denaturation and alters lipid-protein bonds. Fixatives, by their very nature, react with the active sites of enzymes. Loss of enzymes after fixation has been well documented (e.g., Barka and Anderson, 1963; Chayen et al., 1973). Although more workers are attempting to use fresh mineralized tissue, concern over the lability of the soluble enzymes has meant the continued use of fixatives in this field. Given that the histochemical demonstration of enzymes may be possible, the technique has the major drawback in that assessment of whatever enzyme activity is expressed is still only qualitative. The results that are obtained need to be rigorously interpreted with strict controls to minimize the effects of any artefacts produced by histochemical procedures. In light of the limited scope for histochemical and biochemical analysis of the metabolism of mineralized tissues, a new approach to the subject seemed appropriate.

Quantitative Cytochemistry

The best known quantitative cytochemical techniques, and those of particular relevance to this chapter, are the chromogenic reactions for chemically active moieties and enzyme activities.

However, the methodology of cytochemistry is much more extensive (Chayen, 1984). The essence of the approach is to relate biochemical activity to histology using a non-disruptive technique. It is a particularly sensitive technique requiring small amounts of tissue and achieving accurate measurements per cell. The whole approach to quantitative cytochemistry is discussed by Chayen (1984) and Chayen and Bitensky (1987), and the methodology described fully by Chayen et al. (1991). A brief discussion of the techniques will be given here.

The Cytochemical Approach

Chilling and Sectioning of Tissue

The cellular biochemist requires tissue to be hardened for sectioning without the loss of material and chemical and enzyme activity, as can occur with many histological and histochemical procedures. "Freezing" the tissue is a suitable technique but this has to be done in such a way as to minimize ice formation and its consequent effects on the integrity of cellular membranes and organelles (Butcher and Chayen, 1968). The tissue is chilled by precipitate immersion in n-hexane at $-70°C$; once chilled it is not allowed to reach temperatures sufficient to cause ice crystal formation ($-15°C$). The tissue is sectioned on a cryostat microtome in a cabinet at $-25°C$ with the knife cooled with solid carbon dioxide. Transfer of the frozen section from the knife to the glass slide is achieved by bringing the slide close to the knife, and allowing the section to jump the gap. This "flash" dries the section, further preventing ice crystal formation in the tissue.

Validation of the chilling and sectioning procedures has been reported (Chayen and Bitensky, 1968). Ultrastructural evidence of the integrity of such sections has been reported for soft tissues (Altman and Barrnett, 1975; Zoller and Weisz, 1980) as well as for adult bone (Dodds et al., 1988).

The Use of Unfixed Sections

If fixation is used, as in many histochemical procedures, it is not unusual for a loss of 70% of enzyme activity to be found (Chayen et al., 1991). Moreover, the loss of nitrogenous material and soluble enzymes from unfixed sections during incubation has also been demonstrated by many workers (e.g., Jones, 1965; Gahan and Kalina, 1965). However, it was found (Altman and Chayen, 1965) that the use of suitable concentrations of a non-toxic colloid stabilizer, namely, polyvinyl alcohol (PVA), in the reaction medium could prevent this loss of material. The retention of soluble enzymes by various other colloid stabilizers has since been described (Butcher, 1971; Henderson et al., 1978; Altman, 1980).

Cytochemical Reactions

The cytochemical chromogenic reactions are similar to biochemical methods, the main difference being that the cytochemical colored reaction product must be precipitated at or close to the site of the active groups by which they are generated. The same stoichiometry and specificity are required for cytochemistry as for biochemistry. Where it has been applicable, comparisons between the two techniques have demonstrated that equivalent enzyme activity can be measured (Altman, 1969; Olsen *et al.*, 1981). The four essential types of cytochemical chromogenic reaction are (a) production of color in a structural component, e.g., Feulgen nuclear reaction for DNA; (b) simultaneous capture reactions, e.g., for alkaline phosphatase; (c) post coupling reactions, e.g., acid phosphatase; and (d) tetrazolium reactions, e.g., glucose 6-phosphate dehydrogenase. These and other cytochemical methods are discussed fully by Chayen *et al.* (1991).

Measurement of Enzyme Activity

The measurement of the chromophore produced by enzyme activity or by direct staining of the tissue is done with a microdensitometer, which is essentially a spectrophotometer built around a microscope. Most cytochemical reaction products are inhomogeneously distributed in the section, but this is overcome by light of the correct wavelength being passed across the region selected for measurement by means of a flying spot. This spot can be as small as the resolution of the microscope ensuring that each area that is measured is optically homogeneous. An optical mask is selected to define the cell or area to be measured, thus making it possible to correlate exactly the biochemical activity with detailed histology. A full discussion of microdensitometry is given by Bitensky (1980), and Chayen (1982).

Application of Quantitative Cytochemistry to Mineralized Tissue

The methodology and validity of the cytochemical approach has been well documented for soft tissues. Although in theory the advantages of the technique seemed particularly applicable to mineralized tissue, the problems of handling the tissue had to be overcome. Essential to the technique is the use of fresh, unfixed, undecalcified sections of bone.

Sectioning of Undecalcified Bone

The routine sectioning of undecalcified bone has been described by Johnstone (1979). Initially a Bright's cryostat fitted with a Jung 1130 rotary microtome was used. Since that time bone cutting cryostats have become commercially available; at the present time in the author's laboratory a standard Bright's open-top cryostat with a rotary retracting microtome is in use (Fig. 1). The most important feature is the steel knife, tipped with

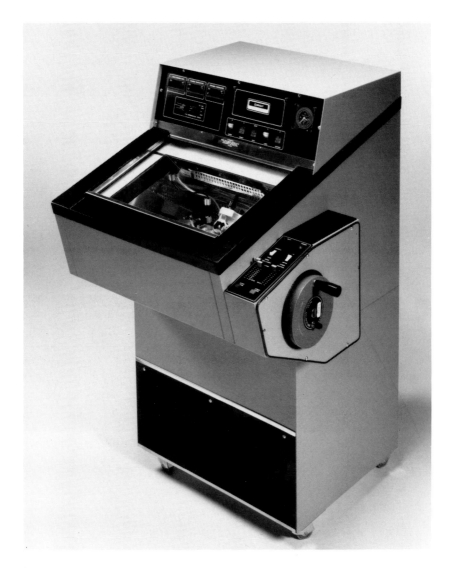

Fig. 1   The Bright's open-top cryostat with tungsten carbide knife for sectioning undecalcified bone.

tungsten carbide. This, together with the automatic drive on the machine, gives excellent reproducibility of sections and the histological preservation needed for the subsequent cytochemical procedures. One further modification of the technique is that the tissue is soaked in 5% polyvinyl alcohol prior to chilling. This facilitates the handling and sectioning of the tissue. Adhesion of the tissue to the microtome chuck is also achieved most satisfactorily with 5% polyvinyl alcohol. There has been some traditional reluctance to section undecalcified bone, and although as with all cryotomy a degree of expertise is called for, if the correct procedure is adhered to at every stage, excellent results can be achieved (Fig. 2).

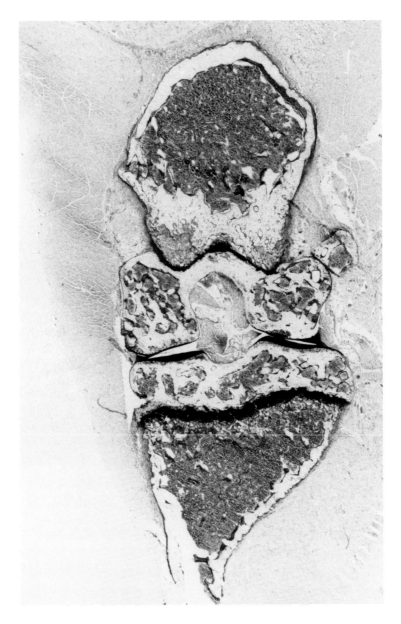

Fig. 2 A section (10 μm) stained with toluidine blue of an intact, undemineralized knee joint of a mouse aged 3 months. (Magnification × 20.) (From Dunham, J. *et al.*, 1988).

The Fracture Callus

The cytochemical approach is particularly suitable for studies on the metabolism of the fracture callus. The callus has an ever changing population of cells and there are obvious advantages in being able to relate quantitative metabolic assessments to histological observations. The author has applied these techniques to the fractured rat metatarsal (e.g., Shedden *et al.*, 1976; Dunham *et al.*, 1977; Dunham, 1978, 1979).

Enzyme Biochemistry of Normal Bone

A detailed review of the histochemistry and enzymology of bone cells has been given by Doty and Schofield in Volume 1 and Doty in Volume 2 of this series. These did not include results obtained from the application of cytochemical techniques which have highlighted some interesting facets in the metabolism of normal bone.

A characteristic feature of bone is the considerable amount of lactate produced under aerobic conditions. This paradox has been investigated in the cells of the epiphyseal plate including osteocytes and osteoblasts (Dunham *et al.*, 1983). The measured activities of a number of oxidative enzymes indicated particularly high glucose 6-phosphate dehydrogenase activity in the osteoblasts, with the osteocytes and chondrocytes having relatively more lactate dehydrogenase activity (Fig. 3). It has been suggested that the contribution of fatty acid oxidation may play a role in the build up of lactate in this tissue (see Table 1).

Most enzymatic studies on bone have relied on easily accessible bone preparations, for example, the growth plate. More recently, Dodds *et al.* (1988) have made direct measurement of metabolic activities of osteoblasts in sections of unfixed, undemineralized iliac crest biopsies of normal bone. They have shown, contrary to the general assumption that trabecular bone is more active than cortical bone, that cortical bone has a higher level of activity per cell, at least with respect to certain oxidative enzymes and alkaline phosphatase (Table 2).

Metabolic activity in the periosteal cells of the rat metatarsal bones has been demonstrated to alter with age (Dunham, 1978). In particular, the activity of the dehydrogenase enzymes of the pentose shunt decreased significantly with the age of the animal. This change was less marked with the enzymes of the glycolytic pathway.

Metabolism of the Fracture Callus

Morphological Studies

A brief morphological description of the fracture callus is needed before considering the metabolism of the constituent cells. Most descriptions of the healing process have involved experimental models but human studies have served to corroborate the main features observed. Some traditional descriptions of fracture healing have been given by Ham and Harris (1971), and McKibbin (1978).

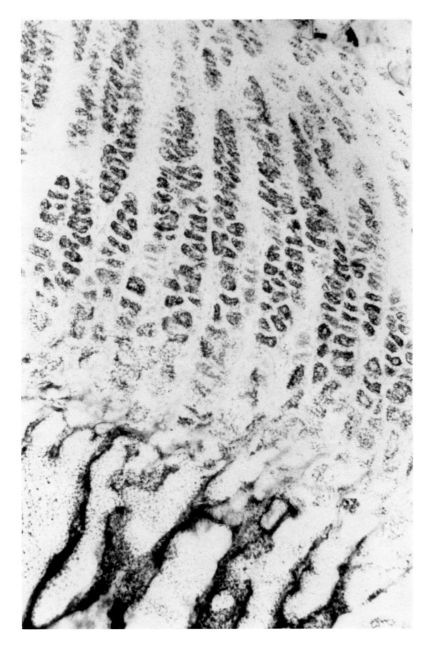

Fig. 3 Glucose 6-phosphate dehydrogenase activity in the cells of the growth plate region of the metatarsal of a young rat. (Magnification × 200.)

The repair process may be summarized as follows. There is an initial inflammatory response to the trauma of the fracture with the formation of a hematoma around the fracture site. This is followed by proliferation and differentiation of pluripotential osteoprogenitor cells to functional fibro-

Table 1.
Enzymatic Activities in the Various Cell Types of the Metatarsal Growth Plate of the Rat
(Mean Integrated Extinction × 100 ± SEM/cell/45 Min Reaction)

			Chondrocytes From		
Enzyme	Osteocytes	Osteoblasts	Hypertrophic Zone	Proliferating Zone	Resting Zone
G6PD	12.0 ± 1.0	54.2 ± 2.6	29.4 ± 0.9	21.0 ± 0.9	13.4 ± 0.6
LDH	32.3 ± 1.0	63.2 ± 1.0	95.6 ± 1.0	81.9 ± 2.0	45.8 ± 1.0
G3PD	14.0 ± 1.0	24.2 ± 1.1	20.7 ± 1.3	11.6 ± 0.9	8.6 ± 2.9
HOAD	8.9 ± 1.9	19.6 ± 1.6	19.6 ± 2.6	14.2 ± 1.5	10.1 ± 3.2
SDH	13.0 ± 0.7	32.0 ± 2.0	9.0 ± 0.6	9.0 ± 0.5	6.0 ± 0.5

G6PD: glucose 6-phosphate dehydrogenase; LDH: lactate dehydrogenase; G3PD: glyceraldehyde 3-phosphate dehydrogenase; HOAD: hydroxyacyl dehydrogenase; SDH: succinate dehydrogenase.

After Dunham et al., 1983b.

Table 2.
Metabolic Activities in Cortical and Trabecular Bone from Human Iliac Crest Biopsies

	Osteoblasts			
Enzyme	Cortical	Trabecular		Ratio
G6PD	73.6 ± 4.6	61.8 ± 4.0	p<0.036	1.2:1
LDH	26.9 ± 1.7	20.5 ± 1.3	p<0.09	1.3:1
G3PD	26.8 ± 1.5	18.3 ± 0.8	p<0.001	1.5:1
HOAD	5.7 ± 0.3	4.7 ± 0.2	p<0.002	1.2:1
SDH	21.3 ± 1.0	19.7 ± 1.1	NS	1.1:1
6PGD	35.6 ± 2.8	24.0 ± 3.2	p<0.02	1.5:1
Alk.P.	89.1 ± 5.6	67.1 ± 5.5	p<0.003	1.3:1

Abbreviations as for Table I. In addition: 6PGD: 6-phosphogluconate dehydrogenase; Alk.P.:
alkaline phosphatase.

After Dodds et al., 1989.

blasts, chondrogenic and osteogenic cells. These cells are said to arise from
the periosteum, endosteum, and marrow stroma (Simmons, 1985). At various stages of the repair process, the callus will consist of granulation tissue,
cartilaginous tissue at different stages of maturity, hypertrophy, and calcification, and new bone. Extensive resorption of the necrotic bone at the
fracture site precedes union with woven bone and remodeling to cortical
bone.

The various stages of morphological transformation of the fracture callus
has been studied in detail in the fractured rat metatarsal (Dunham, 1978;
Dunham et al., 1983; Dodds, 1985; Dodds et al., 1986b). Fractures produced
manually by digital pressure in the metatarsals of the hind limb of mature
Wistar rats achieve full union at around 8 weeks. Typically a cellular callus
consisting largely of relatively undifferentiated cells was established by 5

days. The soft callus was fusiform in shape enveloping the two bony ends. At this stage, the first new sub-periosteal bone was seen on the shaft of the bone some distance behind the fracture. At around 7 days cartilage first appeared adjacent to proliferating periosteum or new bone. By 10 days sufficient resorption of the fractured bone had taken place to reveal a gap between the two bones, the central callus still being filled predominantly with fibroblastic and fibrocartilaginous cells. Cartilage at various stages of maturity and hypertrophy was found adjacent to new woven bone. By 15 days the fracture gap had increased with callus consisting mainly of carti- lage; by 21 days this had undergone ossification with large areas of woven bone within the callus. The external callus then reduced in size and the two bone ends became realigned by 28 days. At around 8 weeks union with woven bone was usually complete (Figs. 4a and b). Although this pattern of healing and the time scale were extremely consistent for this strain of animal it was found to vary with both the strain and age of the rat. For example, Dodds *et al.* (1984) observed that mature Sprague-Dawley rats showed full union of the fractured metatarsal by 6 weeks rather than the 8 weeks seen in the Wistar rat. It was also noted that the dorsal callus was significantly larger than that on the underside of the metatarsal. It is well known that fractures in children heal more rapidly than fractured adult bone. This effect of age has also been shown in the rat, with fractures produced in the metatarsals of young Wistar rats (40 to 50 g) achieving full union in as little as 3 to 4 weeks. Each stage of the healing process occurred earlier with, for example, differentiation of the callus into cartilage by 5 days.

In the experimental rat model the animals are allowed free movement and the only restriction on the fractured metatarsal was that imposed by the close proximity of the adjacent metatarsals. This meant that a large periosteal callus developed. It is known that the mechanical stability of a healing fracture determines the composition and size of the callus and the time taken for union of the bone. In the rat model when the fracture of the metatarsal was incomplete and a greenstick fracture was produced with one of the periosteal surfaces intact, the healing process advanced more rapidly, and only a small callus was formed. This same situation can be achieved artificially, for example, by a metal compression plate. This has the effect of speeding up the whole process of repair. After the initial hematoma develops, only a very thin callus is produced; because the fracture gap is small, healing occurs as a direct result of Haversian remodeling (Ashurst, 1986).

Metabolic Studies

Within the fracture callus there exists a constantly changing population of cells, irregularly arranged and with very varied morphological and bio- chemical characteristics. This heterogeneity, together with the problem of

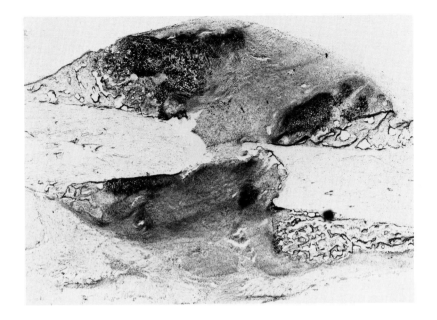

a

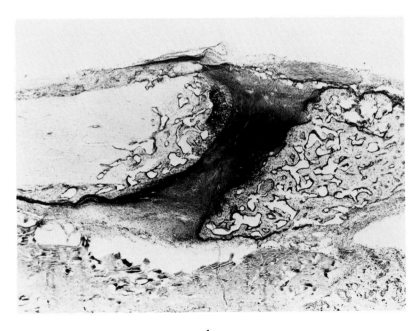

b

Fig. 4 Sections through the rat metatarsal (a) 15 days after fracture (magnification × 25) and (b) 28 days after fracture (magnification × 30). Stained with toluidine blue. (From Dunham, J. *et al.*, 1983a).

processing the mineralized component of the tissue, has resulted in a limited number of metabolic studies being performed on the callus. The biochemists have had to resign themselves to obtaining "relatively homogeneous" populations of cells for conventional biochemical analysis, and with techniques that do not allow the correlation of quantifiable biochemical activity with histology. The histochemists, on the other hand, have been unable to quantify their observations. Even if measurement were to be considered, the known problem of enzyme loss after certain histochemical procedures would make the validity of such quantitation questionable.

Biochemical Studies

Although the number of biochemical investigations that have been done on the fracture callus are relatively few, some examples can be given.

Early biochemical studies (Lénárt et al., 1971, 1972) involved isolation and homogenization of the whole callus. The biochemical analysis required 0.3 g of tissue from the fractured rat tibia. A number of enzymes were evaluated in the callus, but the authors admitted that a severe drawback to the method was the treatment of the tissue as a homogeneous population of cells. Although overall changes in enzyme activity were reported, this took no account of the change in the proportion of cell types within the callus. Two examples of these enzymatic changes were lactate dehydrogenase and alkaline phosphatase, which were shown to decrease with time, although in fact the study was not extended to cover the full transformation of the callus to bone. A similar study by the same authors on enzymatic changes in long bones failed to show any change after fracture. The authors suggested this might indicate an initial reaction in the periosteum, rather than in the cells within the bone matrix but the techniques did not allow the validation of this hypothesis. These studies served to indicate a potential for biochemical evaluation of the fracture callus but the need for histological correlation was all too apparent.

A more detailed and comprehensive biochemical study of the callus of the femoral fracture of the rabbit was done by Kuhlman and Balowski (1975) and is an example of a detailed biochemical investigation in this field. For this study representative callus samples were removed from the fractured femur, frozen sections prepared and lyophylized. From these sections areas of uniform morphology were dissected out, the tissue samples weighing on the order of 1 μg. Seven days after fracture the callus samples could be divided into samples composed of proliferating fibrous tissue, hypertrophic cartilage, and new bone. Prior to this, the callus consisted of hematoma and inflammatory components and unorganized granulation tissue. Eight different enzymes, together with hydroxyproline and inorganic phosphate, were studied at five different times after fracture, in a total of 27 animals. According to the authors, 3000 separate biochemical determinations were made, the number of determinations for each result being between 2 and 38. These details indicate the scale of such studies.

Kuhlman and Balowski concluded that enzymes mediating carbohydrate metabolism were present in considerable amounts in fracture callus, indicating that these pathways provide structural intermediates and energy for the repair process. From their results, lactate and malic dehydrogenases were particularly active in callus, decreasing as new bone was formed. Hexokinase and glucose 6-phosphate dehydrogenase appeared to be present in very small amounts in the callus and virtually absent in new bone. These results are at odds with the findings of Dunham (1979) and Dodds *et al.* (1984). Alkaline phosphatase activity was found to increase with calcification, whereas acid phosphatase was maximal in proliferating cartilage. The levels of acid phosphatase activity reported were low. Kuhlman and Balowski (1975) found in agreement with the present author (Dunham, 1976) that although the proportion of each particular tissue constituent may vary during the process of fracture healing, these areas will have similar biochemical characteristics no matter what the age of the fracture callus. They also reported that once the cells of the callus were established, their enzyme activity resembled that of proliferating and hypertrophic cartilage of the epiphyseal plate (Kuhlman and McNamee, 1970). Many studies have used this similarity as a basis on which to compare the changes in metabolism in the fracture callus.

Ketenjian and Arsenis (1975) reported that in the rabbit tibia the process of differentiation of cartilage was more gradual than that seen in the strict organization of the epiphyseal plate. These authors grouped the cell types into fibrocartilage, proliferating, hypertrophic, and calcified cartilage. These were distinguished and dissected on the basis of texture, color, consistency, and transparency. It was claimed that meticulous free hand dissection could yield relatively homogeneous samples. Comparisons of activities of "aerobic glycolysis" (cytochrome oxidase, citrate synthase) with those of "anaerobic glycolysis" (hexokinase, phosphofructokinase), led the authors to suggest a shift to oxidative glycolysis with maturation of the callus. Hypertrophic and calcified cartilage were analyzed as one region in which lysosomal activity, glucose 6-phosphate dehydrogenase, and alkaline phosphatase were shown to be most active. A more even distribution throughout the callus was shown for 6-phosphogluconic acid dehydrogenase. It was suggested that the higher activities of both anabolic and catabolic enzymes in the callus indicated a faster process of cartilage differentiation in this tissue in comparison with the epiphyseal plate. It must be considered that the differing cellularities of the two tissues could lead to misinterpretation of the biochemical analyses.

It has been suggested by Ashurst (1986) that comparisons between the growth plate and the callus are only valid with respect to the replacement of cartilage by bone. The process of secretion of matrix within the callus is transient with rapid degeneration of the cells in comparison to the continuous growth process of the growth plate.

Histochemical Studies

The majority of metabolic studies on the fracture callus have been done using histochemical techniques. For example, the enzymes of the glycolytic pathway, Krebs cycle, and pentose shunt have been investigated by Balogh and Hajek (1965). They found that the periosteum of the rat long bone showed a striking increase in oxidative enzyme activity after fracture, associated with proliferation. Pentose shunt activity and isocitrate dehydrogenase activity increased in the callus with the maturation of cartilage but decreased as the cells hypertrophied.

Takada (1966) reported an extensive study of the presence and localization of a number of enzymes in the fracture callus of the rat tibia. Enzymes related to the Krebs cycle, pentose phosphate pathway, fatty acid metabolism, and a number of hydrolytic enzymes were demonstrable. He observed that, in general, NADP-dependent dehydrogenases were preferentially active in proliferating and hypertrophic cartilage while NAD-dependent dehydrogenases were more evident in fibrocartilage and calcifying cartilage. It was noted that the appearance of alkaline phosphatase, leucine aminopeptidase, and the NAD-dependent dehydrogenases in the early fibrocartilage resembled that of the early proliferative stage of wound healing in the skin. The later stages of healing in the callus were reported to resemble the metabolic events found in ossification in the growth plate.

Aminopeptidase activity has also been studied in some detail by Mori *et al.* (1975). These workers reported the enzyme to be confined to fibrous and cartilaginous callus and to be absent in ossifying cells. In contrast to the findings of other workers (Byers *et al.*, 1981) osteoclasts and chondroclasts were reported to be devoid of activity, although acid phosphatase and succinate dehydrogenase activities could be demonstrated in these cells. Resting osteocytes have little leucine aminopeptidase activity unless bone resorption is stimulated (Vainio, 1970). The enzyme has been found to be most active in the hypertrophic cartilage cells of the callus (Fullmer, 1966; Takada, 1966; Mostafa, 1979; Dunham, 1981).

Of the other lysosomal enzymes, acid phosphatase has received the most attention. Although originally reported to be confined to the osteoclasts and chondroblasts of the fracture callus (Schajowicz and Cabrini, 1958), this enzyme is also found in undifferentiated callus, osteoblasts, and cartilaginous tissue, particularly hypertrophic cells (e.g., Wergedal and Baylink, 1969; Owen, 1970; Kuhlman and Balowski, 1975; Dunham, 1978). Chondrocyte lysosomes have been shown histochemically to contain acid phosphatase (Matsuzawa and Anderson, 1971) and by biochemical procedures after isolation (Ali and Evans, 1973).

Acid phosphatase, β-acetylglucosaminidase, and β-galactosidase have been shown to increase significantly in the bony callus at the resorptive stage of fracture healing (Brown and Cameron, 1974). β-glucuronidase and nonspecific esterases have been demonstrated in undifferentiated cells, osteoclasts, osteoblasts, and in cartilaginous callus (Fullmer, 1966; Takada, 1966; Mostafa, 1979). As with the other lysosomal enzymes, maximal activity was found in the hypertrophic chondrocytes.

Most workers have included alkaline phosphatase in enzyme studies of the fracture callus. The enzyme has been shown to be most active in regions of hypertrophic cartilage; it is less evident during the stages of maturation, although the early proliferative cells have been shown by some workers to have some activity (Pritchard, 1952; Ketenjian and Arsenis, 1975). Once the new bone formation has taken place the alkaline phosphatase activity declines and osteocytes show little activity. Raekillio and Makinen (1969) demonstrated a loss of both acid and alkaline phosphatase activity in the vincinity of the fracture site, which they regarded as indicative of necrosis, but peripheral to this they found an increase in periosteal and endosteal enzyme activity. This was interpreted as an initial response to injury prior to a more specific regenerative role for the enzyme.

The association of mineralization of the epiphyseal plate cartilage with the presence of matrix vesicles is well known (Bonnuci, 1965; Anderson, 1969; Ali et al., 1970). More recent studies using electron microscopy have emphasized a functional association between alkaline phosphatase activity and endochondral calcification mediated by extracellular vesicles during fracture healing (Volpin et al., 1986). Calcification of cartilage was found to be associated with the degeneration of hypertrophic chondrocytes and to take place within and around alkaline phosphatase containing matrix vesicles formed from early hypertrophic chondrocytes.

Experimental Fracture in the Rat

In the rat metatarsal the initial response to fracture was a proliferation of the periosteum. Enzyme activity was first measured in these periosteal cells at defined distances away from the fracture site. Around 5 days new woven bone was evident on the shaft behind the fracture; the periosteum was elevated and had become indistinguishable histologically. Enzyme activity was then measured in the cells of the newly formed bone and in the constituent cells of the callus.

Enzymatic Changes in the Periosteum

Glucose 6-Phosphate Dehydrogenase Activity

Normal periosteum showed little enzyme activity (Dunham et al., 1977). This increased to measurable amounts of activity within 24 h after fracture in four out of six rats studied. By 5 days all animals were showing significant periosteal activity (Fig. 5). This initial increased enzyme activity was in the cells close to the fracture site, but around 4 or 5 days after fracture high

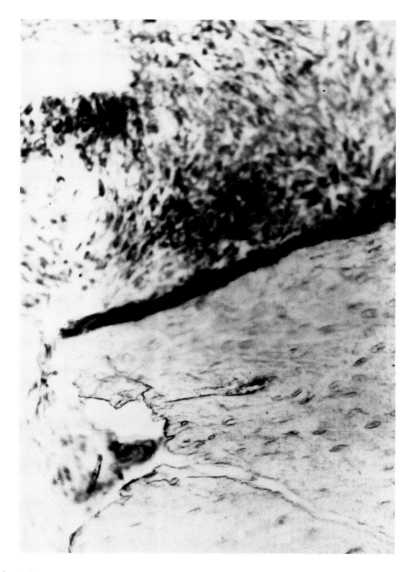

Fig. 5 Glucose 6-phosphate dehydrogenase activity in the periosteal cells of the metatarsal of a 200 g rat 3 days after fracture. (Magnification × 160.)

activity was also seen in the region of new bone formation some distance behind the fracture.

Alkaline Phosphatase Activity

This enzyme is particularly active in periosteal cells. In the rat metatarsal this was remarkably consistent between animals of the same strain and age

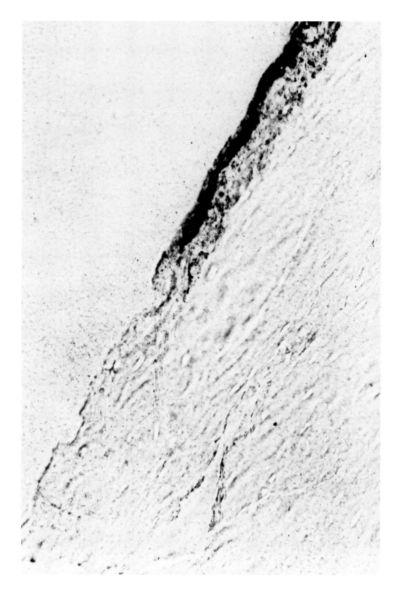

Fig. 6 Alkaline phosphatase activity in the periosteal cells of the metatarsal of a 200 g rat 3 days after fracture. Note the absence of activity close to the fracture site. (Magnification × 160.)

(Shedden *et al.*, 1976). After fracture there was a marked diminution or loss of enzyme activity in the periosteal cells close to the fracture line (Fig. 6). Normal values were found 0.6 to 1.0 mm behind the fracture. This loss of activity was not due to cell death for two reasons. First, serial sections showed strong oxidative activity in this region, and second, in two examples

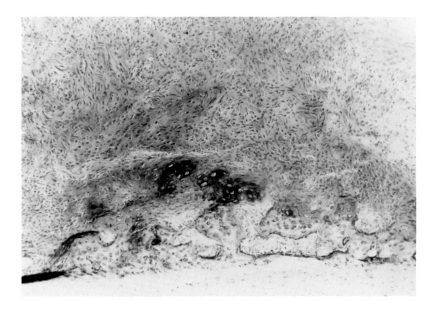

Fig. 7 Heterogeneity of cell types seen in the callus of the rat metatarsal 10 days after fracture. Stained with toluidine blue. (Magnification × 100.) (From Dunham, J. *et al.*, 1983a.)

of greenstick fractures in which the periosteum remained intact this loss of activity was still seen in the region of the fracture line.

Lysosomal Enzyme Activity

Even 1 day after fracture there was strong leucine naphthylamidase activity in the cells of the periosteum in the region of the fracture. Using techniques to determine the fragility of the lysosomes (Bitensky and Chayen, 1977), it was found that although the periosteal cells in unfractured bone showed similar total enzyme activity, the functional state of the lysosomes was greatly altered after fracture so that there was more freely available enzyme activity (Dunham, 1981).

Enzymatic Activity in the Callus

In the rat, the metabolism of the fracture callus from 7 days onwards has been examined (Dunham, 1979; Dunham *et al.*, 1983a). The cell types were defined according to their histological appearance: (a) loose granulation tissue, relatively undifferentiated; (b) cellular granulation tissue (more closely packed, enzymatically more active); (c) mature cartilage; (d) calcified cartilage; (e) osteoblasts of new woven bone; and (f) osteocytes (Fig. 7).

Glucose 6-Phosphate Dehydrogenase

This enzyme was found to be active in the relatively loose granulation tissue which contained cells originating from the proliferating periosteum. As these cells differentiated into chondrogenic and osteogenic cells in the cellular granulation tissue there was a concomitant rise in glucose 6-phosphate dehydrogenase activity. Activity was maintained in cartilage but decreased as the cells calcified. In the osteoblasts of the new woven bone enzyme activity was high, but this diminished as the cells settled as osteocytes within the bone matrix.

Alkaline Phosphatase

Undifferentiated callus cells showed little enzyme activity, but with increasing cellularity and differentiation in the callus this activity increased. Maximum alkaline phosphatase activity was seen in cartilage and persisted as long as the cell type was evident. As the cartilage calcified so enzyme activity decreased. Osteoblasts were active, but as with glucose 6-phosphate dehydrogenase, activity decreased as the cells settled within the matrix as osteocytes.

Thus, in the proliferative stages of fracture healing glucose 6-phosphate dehydrogenase was high while alkaline phosphatase was negligible. In the later stages of differentiation the activity of both enzymes increased: glucose 6-phosphate dehydrogenase activity was maximal in the cellular granulation tissue whereas that of alkaline phosphatase was maximal in regions of cartilage and bone formation (Tables 3a and b).

Other Metabolic Activities

This pattern of activity for glucose 6-phosphate dehydrogenase and alkaline phosphatase has been confirmed by Dodds et al. (1986b) in the analysis of the calluses from a number of rat metatarsals taken 12 days after fracture. In addition to these two enzymes, enzymes of the glycolytic pathway (glyceraldehyde 3-phosphate dehydrogenase and lactate dehydrogenase) and hydroxyacyl dehydrogenase, a marker of fatty acid oxidation, were also measured. In the normal control rat, glyceraldehyde 3-phosphate dehydrogenase was maximal in the cellular granulation tissue. The activity decreased as chondrocytes calcified and, in comparison to other enzymes, appeared relatively low in all other cell types. Lactate dehydrogenase, on the other hand, was active throughout the callus, and was particularly high in the chondrocytes. Hydroxyacyl dehydrogenase activity was low in all cell types (Table 4).

Resorption of the Fractured Bone

It is believed by many workers (Ham and Harris, 1971) that the dead bone at the fracture site is removed prior to union of the cortices. Other workers (McKibbin, 1978; Ashurst, 1986) consider this resorption to depend

Table 3a.
The Activity of Alkaline Phosphatase in the Cells of the Callus at Various Times After Fracture of the Rat Metatarsal (Mean Integrated Extinction × 100 ± SEM)

Days	Granulation Tissue		Cartilage		New Bone	
	Loose	Cellular	Mature	Calcified	Osteoblasts	Periosteum
7	0	0	20 ± 1	—	30 ± 2	50 ± 4
	0	10 ± 1	34 ± 1	—	25 ± 1	
10	0	17 ± 1	41 ± 2	—	40 ± 2	39 ± 3
		18 ± 5	34 ± 5	—	30 ± 2	50 ± 3
15	0	17 ± 2	30 ± 5	17 ± 2	40 ± 2	50 ± 3
		14 ± 2	24 ± 2	15 ± 1	30 ± 2	49 ± 4
21	18 ± 2	61 ± 2	43 ± 4	21 ± 2	50 ± 2	—
28	8 ± 1	29 ± 2	49 ± 2	10 ± 1	60 ± 3	—
35	0	0	57 ± 3	0	50 ± 3	—
49	0	5 ± 1	17 ± 1	—	30 ± 2	—
86	—	—	—	—	40 ± 2	51 ± 3
112[a]	16 ± 1	—	20 ± 1	—	32 ± 2	36 ± 2

[a] An example of nonunion.

From Dunham *et al.*, 1983a.

Table 3b.
The Activity of Glucose 6-Phosphate Dehydrogenase in the Cells of the Callus at Various Times After Fracture of the Rat Metatarsal (Mean Integrated Extinction × 100 ± SEM)

Days	Granulation Tissue		Cartilage		New Bone	
	Loose	Cellular	Mature	Calcified	Osteoblasts	Periosteum
7	51 ± 2	159 ± 5	150 ± 3	—	75 ± 8	92 ± 3
	90 ± 4	180 ± 4	174 ± 4	—	81 ± 4	180 ± 15
10	45 ± 4	120 ± 5	57 ± 4	—	30 ± 2	73 ± 5
	60 ± 9	144 ± 8	150 ± 5	—	69 ± 4	158 ± 8
15	42 ± 2	81 ± 7	30 ± 4	24 ± 1	78 ± 3	153 ± 3
	60 ± 8	216 ± 5	48 ± 3	24 ± 2	81 ± 5	—
21	57 ± 4	117 ± 10	51 ± 3	3 ± 0.03	84 ± 5	—
28	27 ± 2	138 ± 4	15 ± 1	0	60 ± 7	—
35	15 ± 2	168 ± 6	123 ± 6	0	105 ± 7	—
49	0	45 ± 1	81 ± 3	—	78 ± 5	—
86	—	—	—	—	58 ± 4	53 ± 3
112	0	—	0	—	0	0

From Dunham *et al.*, 1983a.

on the mechanical stability of the fracture. If normal alignment is maintained after fracture, the dead bone may be removed as part of the remodeling process.

Resorption of bone is thought to take place through the action of osteoclasts (Chambers, 1985) and they are reported to be seen frequently on the fractured surfaces in the gaps of unstable fractures (Ashurst, 1986).

Table 4.

The Relative Metabolic Activities in the Callus of the Rat Metatarsal 12 Days After Fracture (Mean Integrated Extinction × 100/cell/10 Min Reaction: Mean ± SD)

Enzyme Activity	Loose Granulation Tissue	Cellular Granulation Tissue	Mature Chondrocytes	Calcifying Chondrocytes	Osteoblasts	Number of	
						Bones	Rats
G6PD	10.6 ± 1.8	33.0 ± 9.1	23.7 ± 4.5	6.2 ± 1.3	18.3 ± 4.5	15	7
LDH	15.6 ± 3.3	34.5 ± 9.1	52.9 ± 2.5	15.9 ± 1.1	25.1 ± 2.1	8	4
G3PD	3.1 ± 0.4	10.7 ± 4.7	6.4 ± 3.3	2.2 ± 0.3	4.0 ± 0.5	6	4
HOAD	1.9 ± 0.8	3.5 ± 2.0	3.9 ± 1.5	1.7 ± 0.5	5.2 ± 1.4	8	4
Alk.P.[a]	4.1 ± 2.3	16.9 ± 2.8	27.2 ± 5.0	11.9 ± 4.5	30.1 ± 6.5	15	7

Abbreviations as for Tables I and II.

[a] 3 min reaction.

After Dodds *et al.*, 1986b.

However, in the fractured rat metatarsal model this does not seem to be the case (Dunham, 1981). Whereas large multinucleate cells were obvious in regions where bone remodeling was taking place, no such cells could be observed in the areas of rapid resorption of the fracture ends. In this model, resorption was extensive. Initially in the first 5 days following fracture there was an area of overlap between the fracture bone ends of between 6 to 20% of the total inter-epiphyseal length. In the next 5 days this was reduced to between 2 to 15%. This overlap region disappeared so that between 15 and 35 days there was a gap of 4 to 6% of the total length. Thus the amount of bone that was removed comprised something of the order of a quarter of the whole bone length (Fig. 8). This occurred in the apparent absence of cells with the typical appearance of osteoclasts. As has been discussed above, lysosomal enzyme activity is evident throughout the fracture callus particularly in the hypertrophic chondrocytes. In an attempt to define osteoclastic activity even in the absence of morphologically distinct cells, acid phosphatase and leucine naphthylamidase were used. There was strong activity in the morphologically distinct osteoclasts in the remodeling regions, but these enzymatic activities were not markedly increased in the resorption regions.

Enzymatic Activity in Experimentally Modified Rat Fracture Callus

The influence of a wide variety of agents, including vitamins and hormones, on the speed and integrity of fracture healing has been reviewed by Byers *et al.* (1981).

Two detailed studies on the effects of experimental modification of the enzymatic activity of the callus in the fractured rat metatarsal have been made by Dodds *et al.* (1984, 1986b). In the first, the effects of dicoumarol on ossification have been tested. Dicoumarol inhibits the vitamin K cycle

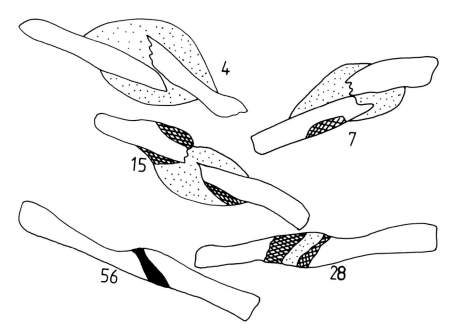

Fig. 8 Outline drawings of images of sections of rat metatarsals at various times after fracture projected through a photographic enlarger.

by blocking the conversion of the vitamin K epoxide. There is considerable evidence that calcification in bone may depend on the conversion of peptide-bound glutamate residues to carboxyglutamate. This involves the vitamin K cycle (Hauschka et al., 1975) in which vitamin K_1 acts only as a carrier of reducing equivalents (NAD(P)H) generated in bone forming cells.

In the fractured rat metatarsal up to 12 days post fracture, dicoumarol markedly delayed the maturation of the callus although the total size of the callus was unaffected. The periosteal activities of glucose 6-phosphate dehydrogenase and alkaline phosphatase were affected, as were those of certain cell types within the callus. The depression of glucose 6-phosphate dehydrogenase activity was most significant in the region of periosteum associated with bone formation and shown to have high activity in the untreated animal. Moreover, dicoumarol depressed glucose 6-phosphate dehydrogenase activity selectively in cells of the callus. Neither alkaline phosphatase activity nor fatty acid oxidation were shown to be affected by dicoumarol in the cells of the callus, although in the periosteum alkaline phosphatase was found to be slightly elevated close to the fracture site.

The retardation of ossification in the callus was considered consistent with an antagonistic effect against vitamin K_1 in the vitamin K cycle. In addition, measurement of glucose 6-phosphate dehydrogenase activity indicated that dicoumarol decreased the amounts of reducing equivalents available for the cycle.

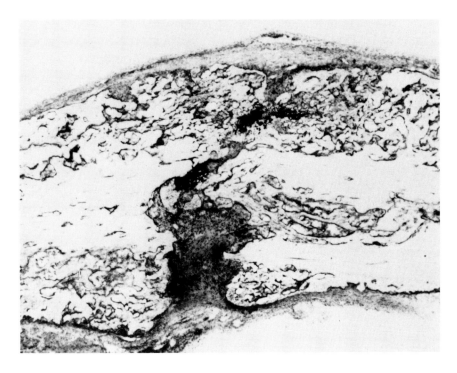

a

Fig. 9 The delay in the maturation of the callus in rats fed a vitamin B_6 deficient diet. (a) Control rat 3 weeks post-fracture with large areas of new bone in the callus and (b) vitamin B_6 deficient rat 3 weeks post-fracture still with a largely cartilaginous callus. Stained with toluidine blue. (Magnification $\times$ 30.) (From Dodds, R. A. *et al.*, 1986.)

Measurements of depressed levels of circulating vitamin K_1 in patients with fractures, suggesting that this vitamin is sequestered from the circulation for use at the fracture site, has given further evidence of the involvement of this vitamin in fracture healing (Hart *et al.*, 1982; Bitensky, 1988).

In the second study the effect of pyridoxine (vitamin B_6) deficiency in the same experimental system was investigated (Dodds *et al.*, 1986b). A deficiency in this vitamin again resulted in a significant delay in the maturation of the callus and union of the bone together with a marked diminution of glucose 6-phosphate dehydrogenase activity in the periosteal region of bone formation and in the developing callus (Fig. 9). Vitamin B_6 deficiency had no effect on the activities of alkaline phosphatase, glyceraldehyde 3-phosphate dehydrogenase, or hydroxyacyl dehydrogenase in any of the cells of the callus. Lactate dehydrogenase was depressed in the chondrocytes and cellular granulation tissue. The predominant effect was on glucose 6-phosphate dehydrogenase which was depressed throughout the callus, particularly in the mature chondrocytes and osteoblasts. It was also suggested that vitamin B_6 deficiency caused changes suggestive of an imbalance in the

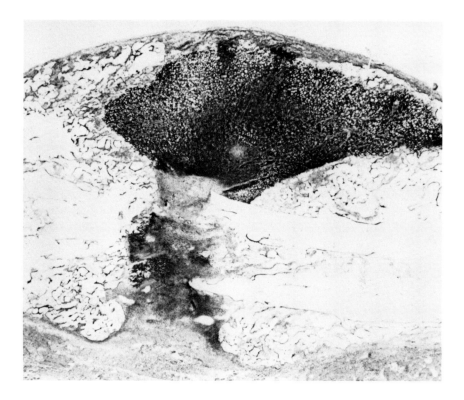

Fig. 9b

coupling between osteoblasts and osteoclasts. The vitamin B_6 status was considered to be important in fracture healing.

Proteoglycans of the Fracture Callus

There have been a number of studies on the chemical composition of the callus, including the involvement of the glycosaminoglycans in the calcification process and bone formation. Quantitative and qualitative variations in the glycosaminoglycans of the callus have been observed (Solheim, 1970). Chondroitin sulfate was found to be the main component with chondroitin 4-sulfate predominating in hyaline cartilage and chondroitin 6-sulfate in fibrocartilage. Whether these differences were prerequisite for a normal mineralization of bone or merely reflected different morphology was unclear. In addition, a minor component of callus was identified as hyaluronic acid and found to be highest in early callus decreasing as the callus matured. Penttinnen (1972) found uronic acids and hexosamines to increase with the appearance and growth of cartilage and to decrease slightly with ossification.

More recently, changes in proteoglycan molecules during initial stages of fracture healing in rats have been characterized (Kopman *et al.*, 1987). The dominant change in the proteoglycan molecules appeared to be disaggregation. It was suggested that the proteoglycans in the callus were similar to those of the growth plate where there is a comparable decrease in aggregate size, reaggregation capacity, and the average monomer size, concomitant with cellular hypertrophy and the onset of calcification. Earlier characterization of the composition of fracture callus showed that the proteoglycan content decreased from the chondroid to the transitional chondroid-osseous stage.

Biochemical studies on the nature of bone proteoglycans have indicated that their structures are very different from those of cartilage. Bone proteoglycans consist of small glycoconjugates with only one or two glycosaminoglycan chains, these being predominantly chondroitin 4-sulfate (Fischer et al., 1983). In hyaline cartilage the most abundant proteoglycan is a high molecular weight aggregating species that contains both chondroitin and keratan sulfate chains. Typically there are 100 to 400 chondroitin sulfate chains both 4- and 6-O-sulfate groups, and 30 to 40 keratan sulfate chains (Hardingham, 1986).

The role of proteoglycans in the transition of cartilage to bone has been examined (Carrino et al., 1985). The extracellular matrix of cartilage is thought to be incapable of mineralization and therefore has to be either modified or removed prior to mineralization. The proteoglycans synthesized during the mineralization process, for example, in the growth plate, have been shown to range from a proteoglycan with large chondroitin sulfate chains and small keratan sulfate chains to a smaller monomer whose chondroitin sulfate chains are similar in size and keratan sulfate chains are larger. In addition a small bone proteoglycan with large highly 4-sulfated chondroitin sulfate chains has been observed in ossifying long bone. The authors (Carrino et al., 1985) proposed that a distinct chondroitin sulfate proteoglycan may be produced by the hypertrophic chondrocytes and that this may alter the extracellular matrix of the cartilage to allow mineralization to occur.

There have been few histochemical studies on the composition of the matrix of the callus. One early example (Ikuta, 1965) used acridine orange fluorescence to detect glycosaminoglycans and concluded that chondroitin sulfate was closely related to calcium deposition in endochondral ossification. It has been observed histochemically that the quantity of glycosaminoglycans increased during the early stages of callus formation (Lindholm, 1974).

The characteristic differences between the glycosaminoglycans of bone and cartilage have been studied with particular reference to the pre-osseous and pre-cartilage cells found within the fracture callus (Dunham, 1983a). Although it is often cited that ossification within the fracture callus is solely endochondral, in the fractured metatarsal of the rat, both endochondral and membranous ossification were demonstrable morphologically. Membranous ossification was seen to occur initially on the side of the shaft, but direct differentiation into osseous tissue was also seen within the callus together with differentiation into chondrocytes.

Why these situations occur has been the subject of much speculation. The generally accepted hypothesis is that differentiation into osteoblasts occurs in areas of high oxygen tension, while differentiation into chondrocytes occurs in areas of low oxygen tension (Ham, 1930; Bassett and Herrmann, 1961; Jargiello and Caplan, 1983). It has been suggested that mechanical stability affects the composition of the callus; cartilage being found only where there is movement or instability at the fracture site (Ashurst, 1986). This movement may be very localized and lead to hypoxic conditions. In the fractured rat metatarsal these two routes of differentiation were seen to occur in close proximity.

The Experimental Rat Fracture

The glycosaminoglycans can be stained quantitatively and selectively using the concept of the "critical electrolyte concentration" (Scott and Dorling, 1965). This feature has been used by the author in an attempt to demonstrate some chemical differences in the relatively undifferentiated cells of the early fracture callus. To do this, the glycosaminoglycan staining pattern of an established callus with both cartilage and bone evident was first determined. This was then compared with the staining pattern of an early callus, cells being distinguished on a descriptive morphological basis. From these studies differences in the chemical composition of the various cell types of the early callus were evident, and it was suggested that this could indicate in which direction the cells would differentiate. Thus, those cells showing a staining pattern akin to that of bone might be those to differentiate directly to bone, whereas others in which the glycosaminoglycan staining pattern was more akin to that of cartilage would go through the process of endochondral ossification (Dunham, 1978).

Conclusion

In conclusion, it seems that studies on the nature of callus and its formation, particularly those of the present author and colleagues, have opened new possibilities of promoting bone healing. The present results (cited above) indicate that healing depends on the stimulation of glucose 6-phosphate dehydrogenase, and, assumably the whole pentose-phosphate shunt, with its formation of both NADPH for biosynthetic pathways and of pentose sugars as are required for new growth.

The NADPH generated by the pentose phosphate pathway can then be used in the vitamin K cycle (Hauschka *et al.*, 1975) as required for the calcification of bone.

However, recent results go even further. They suggest (e.g., Dodds *et al.*,

1986a) that glucose 6-phosphate dehydrogenase can be converted from a weakly active to a strongly active enzyme (Yoshida, 1966) by the action of putrescine. This molecule is generated directly by the activity of ornithine decarboxylase, which depends on pyridoxal phosphate as its coenzyme. The new results, together, suggest that when fracture healing is delayed, it might be reactivated by pyridoxal phosphate (vitamin B_6) together with sufficient vitamin K_1.

References

Ali, S. Y. and Evans, L. (1973). Enzymatic degradation of cartilage in osteoarthritis. *Fed. Proc.*, **32**: 1494.

Ali, S. Y., Sajdera, S. W., and Anderson, H. C. (1970). Isolation and characterisation of calcifying matrix vesicles from epiphyseal cartilage. *Proc. Natl. Acad. Sci. U.S.A.*, **67**: 1513–1520.

Altman, F. P. (1969). A comparison of dehydrogenase activities in tissue homogenates and tissue sections. *Biochem. J.*, **114**: 13–14.

Altman, F. P. (1980). Tissue stabilizer methods in histochemistry. In: *Trends in Enzyme Histochemistry and Cytochemistry*. Ciba Foundation 73. Excerpta Medica, Amsterdam, 81–102.

Altman, F. P. and Barrnett, R. J. (1975). The ultrastructural localization of enzyme activity in unfixed tissue sections. *Histochemistry*, **41**: 179–183.

Altman, F. P. and Chayen, J. (1965). Retention of nitrogenous material in unfixed sections during incubations for histochemical demonstration of enzymes. *Nature (London)*, **207**: 1205–1206.

Anderson, C. (1984). Preparation of calcified tissues for light microscopic histochemistry. In: *Methods of Calcified Tissue Preparation*. Dickson, G. R., Ed., Elsevier, Amsterdam, 57–77.

Anderson, H. C. (1969). Vesicles associated with calcification in the matrix of epiphyseal cartilage. *J. Cell Biol.*, **41**: 59–72.

Ashurst, D. E. (1986). The influence of mechanical conditions on the healing of experimental fractures in the rabbit: a microscopical study. *Phil. Trans. R. Soc. Lond.*, **B313**: 217–302.

Balogh, K., Jr. and Hajek, J. V. (1965). Oxidative enzymes of intermediary metabolism in healing bone fractures. *Am. J. Anat.*, **116**: 429–448.

Barka, T. and Anderson, P. J. (1963). *Histochemistry*. Harper and Row, New York.

Bassett, C. A. L. and Herrmann, I. (1961). Influence of oxygen concentration and mechanical factors on differentiation of connective tissues *in vitro*. *Nature (London)*, **190**: 460–461.

Bitensky, L. (1980). *Trends in Enzyme Histochemistry and Cytochemistry*. Ciba Foundation Symposium 73. Evered D. and O'Connor, M., Eds., Excerpta Medica, Amsterdam, 181–202.

Bitensky, L. and Chayen, J. (1977). Histochemical methods for the study of lysosomes. In: *Lysosomes: A Laboratory Handbook*. 2nd ed., Dingle, J. T., Ed., North Holland, Amsterdam, 209–243.

Bitensky, L., Hart, J. P., Catterall, A., Hodges, S. J., Pilkington, M. J., and Chayen, J. (1988). Circulating vitamin K levels in patients with fractures. *J. Bone Jt. Surg.*, **70B**: 663–664.

Bonnucci, E. (1967). Fine structure of early cartilage calcification. *J. Ultrastruct. Res.*, **20**: 33–50.

Brown, R. M. and Cameron, D. A. (1974). Acid hydrolases and bone resorption in the remodelling phase of the development of bony fracture callus. *Pathology*, **6**: 53–61.

Butcher, R. G. (1971). Tissue stabilization during histochemical reactions: the use of collagen polypeptides. *Histochemie*, **28**: 231–235.

Butcher, R. G. and Chayen, J. (1968). The value of intact tissue sections for studying metabolic inter-actions between the cytoplasm and mitochondria. *Exp. Cell Res.*, **49**: 656–665.

Byers, P. D., Gray, J. C., Mostafa, A. G. S. A., and Ali, S. Y. (1981). The healing of bone and articular cartilage. In: *Handbook of Inflammation*. Vol. 3, Glynn, L. E., Ed., Elsevier/North Holland, Amsterdam, 343–368.

Carrino, D. A., Weitzhandler, M., and Caplan, A. I. (1985). Proteoglycans synthesized during the cartilage to bone transition. In: *The Chemistry and Biology of Mineralized Tissues*. Butler, W. B., Ed., EBSCO Media, Birmingham., 197–208.

Chambers, T. J. (1985). The pathobiology of the osteoclast. *J. Clin. Pathol.*, **38**: 241–252.

Chayen, J. (1982). Scanning microdensitometry. In: *Handbook of Clinical Chemistry*. Vol. 1, Werner, H., Ed., CRC Press, Boca Raton, FL, 529–535.

Chayen, J. (1984). Quantitative cytochemistry: a precise form of cellular biochemistry. *Biochem. Soc. Trans.*, **12**: 887–898.

Chayen, J. and Bitensky, L. (1968). Multiphase chemistry of cell injury. In: *The Biological Basis of Medicine*. Vol. 1, Bittar, E. and Bittar, N., Eds., Academic Press, London, 337–368.

Chayen, J. and Bitensky, L. (1987). Quantitative cytochemistry. In: *Drug Metabolism—From Molecules to Man*. Benford, D. J., Bridges, J. W., and Gibson, G. G., Eds., Taylor & Francis, London, 275–284.

Chayen, J. and Bitensky, L. (1991). *Practical Histochemistry*. 2nd ed., John Wiley & Sons, New York.

Dodds, R. A. (1985). Structural and Metabolic Studies on Normal and Pathological Bone. Ph.D. thesis, Brunel University, London.

Dodds, R. A., Catterall, A., Bitensky, L., and Chayen, J. (1984). Effects of fracture healing of an antagonist of the vitamin K cycle. *Calcif. Tissue Int.*, **36**: 233–238.

Dodds, R. A., Dunham, J., Bitensky, L., and Chayen, J. (1986a). Putrescine may be a natural stimulator of glucose 6-phosphate dehydrogenase. *FEBS Lett.*, **201**: 105–108.

Dodds, R. A., Catterall, A., Bitensky, L., and Chayen, J. (1986b). Abnormalities in fracture healing induced by vitamin B_6-deficiency in rats. *Bone*, **7**: 489–495.

Dodds, R. A., Shore, I., and Moss, J. (1988). Electron microscopy of undecalcified human bone. *J. Clin. Pathol.*, **41**: 465–466.

Dodds, R. A., Emery, R. J. H., Klenerman, L., Bitensky, L., and Chayen, J. Comparative metabolic enzyme activity in trabecular as against cortical osteoblasts. *Bone* (in press).

Dunham, J. (1978). Cellular Biochemistry of Undecalcified Bone and the Response to Fracture. Ph.D. thesis, Brunel University, London.

Dunham, J. (1979). Metabolism of the fracture callus. In: *Quantitative Cytochemistry and its Applications*. Pattison, J. R., Bitensky, L., and Chayen, J., Eds., Academic Press, London, 213–220.

Dunham, J. (1981). Measurement of bone resorption with no demonstrable osteoclasts following fracture of rat metatarsals. *Calcif. Tissue Int.*, **33**: 91A.

Dunham, J., Shedden, R. G., Catterall, A., Bitensky, L., and Chayen, J. (1977). Pentose shunt oxidation in the periosteal cells in healing fractures. *Calcif. Tissue Res.*, **23**: 77–81.

Dunham, J., Catterall, A., Bitensky, L., and Chayen, J. (1983a). Metabolic changes in the cells of the callus during fracture healing in the rat. *Calcif. Tissue Int.*, **35**: 56–61.

Dunham, J., Chambers, M. G., Jasani, M. K., Bitensky, L., and Chayen, J. (1988). Changes in oxidative activities of chrondocytes during the early development of natural murine osteoarthritis. *Br. J. Exp. Pathol.*, **69**: 845–853.

Dunham, J., Dodds, R. A., Nahir, A. M., Frost, G. T. B., Catterall, A., Bitensky, L., and Chayen, J. (1983b). Aerobic glycolysis of bone and cartilage: the possible involvement of fatty acid oxidation. *Cell Biochem. Funct.*, **1**: 168–172.

Fell, H. B. and Canti, R. B. (1935). Experiments on the development *in vitro* of the avian knee joints. *Proc. R. Soc. Lond. Ser. B.*, **161**: 316–351.

Fell, H. B. and Robison, R. (1929). Growth: development and phosphatase activity of embryonic avian femora and limb buds cultivated *in vitro*. *Biochem. J.*, **23**: 767–784.

Fischer, L. W., Termine, J. D., Dejter, S. W., Jr., Whitson, S. W., Yanagishita, M., Kimura, J. H., Hascall, V. C., Kleinman, H. K., Hassel, J. R., and Nilsson, B. (1983). Proteoglycans of developing bone. *J. Biol. Chem.*, **258**: 6588–6594.

Fullmer, H. M. (1966). Enzymes in mineralized tissues. *Clin. Orthop. Rel. Res.*, **48**: 285–295.

Gahan, P. B. and Kalina, M. (1965). The validity of using neotetrazolium for studying labile, NADP-linked dehydrogenases in histological sections: a quantitative study. *Biochem. J.*, **96**: 11.

Gothlin, G., Arborgh, B., Ericsson, J. L. E., and Helminen, H. (1973). Histochemical and biochemical studies on the localization and activities of lysosomal enzymes in fracture callus. *Histochemie*, **35**: 97–110.

Ham, A. W. (1930). A histological study of the early phases of bone repair. *J. Bone Jt. Surg.*, **12**: 827–844.

Ham, A. W. and Harris, W. R. (1971). Repair and transplantation of bone. In: *The Biochemistry and Physiology of Bone*. Vol. 3, 2nd ed., Bourne, G. H., Ed., Academic Press, New York, 337–399.

Hardingham, T. E., Beardmore-Gray, M., Dunham, D. G., and Ratcliffe, A. (1986). *Functions of the Proteoglycans*. Ciba Foundation Symposium 124. John Wiley & Sons, Chichester, 30–46.

Hart, J. P., Nahir, A. M., and Chayen, J. (1982). Determination of vitamin K₁ in plasma by differential pulse polarography and its possible clinical application. *Analyt. Chim. Acta*, **144**: 267–271.

Hauschka, P. V., Lian, J. B., and Gallop, P. M. (1975). Direct identification of the calcium-binding amino acid and γ-carboxyglutamate in mineralized tissue. *Proc. Natl. Acad. Sci. U.S.A.*, **72**: 3295.

Henderson, B., Loveridge, N., and Robertson, W. R. (1978). A quantitative study of the effects of different grades of polyvinyl alcohol on the activities of certain enzymes in unfixed sections. *Histochem. J.*, **10**: 453–463.

Ikuta, H. (1965). Histochemical study of the experimental callus. *Kurume Med. J.*, **12**: 92–107.

Jargiello, D. M. and Caplan, A. I. (1983). The establishment of vascular-derived microenvironments in the developing chick wing. *Dev. Biol.*, **97**: 364–374.

Johnstone, J. J. A. (1979). The routine sectioning of undecalcified bone for cytochemical studies. *Histochem. J.*, **11**: 359–365.

Jones, G. R. N. (1965). Losses of nitrogenous material occurring from frozen sections of rat liver during incubation in an aqueous medium. *Biochem. J.* **96**: 10.

Ketenjian, A. Y. and Arsenis, C. (1975). Morphological and biochemical studies during differentiation and calcification of fracture callus cartilage. *Clin. Orthop. Rel. Res.*, **107**: 266–273.

Kopman, C. R., Boskey, A. L., Lane, J. M., Pita, J. C., and Eaton, B. (1987). Biochemical characterization of fracture callus proteoglycans. *J. Orthop. Res.*, **5**: 7–13.

Kuhlman, R. E. (1980). Functioning enzyme systems present in skeletal tissue and their relationship to structure. In: *Fundamental and Clinical Bone Physiology*. Urist, M. R. Ed., J. B. Lippincott, Philadelphia, 172–207.

Kulhman, R. E. and Balowski, M. (1975). The biochemical activity of fracture callus in relation to bone production. *Clin. Orthop. Rel. Res.*, **107**: 258–265.

Kuhlman, R. E. and McNamee, M. J. (1970). The biochemical importance of the hypertrophic cartilage cell area to enchondral bone formation. *J. Bone Jt. Surg.*, **52A**: 1025–1032.

Lénárt, G., Pinter, J., and Kery, L. (1972). Callus: physical and biochemical studies. *Acta Chir. Acad. Sci. Hung. Tomus*, **13**: 395–401.

Lénárt, G., Széll, V., and Csorba, E. (1971). Comparative investigations on bone and callus enzymes. *Acta Biochim. Biophys. Acad. Sci. Hung.*, **6**: 243–250.

Lindholm, T. S. (1974). Bone resorption and remodelling. *Acta Chir. Scand. Suppl.*, **449**: 7–18.

Matsuzawa, T. and Anderson, H. C. (1971). Phosphatases of epiphyseal cartilage studied by electron microscopic cytochemical methods. *J. Histochem. Cytochem.*, **19**: 801–808.

McKibbin, B. (1978). The biology of fracture healing in long bones. *J. Bone Jt. Surg.*, **60B**: 150–162.

Mori, M., Okta, T., Okada, Y., Makino, M., and Murakami, M. (1975). Aminopeptidase histochemistry in healing bone fractures. *Acta Histochem. Cytochem.*, **8**: 8–17.

Mostafa, A. G. S. A. (1979). Histology and Histochemistry of Fracture Repair. Ph.D. thesis, University of London, London, U.K.

Olsen, I., Dean, M. F., Harris, G., and Muir, I. H. (1981). Direct transfer of a lysosomal enzyme from lymphoid cells to deficient fibroblasts. *Nature (London)*, **291**: 244–247.

Owen, M. (1970). The origin of bone cells. *Int. Rev. Cytol.*, **28**: 225–228.

Penttinen, R. (1972). Biochemical study of fracture healing in the rat, with special reference to oxygen supply. *Acta Chir. Scand. Suppl.*, **432**: 1–32.

Pritchard, J. J. (1952). A cytological and histochemical study of bone and cartilage formation in rats. *J. Anat. (London)*, **86**: 259–277.

Raekallio, J. and Makinen, P.-L. (1969). Alkaline and acid phosphatase activity in the initial phase of fracture healing. *Acta Pathol. Microbiol. Scand.*, **75**: 415–422.

Raisz, L. G. (1965). Bone resorption in tissue culture. Factors influencing the response to parathyroid hormone. *J. Clin. Invest.*, **44**: 103–116.

Schajowicz, F. and Cabrini, R. L. (1958). Histochemical localization of acid phosphatase in bone tissue. *Science*, **127**: 1447–1448.

Scott, J. E. and Dorling, J. A. (1965). Differential staining of acid glycosaminoglycans by Alcian blue in salt solution. *Histochemie*, **5**: 221–233.

Shapiro, I. M., Kakuta, S., and Golub, E. E. (1984). Methods for measurements of energy metabolism in calcified tissue. In: *Methods of Calcified Tissue Preparation*. Dickson, G. R., Ed., Elsevier, Amsterdam, 587–605.

Shedden, R., Dunham, J., Bitensky, L., Catterall, A., and Chayen, J. (1976). Changes in alkaline phosphatase activity in periosteal cells in healing fractures. *Calcif. Tissue Res.*, **22**: 19–25.

Sheehan, D. C. and Hrapchak, B. B. (1980). *Theory and Practice of Histotechnology*. C. V. Mosby, London.

Silbermann, M. and Maor, G. (1984). Organ and tissue culture of cartilage and bone. In: *Methods of Calcified Tissue Preparation*. Elsevier, Amsterdam, 467–530.

Simmons, D. J. (1985). Fracture healing perspectives. *Clin. Orthop. Rel. Res.*, **200**: 100–113.

Solheim, K. (1970). The glycosaminoglycans in callus during fracture repair. *Calcif. Tiss. Res.*, **4 (Suppl)**: 112 114.

Takada, K. (1966). Enzyme histochemistry in bone tissue. II. Histochemical detection of hydrolytic and oxidative enzymes in callus tissue. *Acta Histochem. Bd.*, **23**: 53–70.

Vainio, V. (1970). Leucine aminopeptidase in rheumatoid arthritis. Localization in sub-chondral bone and in synovial fluid cells. *Ann. Rheum. Dis.*, **29**: 434–438.

Volpin, G., Rees, J. A., Ali, S. Y., and Bentley, G. (1986). Distribution of alkaline phosphatase activity in experimentally produced callus in rats. *J. Bone Jt. Surg.*, **68B**: 629–634.

Wergedal, J. E. and Baylink, D. J. (1969). Distribution of acid and alkaline phosphatase activity in undemineralized sections of the rat tibial diaphysis. *J. Histochem. Cytochem.*, **17**: 799–806.

Wong, G. L. (1980). Bone cell cultures as an experimental model. *Arthrit. Rheuma.*, **23**: 1081–1085.

Yoshida, A. (1966). Glucose 6-phosphate dehydrogenase in human erythrocytes. *J. Biol. Chem.*, **421**: 4966–4976.

Zoller, L. C. and Weisz, J. (1980). The demonstration of regional differences in lysosome membrane permeability in the membrane granulosa of graafian follicles in cryostat sections of the rat ovary: a quantitative cytochemical study. *Endocrinology*, **106**: 871–877.

2

Stress Dependence of Synovial Joints

WAYNE H. AKESON, DAVID AMIEL, MICHAEL KWAN, JEAN-JACQUES ABITBOL, and STEVEN R. GARFIN
Division of Orthopaedics and Rehabilitation
University of California, San Diego
San Diego, California

Introduction

Cells adapt to environmental conditions. Of the myriad of influences to
which cells must respond, none are more universal than mechanical forces.
Yet until recently the importance of mechanical forces for tissue homeostasis
has received relatively little attention. Virtually nothing is known about the
mechanisms of signaling by which mechanical forces induce cellular responses. A recently described array of cell membrane receptors called integrins are employed by cells to achieve adherence to other cells or to adjacent
extracellular matrices (Hemler *et al.*, 1987). Integrins provide the linkage
between the cytoskeleton and adjacent extracellular matrices, and between
the cytoskeleton within the cell and the extracellular matrix without. Integrins are probably also an element of the communication system of the
mechano-receptor complex. Details of this complex remain to be described,
but for the present the new technologies of cellular biomechanics coupled
with molecular biology and immunohistochemistry offer opportunities for
study and better understanding of the manner by which cells interact with
their physical environment.

The basic cellular response issues discussed in this chapter are not solely
of theoretical interest. In fact, therapeutic choices of use vs. rest arise daily
in management of the ills of the musculoskeletal system. The rapid deterioration of synovial joint tissues under conditions of stress deprivation has
been described in detail in the past two decades (*vide infra*). The slow
recovery from those effects has also become painfully clear. Because of these
observations, the needs of active motion for synovial joint homeostasis have
been well accepted as the means of prevention of stress deprivation effects.
Due to their overriding importance, the resulting concepts have been incorporated into virtually every aspect of management of injuries and disorders
of the spine and appendicular skeleton. Examples of such applications
abound, including the importance of early mobilization of extremities via
aggressive stabilization of fractures in the multiply-injured patient, the importance of aggressive rehabilitation of the anterior cruciate reconstructed
knee, the widespread use of braces rather than casts, early passive motion
of repaired tendon lacerations, the whole concept of continuous passive
motion, etc. Shortened hospitalizations and consequent economics of health
care costs have been an important by-product of this approach. The reve-

lation that early activity enhances healing as well as facilitating functional recovery has placed modern rehabilitation of musculoskeletal injuries on the fast track of the therapeutic decision tree.

More complete understanding of these interactions can be expected to find application in placing treatment of injuries and disorders of the musculoskeletal system on a more completely rational basis than has been possible in the past.

The Stress Dependence of Connective Tissue

The interrelationship between skeletal form and function has long been accepted. The most explicit expression of the relationship was, of course, Wolff's Law, which states that bone adapts to applied stresses. In more recent years, the expression has been found to apply equally importantly to joint composite, including articular cartilage, ligament, tendon, capsule, and synovial membrane as to bone (Von Reyler, 1874; Weichselbaum, 1878; Parker and Keefer, 1935; Satter and Field, 1960). This broader expansion of Wolff's Law is probably best simply recognized with slight editorial license as Wolff's Law of connective tissue, although others, as is more often the rule in science, may have priority in recognition of the broader application of the general interrelationship between form and function as applied to fibrous connective tissue and the joint composite (Frank et al., 1984).

The following narrative summarizes present understanding of the effects of stress enhancement and stress deprivation on synovial joints. Generalizations are possible to a certain extent, but it is important to remember that specialized connective tissues retain unique characteristics which modulate responses to mechanical influences. As will be pointed out, even fibroblasts from site to site may not respond uniformly.

Anatomic Pathology

It is instructive to review the protean manifestations of stress deprivation on synovial joints in order to put therapeutic decison-making into perspective. There are enough gross and microscopic observations on human anatomic pathology to feel confident that reported experimental animal and human changes are closely similar. The changes are conveniently divided into (1) periarticular and synovial tissue changes, and (2) articular cartilage and subchondral bone changes.

Periarticular and Synovial Tissue Changes

A consistent feature of the gross appearance of the periarticular and synovial tissues of immobilized joints is a fibro-fatty connective tissue proliferation within the joint space (Evans *et al.*, 1960; Enneking and Horowitz, 1972). In knee immobilization models, this phenomenon is seen prominently in the intercondylar notch, but it is also observed in other joint recesses. The proliferative fibro-fatty connective tissue covers exposed intra-articular soft tissue structures such as the cruciate ligaments and the under-surface of the quadriceps tendon. It also blankets the non-articulating cartilage surfaces. With the passage of time, adhesions develop between the exposed tissue surfaces as the fibro-fatty connective tissue is transformed into more mature scar. The proliferation of this type of tissue is similar in such diverse species as the rabbit, rat, dog, and primate. Similar changes are also prominent in human posterior intervertebral joints and in human knee joints (Enneking and Horowitz, 1972).

Articular Cartilage

The changes which occur secondary to immobility affecting articular cartilage can be separated into those in non-contact areas, and those in contact areas. The changes in non-contact areas are thought to be in part secondary to the fibro-fatty connective tissue proliferation described above. The ingrowth of connective tissue which fills the joint space soon covers the joint surfaces. In the rat model studied by Evans *et al.*, (1960) in which the process was evaluated on a progressive time base, there was coverage of the articular surfaces by 30 days. The connective tissue became more dense and adherent during the subsequent month and remained relatively constant thereafter. The surface cartilage cells gradually became confluent with the overlying connective tissue. By 60 days the tangential layer of cartilage cells was lost in many of the animals. There was consistent evidence of gross thinning of the cartilage beginning peripherally where the adhesions first occurred. Fibrillation of the cartilage was also seen and variable loss of staining of matrix was observed. Staining changes were also described by Baker *et al.* (1969) in human spinal facet joints after anterior spine fusion. These changes included first a zone of loss of staining around the cells peripheral to the cellular lacunae. Ultimately, loss of definition of lacunae occurred, and the cartilage cells became stellate with poorly defined margin. Such change in staining characteristics of cartilage matrix had been described much earlier by von Reyher (1874). Baker *et al.* (1969) described similar changes and termed them "Weichselbaum's space" (Weichselbaum, 1878). Parker and Keefer (1935) observed this process in cartilage beneath rheumatoid pannus and proposed that it represented a metaplastic process of cartilage cells transformed into fibroblasts, a view which Baker *et al.* (1969) endorsed.

In the contact areas of opposed articular surfaces, mild to severe changes of articular cartilage are observed depending on the rigidity of immobilization, the position of immobilization, and most importantly, the degree of compression. Typically, the mild changes consist of loss of intensity of staining of the matrix. In areas of greater compressive forces there are varying degrees of destruction up to and including full thickness ulceration of cartilage with cellular distortion and necrosis, fibrillation of matrix, and erosion of matrix down to subchondral bone (Salter and Field, 1960; Thaxter *et al.*, 1965).

The major areas of alteration in the subchondral bone occur beneath cartilage lesions in joints immobilized 60 days or longer. Hyperemia in the subadjacent marrow spaces is noted with proliferation of connective tissue. In some areas this tissue penetrated the subchondral plate and entered the calcified layer of articular cartilage. Trabecular atrophy and resorption in the areas subadjacent to cartilage lesions are also seen. Subchondral cysts sometimes develop in this location in animals followed for longer periods.

Not surprisingly, such profound alterations in gross and microscopic architecture are associated with significant biomechanical and biochemical changes.

Experimental Models of the Fibrous Connective Tissue Response to Stress Alteration

Changes in capsular and ligamentous structures of immobilized limbs have been the subject of considerable interest with respect to the underlying processes involved, and with respect to the possibility of modifying the responses through the use of drugs or hormones. In an experimental model designed to evaluate the soft tissue response to immobility in our laboratory, the hind limbs of dogs (Akeson, 1961) and rabbits (Akeson *et al.*, 1963) were immobilized using internal fixation procedures for up to 12 weeks, and periarticular connective tissues were examined.

Casts or internal fixation of the flexed knee with a threaded pin placed through the tibia and femur well posterior to the knee joint give similar results. The latter technique has generally been preferred to obviate pressure sores from cast compression and friction.

Biomechanical Changes of the Knee Composite

Knee contracture can be assessed immediately after sacrifice utilizing an apparatus called an "arthrograph" (Woo *et al.*, 1975). The arthrograph is designed to measure joint stiffness in knees in terms of a torque-angular deformation (T-O) diagram.The knees of the experimental and control from each animal were mounted on the arthrograph and cycled at a frequency of 0.2 Hz. Two ranges of motion, five cycles each, were used in sequence: the first was 50 to 80°, and the second 45 to 95° of knee angles. Each cycle of flexion and extension was recorded on the X-Y recorder. Recording of the first cycle of the contracture knee is particularly important because subsequent cycles required substantially less energy. In addition, the amount of torque required to extend the knee from 50 to 65% from acute flexion during the first cycle is also significantly higher than that of subsequent cycles. The increases in torque and area of hysteresis are used as measures of increase in joint stiffness of severity of joint contracture. A progressive increase in the strength of contracture is observed on serial evaluations between 2 and 12 weeks. Detailed descriptions of the apparatus and technique are given in several earlier papers (Akeson *et al.*, 1973; Woo *et al.*, 1975). The arthrograph permits evaluation of the efficacy of therapeutic modalities such as drug or hormone injections. Interestingly, hyaluronic acid has been shown to significantly inhibit contracture development under stress deprivation conditions (Amiel *et al.*, 1975).

Biomechanical Changes in Ligaments

Following 9 weeks of immobilization, the linear slope, ultimate load, and energy absorbing capabilities of the rabbit MCL-bone complex during tension decrease to approximately one third that of the contralateral nonimmobilized control. The load-strain characteristics of the MCL substance deteriorates. Further immobilization of up to 12 weeks causes additional degradation of the MCL substance (Woo *et al.*, 1979). These data are obtained with the aid of the video dimensional analyzer system, where the mechanical properties of ligament substance and structural properties of the bone-ligament complex can be simultaneously evaluated (Woo *et al.*, 1983).

The failure mode is altered in this model; failure load and modules of elasticity are reduced. Bone resorption at the ligament insertion site causes failure by avulsion at the insertion site, a problem noted by several investigators (Laros *et al.*, 1971; Cooper and Misel, 1970; Tipton *et al.*, 1978).

These mechanical alterations occur after a relatively brief stress deprivation period compared to common clinical treatment programs for fractures and joint injuries. They have important implications to the rationale for selection of treatment options and, as we will see, equally dramatic implications for rehabilitation following recovery from the initial injuries.

Exercise Effects on Specialized Connective Tissue Structure

An animal model has been used to evaluate effects of exercise on bone, tendon, and ligament in normals. In one study, miniature swine were exercised at intervals on a track over 1 year on a schedule which created cardiac hypertrophy and increased cardiac output (Woo *et al.*, 1980a). At the end of 1 year, cortical bone showed improved structural properties of about one third, indicative of cortical hypertrophy. The material properties were unchanged, indicating that the changes observed were entirely due to bulk change rather than qualitative improvement. Similar changes were observed for digital extensor tendons. The cross-sectional areas 12 months after onset of the exercise period were increased 21% and the load to failure increased 62% (Woo *et al.*, 1980b). It is important to observe that, at 3 months after onset, changes in bone and extensor tendon were not significant, indicating that a long time and great effort are required for improvement in structural properties. Furthermore, site- and tissue-specific factors are involved, since digital flexor tendons and ligaments were less responsive to the exercise program than were bone and extensor tendon.

Recovery from Stress Deprivation

It is of interest that recovery of the MCL properties following immobilization may be quite rapid. The load strain curve properties of the MCL from the experimental knee of 9-week immobilized animals recovers to that of the control after 12 weeks of cage activity. The recovery curve for the 12-week immobilized knees remains slightly inferior after a cage-activity recovery period of 12 weeks (Woo *et al.*, 1987). The experimental knee ligaments continue to have inferior structural properties as compared to those of the control knees. The P_{max} and the A_{max} for the experimentals are approximately two thirds that of the controls. The slower recovery of strength of the bone-ligament junction confirms findings obtained by other investigators (Laros *et al.*, 1971; Tipton *et al.*, 1978; Noyes *et al.*, 1974).

The surprising finding, however, is that following remobilization there is a rapid recovery of properties of the MCL substance in the functional range (up to 5% ligament strain), although the ultimate load and energy absorbing capability of the MCL-bone complex are still considerably inferior (Woo *et al.*, 1987). Tibial insertion sites continue to be the weakest link. These results are consistent with the earlier conclusion of Noyes *et al.*, (1974) who showed that up to 1 year of reconditioning is required to regain the strength of ACL-bone complex following 8 weeks of immobilization. Additionally, our data indicate that the ligament substance will recover rapidly during remobilization and the ligament itself can function normally in the physiologic range.

The implications for treatment are that prevention of stress deprivation effects are paramount to the success of rehabilitation efforts. This conclusion forms the central basis of the scientific rationale of invocation of rehabilitation therapies at the earliest possible juncture.

Biochemical Events Consequent to Stress Deprivation

The biochemical changes of periarticular connective tissue matrix are manifold. Space does not permit a detailed exposition of those changes. However, a summary will follow, along with key references to the literature. An important point which has evolved from our laboratory is that there are notable differences between cellular and biochemical matrix characteristics of ligaments and tendons and, furthermore, there are differences between particular ligaments. The functional implications of these differences are not yet entirely clear and require further study.

Extracellular Fluid Volume Changes

The water content of fibrous connective tissues is in the range of 65 to 70%. As the population of cells is relatively sparse in this tissue, the majority of this water is perforce in the extracellular space. On gross inspection, the dissected tissues from an immobilized limb appear less glistening and more "woody" in texture. Chemical analysis shows a significant decrease in water content of 4 to 6% as compared to the control side (Akeson et al., 1973). It seems likely that this amount of water loss is functionally significant. Fluid movement, which plays such an important role in articular cartilage load-bearing and lubrication, is equally important in fibrous connective tissue in importing viscoelastic properties. It has been established that hyaluronic acid and its attached or entrapped water is the principal fibrous connective tissue lubricant (Swann et al., 1974).

It is presumed that the interstitial fluid in a densely fibrous "connecting" anatomical structure serves as a spacer between individual collagen fibers or fibrils, permitting discrete movement of one fiber or fibril past the adjacent fibers. The importance of interstitial fluid to tissue rheology is obvious as the concept of viscoelasticity of connective tissue rests upon the dual fluid and solid nature of these systems.

Glycosaminoglycan Changes

The largest change found in the composition of the stress deprived periarticular connective tissue is reduction in the concentration of glycosaminoglycans (GAG) (Akeson et al., 1967). The decreases in chondroitin-4- and -6-sulfate (30%) and hyaluronic acid (40%) are statistically significant, while the percent change of dermatan sulfate thought to be associated with fibers is smaller. Decreased concentration of GAG and water would be expected to alter the plasticity and pliability of connective tissue matrices, and to reduce lubrication efficiency. Biochemical analyses of articular cartilage and meniscus from the immobilized knees also show a reduction of 24 and 31%, respectively, of GAG content in these tissues (ibid).

Water content appears to parallel the GAG ranges in concert with the known facts concerning the high water binding capacity of GAG. The preferential loss of GAG is also consistent with known rapid turnover half-life (1.7 to 7 days) (Schiller et al., 1967) as compared with collagen (half-life of 300 to 500 days) (Neuberger and Slack, 1953). Turnover studies utilizing tritium-labeled acetate show that the decrement in specific activity of hyaluronic acid with time after preliminary labeling is the same for control and immobilized limbs. The conclusion is therefore that there is not acceleration of degradation, but rather a reduction in the synthesis of hyaluronic acid in the immobilized extremities. Fibroblasts of the fibrous connective tissue matrix apparently respond to physical forces by a homeostasis feedback loop to maintain the proper balance of connective tissue constituents.

A gel-like structure created by the interaction between water and glycosaminoglycans is currently well accepted by physiologists working with interstitial fluid flow questions (Guyton *et al.*, 1980). Clearly, the gel structure is severely compromised in connective tissue deprived of mechanical stimulation. It is postulated that the GAG and water changes are permissive insofar as qualitative changes in collagen are concerned, as fiber-fiber distances must be reduced when water and GAG volumes are reduced.

It is presumed that the lubricating and volume separating effects provided by hyaluronic acid and water permit the independent gliding of microfibrils past one another, facilitating tissue adaption to motion permitted by the particular connective tissue weave pattern. Loss of this volume-separating and lubricating property provides for fibril-fibril friction as well as the potential for adhesions or cross-linking between adjacent collagen fibrils. Any newly synthesized collagen is apt to be randomlydispersed and to create interference with the functional gliding between fibers necessary for normal mobility. This is particularly so, since in the stationary attitude maturation processes may encourage fibril growth in diameter by including these newly synthesized random fibrils within the fiber structural units. Such mismatch with respect to functional elongation needs without regard to the usual physical force and motion probably is central to the pathomechanics of joint stiffness.

Collagen Changes

The processes seen in the studies described above, which rely on the techniques of anatomic pathology, suggest that connective tissue proliferation or simple granulation tissue production is the basis of joint contractures. However, collagen turnover studies are difficult to reconcile with this concept at first examination. For example, the studies by Brooke and Slack (1959) showed that collagen precursor uptake was actually reduced in denervated rat limbs compared to controls. However, collagen synthesis did proceed, but at a reduced level. Peacock (1963) used saline solubility of collagen to estimate the amount of new collagen synthesized and found no differences in immobilized and control joints except for the posterior capsular area where there was increased collagen solubility. However, as he used pin fixation with a placement proximate to the posterior capsule, the significance of finding total collagen mass changes became uncertain. Our laboratory was able to demonstrate reduction in total collagen of only 10% by total joint mass evaluation using the whole periarticular connective tissue unit (Amiel *et al.*, 1980). Studies of Klein *et al.*, (1977) using long-term labeling techniques which are more sensitive for this purpose, found small increases in collagen mass in denervated limbs.

We feel that strategic placement of anomalous cross-links of newly synthesized collagen fibrils in the contracture process is of importance. These cross-links can act as bridges between existing functionally independent fibers with divergent tracking patterns.Using a simplified model, i.e., the Chinese finger trap mechanism, it can be seen that fixed contact at just a few nodal points defects the functional gliding of the whole apparatus. Demonstration of such changes within the weave of the joint capsule is quite difficult because of right to left variability in micro-architecture and the small degree of change necessary to effect a mechanical impediment. However, it is easy to be convinced that such a process must play a role in the synovial joint contracture process. Disorganization which occurs in the cruciate ligament of a rabbit after 9 weeks of immobilization has been demonstrated in our previous work (Akeson et al., 1978). The pattern of cellular alignment becomes distorted as well, almost certainly reflecting a more random matrix organization.

Collagen Cross-Link Alterations. The studies of quantitative changes in the cross-linking of collagen from the immobilized rabbit knees periarticular connective tissue show significant increases in sodium borohydride reducible intermolecular cross-links (Akeson et al., 1977). A typical radioactive elution profile from column 1 of a $3N$ p-toluene sulfonic acid hydrolysate of [3H]NaBh$_4$ reduced periarticular connective tissue from control and immobilized joints and rechromatography on an extended basic column of the aldolhistidinedihydroxylysinonorleucine peaks show a twofold increase in DHLNL on the immobilized side. It was shown that dihydroxylysinonorleucine (DHLNL), hydroxylysinonorleucine (HLNL), and histidinohydroxymerodesmosine (HHMD) are the major cross-links which increase following immobilization. No change in hydroxylysine/lysine ratio between the immobilized and control periarticular connective tissue collagen was detected.

It can be speculated that the increased intra- and intermolecular collagen cross-links are important in the contracture process. How do such cross-links interact at a molecular level? To begin with, it is unlikely that a fiber to fiber distance is bridged by a lysine-lysine or lysine-hydroxylysine reaction. The distances are much too great and the forces too small to create the nodal fiber to fiber cross-link which is proposed to hamper joint motion. Rather, it is presumed that the nodal fiber-to-fiber cross-links are brought about by aggregation of new fibrils with pre-existing fibers of the matrix. The process may proceed in the usual manner of aggregation of fibrils into fibers, then incorporating bridges of newly synthesized collagen fibril elements into pairs of existing fibers. Such structures become mechanically constraining at the time when the joint is freed from constraining devices.

Collagen Type Changes. Since the formation of reducible cross-links follows collagen synthesis (Bailey and Robins, 1973), and since the presence and relative amounts of these cross-links may, in part, depend upon the type of collagen being synthesized (Jackson and Mechanic, 1974), it is important to examine the type or types of periarticular connective tissue collagen synthesized during the period of immobilization. Examination of densitometric scans of the SDS gel of the CNBr-cleaved peptides from control and immobilized tissue reveals no alteration in the type of collagen being synthesized during the period of immobilization (Amiel *et al.*, 1980). The peptides α_1 [III] CB3 and CB6 characteristic of Type III collagen are absent in the CNBr-digest of control and immobilized periarticular connective tissue collagen. Furthermore, these results are confirmed by amino acid analysis and SDS gel electrophoresis performed on intact components separated by CM cellulose chromatography. These results provide additional supportive evidence that only type I collagen is found in the dense fibrous structures of normal and contracture knees.

The significance of the changes in collagen type ratios and cross-linking patterns observed secondary to stress deprivation probably reflects the effects of increased collagen turnover. The altered mechanics, in turn, most probably result from the random orientation of newly synthesized fibrous matrix constituents. These new fibrils are disposed without regard to mechanical requirements because of the lack of input from the mechanical signals which are normally operative.

The Development of Concepts of Passive Motion

The events described above indicate a disturbing and very harmful outcome of stress deprivation on synovial joints which threatens the success of rehabilitation after treatment with casts or splints for trauma or other disorders requiring immobilization. It was not unexpected, therefore, to observe the development of new concepts of treatment emphasizing early motion. The controversy about early motion had, in fact, erupted earlier still. The archetypical protagonists commonly identified as providing leadership for the motion vs. rest camps in the century passed were Hugh Owen Thomas, called "Hugh the rester" and Championniere, whose philosophy of treatment was exemplified by his phrase "in motion there is life". The historical advocates of rest vs. motion schools relied almost entirely on empirical observation and appeals to authority for the basis of therapeutic decisions. It remained for the clarification of effects of stress on synovial joints to properly prioritize the therapeutic decision on rehabilitation. Equally important in the evolution of modern rehabilitation philosophy were fundamental studies on the influence of stress and motion on repair of bone, tendon, ligament, and cartilage. Furthermore, studies on stress and motion effects on disorders of the synovial joint composite have provided a foundation for musculoskeletal management decisions which are approaching a more logical construct. Technological advances have occurred which, hand in hand with these observations, have provided new avenues for treatment which could be coupled with the early motion philosophy of rehabilitation.

In fracture management, for example, it has been possible to achieve improved fracture stability with biomechanically sound internal fixation devices. These devices applied very early in the post injury period have permitted not only early joint mobility (Baxendale *et al.*, 1985; Mooney and Stills, 1987), but mobilization of the total patient. The ability to mobilize patients after multiple trauma has resulted in a marked improvement in the survival rates in the critically injured patient—a tribute to the modern trauma management system—and a tribute to the philosophy of early mobilization.

The philosophy of early mobilization has adapted passive motion in several forms: (1) occasional, (2) interrupted, and (3) continuous, with various combinations thereof, to the early post injury or postoperative state where patient compliance with active motion programs cannot reasonably be expected because of postoperative pain or weakness.

For successful application of passive motion to the post injury state, the integrity of the repair—bone, ligament or tendon—must be maintained. Details of specific applications await further contributions from basic and clinical science. However, enough is known that it is possible to develop an understanding of some of the general principles of application which should find universal utility in musculoskeletal rehabilitation for the foreseeable future. What follows is a brief outline of the evidence of efficacy of passive motion in a variety of clinical applications and of the scientific basis of those applications.

Synovial Joint Space Clearance During Continuous Passive Motion

Studies on clearance rates from synovial joints have demonstrated the value of passive motion in facilitating transport of intrasynovial contents. Cyclical changes in intra-articular pressure during CPM have been documented (Pedowitz *et al.*, 1989; Baxendale *et al.*, 1985; Caughey and Bywaters, 1963). The clearest example of this application is the paperof O'Driscoll and colleagues (1983) on the clearance of blood from the joint space. These data demonstrated convincingly that hemarthrosis in a model system treated by CPM was more rapidly cleared than in contralateral mobilized joints. The clearance rate of indium-III-oxine-labeled erythrocytes was double that seen in the immobilized joints. After 1 week there was significantly less blood remaining in the joints treated with CPM. These results were supported by Danzig *et al.*, 1987.

This effect was seen indirectly in a paper by Skyhar *et al.*, (1985) using $^{35}SO_4$ to study nutrition of anterior cruciate knee ligaments under conditions of CPM and rest. It was demonstrated that in CPM knees there was less $^{35}SO_4$ uptake than in a cage activity group. The effect of CPM on synovial fluid clearance was so large that the uptake of $^{35}SO_4$ in the CPM treated knees was less than that in the immobilized knees, suggesting, at first, poor diffusion under conditions of CPM—but actually indicating that clearance of isotope occurred before diffusion into the ligament could occur.

These experiments demonstrate the importance of the convection effect of activity to the nutritional support of synovial joint components, especially articular cartilage and ligaments. Furthermore, the clinical application of CPM in the postoperative state is emphasized as a practical step in improved patient care postoperatively or post trauma. The clearance of blood from the joint space is of undisputed advantage knowing the harmful effects of chronic hemarthrosis in states such as hemophilia.

Continuous Passive Motion in Treatment of Septic Arthritis

The use of motion to favorably influence the outcome of septic arthritis has been demonstrated in papers by Salter et al., (1981) and O'Driscoll and Salter (1984) in a model system. The beneficial effect was most prominently seen in articular cartilage, where the damage of the septic process from proteolytic enzymes was reduced by the imposition of a passive motion program. Presumably, clearance of the deleterious lysosomal enzymes which accumulate in joint fluid in septic arthritis was facilitated by motion induced convection effects. The articular cartilages of joints treated by the activity protocols were presumably spared exposure to high levels of matrix destructive enzymes by the acceleration of clearance of those products from the joint space by CPM. Clinical support for this application has recently been presented by Mooney and colleagues (Mooney and Stills, 1987).

Passive Motion Effects on Repair

Several repair models have been studied under the influence of one of the passive motion modalities. In several applications the quality of repair appears to be improved under motion conditions as compared to immobility. These applications require stability of the repair line in order for healing to proceed successfully. This is seen most clearly in flexor tendon repair, where failure of the suture line in the early postoperative state can result in tendon disruption. However, if the suture line is maintained, improved outcome has been observed in several respects (Gelberman et al., 1982). In certain circumstances intermittent passive motion has resulted in a successful outcome. In the case of ligament, cage activity has been shown to be superior to immobilization (Inoue et al., 1980). In still other circumstances, especially in cartilage healing, CPM was shown to provide a superior outcome (Salter et al., 1980). Generally speaking, the experimental models have indicated improved healing rates of bone, tendon, ligament, and cartilage under motion conditions and also improved quality of repair. Indeed, in the flexor tendon case within the flexor tendon sheath, it has been shown that healing proceeds by different mechanisms under motion conditions (intrinsic healing) as compared to immobilization (extrinsic healing—the one wound concept) (Gelberman et al., 1982). The available data is insufficient to describe optimum clinical protocols of frequency, intensity or duration of passive motion. We have spoken of the problem as analogous to the drug dose/response curve. In fact, the optimum values for passive motion may be found to vary in the spectrum of specific applications. Until those data are available, empirical rules will apply.

The examples below, however, will provide insights into the range of potential applications of passive motion to the problems of specialized connective tissue healing and the broad principles which underly these uses.

Continuous Passive Motion Influence on Cartilage Healing

The interaction between healing of the joint surfaces and motion had beginnings with the early concepts of cup arthroplasty. It was recognized that conversion of the new arthroplasty surface to fibrocartilage following debridement of the degenerative hip and reaming to a concentric sphere of bleeding bone required motion. Without motion the surface contained only fibrous tissue. In a few instances there was the opportunity to observe surfaces in patients who had not been able to move the hip for unrelated medical reasons. In these patients conversion of fibrous tissue to fibrocartilage was not observed. Mooney et al., (1966) showed this effect in the rabbit metatarsophalangeal joint where immobilized segments did not develop fibrocartilage surfaces as well as mobilized joints. Hohl and Luck (1956) were able to demonstrate superior healing in drill hole defects in femoral cartilage of primates if motion occurred. Convery and Akeson (1972) studied varying size drill hole defects of femoral condyles of horses on pasture grazing activity and observed that relatively small defects ($^1/_8$ in diameter) healed readily, but larger defects ($^1/_4$ to $^7/_8$ in) did not heal. The dimensional aspect of cartilage healing is important to recognize, because with or without motion regimens large defects ($^1/_4$ in or larger) simply do not heal by restoration of hyaline cartilage. Nor do arthroplasty surfaces heal with hyaline cartilage. The composition of the articular surface replacement matrix is that of fibrocartilage, not hyaline cartilage. This conclusion has been demonstrated convincingly by histological and biochemical methods. These factors have obvious functional and clinical implications which must temper the interpretation of CPM effects on cartilage healing.

Salter and colleagues have been important contributors to the studies of facilitation of cartilage healing under the influence of CPM. They have shown convincingly that small defects of rabbit femoral articular cartilage of the order of magnitude of $^1/_8$ in diameter will heal with hyaline cartilage in a significant percentage of knees mobilized by CPM. This is an important observation which relates to several clinical circumstances in which small defects in hyaline cartilage of the joint surface occur such as cracks in articular surfaces seen commonly in fracture patterns. It is important to note that the facilitation of repair of primitive mesenchymal cells to hyaline cartilage occurs in *only* the very small defects, not in large or full surface defects.

Continuous Passive Motion Influences on Periosteal and Perichondrial Grafting of Cartilage Defects

The fact that only very small cartilage defects heal with a satisfactory extracellular matrix of hyaline cartilage has led several investigators to search for improved techniques of treatment of such defects. Ohlsen (1978), and Engkvist (1979) studied rib perichondrial tissue as a potential source of primitive cells with chondrogenic potential for this purpose. The work was later confirmed by Coutts et al. (1983), Salter (1989), Zarnett and Salter (1989), O'Driscoll et al. (1988), and Shimizu et al. (1987). Because experimental studies indicated considerable promise, pilot clinical perichondrial arthroplasty studies for small joints of the hand were soon thereafter performed with some success (Engkvist and Johansson, 1980). Poussa et al. (1981) showed similar chondrogenic potential of periosteal grafts. O'Driscoll and Salter (1984) confirmed Poussa's work in a rabbit knee joint model. They were able to improve the result from 8% success in immobilized knees to 59% success in knees managed by CPM. Fixation of the periosteal or perichondrial membrane is crucial to the successful outcome of periosteal or perichondrial grafting. O'Driscoll et al. (1984, 1988), Zarnett and Salter (1989), and Salter (1989) developed a method of stretching the periosteal membrane over a bone plug sized to fit the defect to be filled. This technique has worked effectively in the experimental application, but different methodology will probably be required for clinical application.

Continuous Passive Motion Influence on Fracture Healing

The development of modern biomechanical devices and modern principles of application of those devices to fracture fixation permits the use of CPM early in the post injury states (Mooney and Stills, 1987). CPM is most effectively applied in intra-articular fractures where fracture lines through subchondral bone and articular cartilage are commonly observed. Following the observations of Salter (1989), it will frequently be the case that the width of the gap between fracture fragments after reduction is less than $1/8$ in. If congruence of the joint is established and the cartilage fracture gaps are narrow, CPM may facilitate the cartilage healing process. Additional benefits should be anticipated in terms of facilitation of the rehabilitation program by lessening stress deprivation effects and by providing stress enhancement to guide deposition of matrix components in an orderly and functionally desirable alignment.

Intermittent Passive Motion Effects on Tendon Healing

The application of passive motion to flexor tendon healing in "no man's land" in the flexor tendon sheath has been slow to evolve for two reasons: (1) concern about integrity of the suture line and (2) concern about the mechanism of tendon healing requiring ingrowth of connective tissue from the flexor tendon sheath. The paradox of the latter process, termed the "one wound concept" by Peacock (1963), is that the very tissue ingrowth which caused healing also caused the tendon to be locked against the flexor sheath, thus limiting functional tendon excursion. Indeed the major failures in tendon surgery are not with tendon healing, but with tendon adhesions which markedly reduce the range of motion of the tendon and affected joints. The fundamental studies of Gelberman *et al.* (1982) reversed this thinking by demonstrating clearly that tendon healing could occur by an intrinsic mechanism of proliferation of epitenon and endotenon cells when the extrinsic mechanism is blocked by intermittent passive motion. The canine forepaw model was used for these flexor tendon studies. Not only did the tendon heal by the intrinsic route with passive motion application, but the healing occurred more rapidly and with greater mechanical strength while simultaneously preserving mobility of tendon and the joints of the affected finger.

It is important to note that the motion required for this effect is not of great duration. The mobilization schedule used in the studies mentioned above was only 5 min of careful manual passive motion conducted by a technician twice a day. The remainder of the time the limb was immobilized in a fiberglass cast. This "mini" passive motion schedule recognized the concerns about the potential of rupture of the suture line if a more aggressive passive motion protocol were used.

In this instance, passive motion therapy was able to convert the healing mode from extrinsic to intrinsic, while simultaneously providing improved healing strength and improved mobility — a string of therapeutic bonuses which are seldom so clearly identified after modification of a postoperative treatment protocol.

Salter and colleagues have shown, in the patellar tendon laceration model, similar effects of improved healing associated with continuous passive motion. In this case, repair involves both extrinsic and intrinsic mechanisms due to the anatomical differences between patellar and flexor tendons.

Intermittent Active Motion Effects in Ligament Healing

The discussion of ligament healing is confounded by the diversity of structures under the ligament classification with respect to unique anatomical and physiological features. For example, the anterior cruciate ligament (ACL) of the knee will not heal for reasons not precisely known, although the "hostile" synovial environment in which the ACL resides is widely presumed to be an important or even decisive factor in the outcome. The ACL receives significant nutrition from synovial fluid and that nutritional source may not be adequate to support fibroblastic proliferation (although it will support a healing response in the case of flexor tendon). Recently it has been demonstrated in our laboratory that the cells of the ACL have fibrocartilage characteristics. Failure of fibrocartilage structures to heal is well known. However, whether the cellular morphology of the ACL is the explanation for the poor healing of the ACL is unproven. The enigma remains. Nevertheless, CPM is used by many clinicans in the postoperative period following replacement of the ACL by a grafting technique employing a tendon or a bone-tendon-bone unit. Burks and colleagues (1984) have cautioned that CPM can cause failure of the tendon graft if the graft is not isometric and is not firmly secured. However, if those conditions prevail, the graft is unlikely to survive in a rehabilitation setting whether CPM is used or not. Clinical studies by Noyes and colleagues (1987) support the conclusion that CPM is a safe modality when surgery is properly performed. Tendon grafts actually become very weak structurally 3 to 6 weeks after insertion. Nevertheless, the best clinical successes have been shown to occur with early and aggressive rehabilitation protocols.

Experimental studies have shown that tendon cells of the ACL graft undergo autolysis in the intrasynovial environment (Amiel et al., 1986) and are replaced by cells from synovial sources. The matrix of the graft is gradually remodeled and assumes the matrix characteristics of ACL (Amiel et al., 1986). None of the animal studies has shown recovery of mechanical strength of the ACL graft substitute to the original tissue mechanical and structural properties.

Better experimental and clinical results can be reported for most other ligaments. The medial collateral ligament of the knee, for example, has an abundant surrounding soft tissue blood supply which offers ample nutritional and cellular support of the needed fibroplasia. In this case, the recent work of Inoue et al. (1986) has provided strong evidence supporting the concept of early active motion of the knee. When compared to knees immobilized for the entire postoperative period, or knees immobilized for the first half of the postoperative period, the early activity group clearly showed superior mechanical and structural strength at the end of 12 weeks. Others have shown a favorable effect of CPM on reorganization of the fibrils of the scar into parallel arrays (Fronek et al., 1983). It is to be emphasized that in these models the cruciate ligaments are intact, thus providing stability necessary for early ambulation or CPM.

Continuous Passive Motion After Total Knee Replacement

The total knee replacement procedures now frequently performed for degenerative or rheumatoid arthritis have provided a challenging problem for the application of CPM. Early achievement of a nearly full range of motion postoperatively is important in the rehabilitation of these patients. Slow recovery of flexion is commonly observed postoperatively, sometimes requiring forceful manipulation under anesthesia.

A multi-institutional study of over 100 total knee replacement cases treated traditionally and compared to similar cases treated with CPM has provided data which clarifies the effectiveness of CPM in a clinical rehabilitation setting (Coutts et al., 1983). The patients treated with CPM had a more rapid gain in knee motion and a shorter hospital stay than patients treated traditionally, a finding supported by other studies (Romness et al., 1988; Lynch et al., 1988; Vince et al., 1987). Data in Coutts' series showed a lower pain medication requirement than in the traditionally treated series. The theory commonly employed to explain the surprising tolerance of postoperative patients for passive motion is the "gate" theory of Melzack and Wall (1970), which postulates that nonpainful afferent input into spinal cord ganglia can overwhelm pain fiber input, thereby blocking a part of the pain perception otherwise experienced. CPM provides considerable afferent input due to effects of motion on proprioceptive receptors. There is no universal acceptance of this effect in postoperative applications of CPM, but at least it seems clear that CPM does not increase pain medication requirements.

Continuous Passive Motion and Wound Healing

CPM in the postoperative patient does not inhibit wound healing. No wound disruptions have been reported from application of CPM postoperatively, and furthermore, postoperative swelling and joint effusions were reduced (Coutts et al., 1983). In total, the benefits of a relatively brief few days of application of CPM postoperatively in this application appear to significantly outweigh questions of cost or of risk.

Continuous Passive Motion Prophylaxis Against Thrombophlebitis

The use of CPM in the variety of clinical applications described above has evoked interest in its use in prophylaxis against thrombophlebitis in the postoperative period of high risk (Fisher et al., 1985). The proposed physiological basis of the desired effect is the cycling of intramuscular pressure which occurs during passive motion as the muscles of the limb are lengthened and shortened passively (Coutts, personal communicaton). The passive pressure alteration almost certainly has the same functional effect as active muscle contraction in propelling venous blood back to the heart. Since venous stasis is presumed to be an important factor in venous thrombosis, the utilization of CPM, which would significantly reduce venous stasis, would be expected to have a salutary effect on reducing the rate of complications of postoperative thrombophlebitis and pulmonary embolism.

Preliminary results suggesting the validity of this line of reasoning have been presented by Lynch et al. (1984), and by Vince et al. (1987), but other studies showed no prophylaxis with respect to incidence of deep venous thrombosis as visualized by venogram (Romness and Rand, 1988; Lynch et al., 1988). Several centers have ongoing studies on this problem and considerable information will be forthcoming in the near future to document the degree of effectiveness of CPM in this application. As is typical of other studies of DVT postoperatively, the clinical series size must be very large in order to have the statistical power to be valid.

Other Uses of Continuous Passive Motion

An almost infinite variety of conditions can be treated by CPM. These include use in treatment of elbow contractures post surgical release (Breen *et al.*, 1988), treatment of hemophiliac joints post synovectomy (Limbird and Dennis, 1987), and treatment of knee contractures post arthroscopy (Parisien, 1988). Recent review articles by Salter (1989) and by Mooney and Stills (1987) highlight other related clinical applications. The principles of application of CPM are so fundamental as to preclude boundaries with respect to potential future applications, including application to the spine.

New Observations on Mechanisms of the Cellular Response to Mechanical Stimuli

The tissue adaptation to mechanical forces varies dramatically depending on whether the forces are compressive or tensile. Areas where forces are primarily tensile develop fibrous characteristics. Areas where forces are primarily compressive generally develop cartilaginous characteristics. The obvious example of cartilaginous adaptation, of course, is articular cartilage covering the joint surfaces at the ends of long bones. In other areas where the compressive and tensile forces are mixed, fibrocartilaginous tissue develops; examples include annulus fibrosus of the intervertebral disc and the meniscus of the knee. These structures share load bearing of longitudinal compressive forces and simultaneously accept considerable tensile load via hoop stresses. Recently the presence of primarily fibrocartilaginous cells in the anterior cruciate ligament has been described. Whether this results from the ligament during flexion and extension of the knee or from other causes such as nutritional factors of meager blood supply is not clear.

Cartilaginous and fibrocartilaginous tissues lack a significant blood supply, relying on diffusion and convection of fluid, ions, and small molecules for nutrition and homeostasis. Compressive forces undoubtedly force an adaption toward avascularity because of the tendency of those forces to collapse small vessels and capillaries. However, the adaptation has a large price—the inability of these tissues to achieve intrinsic healing. The lack of vessels and associated primitive perivascular cells denies the possibility of scar production following injury. Major clinical effects result from the lack of a healing response of cartilaginous and fibrocartilaginous tissues are manifold; failure of healing of intervertebral discs, of meniscus and anterior cruciate ligament of the knee, of the Bankhart lesion of the shoulder, etc.

Cellular Differences Between Ligament

Ultrastructural, histological, biochemical, and biomechanical differences have been described between the ACL and MCL, tissues with strikingly different capacities for healing (Amiel *et al.*, 1984; Lyon *et al.*, 1989). Light microscopy of the MCL reveals spindle-shaped cells aligned with the long axis of the ligament and interspersed throughout the collagen fiber bundles (Amiel *et al.*, 1984). The ACL cells are oval shaped and aligned in columns between fiber bundles. Ultrastructurally, MCL collagen fibers are uniformly of large diameter (Lyon *et al.*, 1989). The fibroblasts have long cellular processes in close apposition to surrounding collagen fibrils. The ACL has a more heterogeneous population of fibril diameters. Oval-shaped cells are surrounded by an amorphous ground substance and have small micropro-cesses which are not in close apposition to collagen fibrils.

It appears that a spectrum of fibroblast phenotypes exists between the spindle-shaped connective tissue fibroblast of dermis, tendon, and fascia on the one hand, and the rounded, nested fibroblast of fibrocartilage on the other. The ACL fibroblast seems to exist near the fibrocartilaginous end of the spectrum in terms of morphologic features. Quite possibily the morpho-logical features of these fibroblasts are interrelated with cellular function, and play a determinate role in their response to injury. The form/function suitable for survival in a synovial environment may not be sufficient for mounting and sustaining an effective healing response. The concept that the shape of a cell and its orientation with respect to the surrounding matrix are important factors in modulating its proliferative response to mitogens was mentioned by Wessels (1977) in studies on skin. These observations were expanded by Gospodarowicz *et al.*, (1986) in a paper entitled "Cellular Shape is Determined by the Extracellular Matrix and is Responsible for the Control of Cellular Growth and Function".

Fibronectin

Fibronectins (FNs) are a class of high molecular weight glycoproteins proposed as a key element in the structural interrelationship of cells to matrix and to other cells (Ruoslahti and Pierschbacher, 1986, 1987). They are associated with an array of cellular functions, including cellular adhesion (both cell-to-cell and cell-to-substratum), intra- and extracellular matrix morphology, cell migration, and reticuloendothelial system function (i.e., phagocytosis and chemotaxis). By having adhesive domains specific to fi-brin, actin, hyaluronic acid, collagen, heparin, and cell surface factors, they function to attract and couple key elements in normal, healing, and growing organized tissue. In fact, FN has been shown to facilitate wound healing (Nagelschmidt *et al.*, 1987) and to be required for normal collagen organi-zation and deposition by fibroblasts *in vitro* (McDonald *et al.*, 1982).

The ACL, MCL, and meniscus have stained positive for FN. The FN is heavily concentrated in the amorphous ground substance surrounding the ACL cells and meniscal cells, whereas in the MCL the distribution of FN is spread evenly over the cell membrane, even out along the long cellular processes.

The amount of FN in rabbit periarticular soft tissues has also been quantitated (Amiel et al., 1990). The amounts of total extractable FN found to be present in ACL, PCL, MCL, and PT, respectively, were 2.0, 1.9, 0.8, and 0.7 μg/mg of dry tissue. While the FN quantities in ACL and PCL were found to be similar, they were over twice as high as the amounts found in either MCL or PT.

Our laboratories have shown that prolonged disuse of the knee joint in a rabbit model, i.e., 9 and 12 weeks of stress deprivation, resulted in significant alterations in fibronectin concentration in the periarticular connective tissues (PCTs) (ACL, MCL, and PT).

The concentration of FN was measured by competitive enzyme-linked immunosorbant assay (ELISA: Amiel et al., 1990). Decreases of 54.0 and 663.7% occurred in the ACL after 9 and 12 weeks. The PT, being tonically stressed by the quadriceps muscles, showed no statistical change. The decreases in total FN concentration observed in this study may reflect increased activity in enzymes that can degrade FN, such as stromelysin. It should also be stated that the decrease in FN following stress deprivation could be explained by biochemical alterations of the PCTs, i.e., ligaments and tendons.

The loss of GAG- and collagen-bound FN following stress deprivation could also be related to degradation of the GAGs and the collagen observed in these PCTs.

While FN levels have been observed to increase in healing tissue (Kurkinen et al., 1980; Lehto et al., 1985; Williams et al., 1984), it is not known whether differences in the baseline levels of FN affect the healing potential of a tissue such as cruciate ligament. Baseline levels in the cruciates are high compared to other periarticular tissues which have a better healing response. While the importance of FN in various connective tissues is increasingly becoming more evident, further studies are required to clarify its role in normal ligament structure and in the ligament healing response.

Adhesive Protein Receptors

Recently a superfamily of adhesion-mediating cell surface glycoproteins (the integrins) has been identified and partially characterized (Dahners, 1986). A major subfamily called the "very late antigens" (VLA) appear to play a primary role in adhesion of cells to components of the extracellular matrix including FN, collagen, and laminin.

VLAs are transmembrane glycoproteins expressed on a wide variety of cells including fibroblasts, epithelial, and hematopoietic cells. A number of functional roles have been assigned to these adhesive protein receptors, including cell migration cell-matrix adhesions, wound contraction, and ligament "tensioning" (Roberts et al., 1988).

The adhesive protein receptors of ligament tissue have received little attention to date. Generalizing from other fibroblast-containing structures, it is reasonable to expect that these receptors exist on cells of the cruciate ligaments and other periarticular tissues. Recently TGF_β has been found to regulate the cell-surface display of VLAs on a variety of cell types, and to modulate the interaction of cells with the extracellular matrix (Roberts *et al.*, 1988; Ignotz and Massague, 1987). These studies lead us to believe that cell surface receptor distribution and expression may have profound effects on ligament healing capacity. Fundamental studies on these receptors are in progress in several laboratories with respect to distribution in various connective tissue cells and to alteration of expression during the healing process.

Conclusions

This review summarizes existing knowledge on the importance of stress and motion to synovial joint homeostasis. The deleterious effects of stress deprivation occur rapidly and are profound, influencing joint mechanics, biochemistry, and physiology in fundamental ways. Recovery from this process is not symmetrical, requiring many months, rather than weeks, to reestablish near normal values. In fact, mechanical strength of composite ligament structures have not regained normal strength even after 12 months of resumption of activity.

Exercise at a level producing cardiac hypertrophy and increased cardiac output causes hypertrophy of specialized fibrous connective tissues such as tendons and ligaments. However, that effect occurs slowly at great effort; it requires 1 year to produce hypertrophy which is at nominal levels of significance.

The use of CPM to bypass some of the deleterious effects of stress deprivation and its application to repair of cartilage, tendon, ligament, and fractures were described. Clinical use in the postoperative management of total joint replacement seems solidly in place and is widely applied to facilitate rehabilitation of the joint affected, to reduce swelling and joint effusion, possibly to reduce incidence of thrombophlebitis and to shorten the hospital stay. Passive motion places in effect such fundamental cellular and tissue processes that we are probably observing only the infancy of its development. The next decade should see a dramatic increase in its application to problems in the field of synovial joint rehabilitation.

The manner in which cells interpret physical signals will be a lively field for fundamental science in parallel with, and in support of, the clinical efforts. Although more and better clinical studies in this field are imperative, the clinical utility of exercise as a therapeutic adjunct for rehabilitation of supporting connective tissues is on the threshold of a rapid expansion due to successes in the several applications described. Facilitation of repair processes by early motion seems an almost universal observation for tendon, ligament, cartilage, and bone. The utility of the early motion concept to treatment of such widely divergent problems as septic arthritis, hemarthrosis, total joint replacement, and tendon repair indicates the breath of applications currently employed clinically. The key appears to be the importance of mechanical stimuli as signals to cell receptors which control synthesis of matrix components and other factors which guide extracellular organization of those components. Clearly, additional efforts are required to provide more complete documentation of the importance and relevance of these principles. The primacy of application of early motion as a fundamental rehabilitation principle in the treatment of injuries and other disorders of the musculoskeletal system is likely to be followed even more aggressively in the future.

References

Akeson, W. H. (1961). An experimental study of joint stiffness. *J. Bone Jt. Surg.*, **43A**: 1022.

Akeson, W. H., Amiel, D., and LaViolette, D. (1967). The connective tissue response to immobility. A study of chondroitin 4 and 6 sulfate and dermatan sulfate changes in periarticular connective tissue of control and immobilized knees of dogs. *Clin. Orthop. Rel. Res.*, **51**: 183.

Akeson, W. H., Amiel, D., and Woo, S. L.-Y. (1980). Immobility effects on synovial joints: the pathomechanics of joint contracture. *Biorheology* **17**: 95.

Akeson, W. H., Amiel, D., Mechanic, G. L., Woo, S. L.-Y., and Harwood, F. L. (1977). Collagen cross-linking alterations in joint contractures: changes in the reducible cross-links in periarticular connective tissue collagen after nine weeks of immobilization. *Connect. Tissue Res.*, **5**: 15.

Akeson, W. H., Amiel, D., Woo, S. L.-Y., and Harwood, F. L. (1978). Mechanical imperatives for synovial joint homeostasis: the present potential for their therapeutic manipulation. *Proc. Third Int. Congr., Biorheol.*, 47.

Akeson, W. H., Woo, S. L.-Y., Amiel, D., Coutts, R. D., and Daniel, D. (1973). The connective tissue response to immobility: biochemical changes in periarticular connective tissue of the immobilized rabbit knee. *Clin. Orthop. Rel. Res.*, **93**: 356.

Akeson, W. H., Woo, S. L.-Y., Amiel, D., and Frank, C. B. (1984). The biology of ligaments. In: *Rehabilitation of the Injured Knee*, Hunter, L. and Funk, F., Eds., C.V. Mosby, St. Louis.

Alm, A. and Stromberg, B. (1974). Vascular anatomy of the patellar and cruciate ligaments. A microangiographic and histologic investigation in the dog. *Acta Chir. Scand. Suppl.*, **445**: 25–35.

Amiel, D., Abel, M. F., Kleiner, J. B., Lieber, R. L., and Akeson, W. H. (1986). Synovial fluid nutrient delivery in the diarthrial joint: An analysis of rabbit knee ligaments. *J. Orthop. Res.*, **4**: 90–95.

Amiel, D., Akeson, W. H., Harwood, F. L., and Mechanic, G. L. (1980). Effect on nine week immobilization of the types of collagen synthesized in periarticular connective tissue from rabbit knees. *Connect. Tissue Res.*, **8**: 27–32.

Amiel, D., Foulk, R. A., Harwood, F. L., and Akeson, W. H. (1990). Quantitative assessment by competitive ELISA of fibronectin (fn) in tendons and ligaments. *Matrix*, **9(6)**: 421–427.

Amiel, D., Frank, C., Harwood, F., Fronek, J., and Akeson, W. H. (1984). Tendons and ligaments: a morphological and biochemical comparison. *J. Orthop. Res.*, **1(3)**: 257.

Amiel, D., Frey, C., Woo, S. L.-Y., Harwood, F., and Akeson, W. H. (1985). Value of hyaluronic acid in the prevention of contracture formation. *Clin. Orthop. Rel. Res.*, **196**: 22.

Amiel, D., Kleiner, J., and Akeson, W. H. (1986). The natural history of the anterior cruciate ligament autograft of patellar tendon origin. *Am. J. Sports Med.*, **14(6)**: 449–462.

Andrish, J. and Holmes, R. (1979). Effects of synovial fluid on fibroblasts in tissue culture. *Clin. Orthop.*, **138**: 279–283.

Arnoczky, S. P., Rubin, R. M., and Marshall, J. L. (1979). Microvasculature of the cruciate ligaments and its response to injury. *J. Bone Jt. Surg.*, **61A**: 1221.

Bailey, A. J. and Robins, S. P. (1973). Development and maturation of the cross-links in the collagen fibers of skin. *Frontiers Matrix Biol.*, **1**: 130.

Baker, W. C., Thomas, T. G., and Kirkaldy-Willis, W. H. (1969). Changes in the cartilage of the posterior intervertebral joints after anterior fusion. *J. Bone Jt. Surg.*, **51B**: 737.

Baxendale, R. H., Ferrell, W. R., and Wood, L. (1985). Intra-articular pressures during active and passive movement of normal and distended human knee joints. *J. Physiol.*, **396**: 179P.

Breen, T. F., Gelberman, R. H., and Ackerman, G. N. (1988). Elbow flexion contractures: treatment by anterior release and continuous passive motion. *J. Hand Surg.*, **13(3)**: 286.

Brooke, J. S. and Slack, H. G. B. (1959). Metabolism of connective tissue in limb atrophy in the rabbit. *Ann. Rheum.*, **18**: 129.

Burks, R., Daniel, D., and Losse, G. (1984). The effect of continuous passive motion on anterior cruciate ligament reconstruction stability. *Am. J. Sports Med.*, **12**: 323.

Butler, D. L., Noyes, F. R., Grood, E. S., Olmstead, M. L., and Hohn, R. B. (1983). The effects of vascularity on the mechanical properties of primate anterior cruciate ligament replacements. *Trans. Orthop. Res. Soc.*, **8**: 93.

Cabaud, H. E., Rodkey, W. G., and Feagin, J. A. (1979). Experimental studies of acute anterior cruciate ligament injury and repair. *Am. J. Sports Med.*, **7**: 18–22.

Caughey, D. E. and Bywaters, E. G. L. (1963). Joint fluid pressure in chronic knee effusions. *Ann. Rheum. Dis.*, **22**: 106.

Cheung, H. S., Halverson, P. B., and McCarty, D. J. (1981). Release of collagenase neutral protease, and prostaglandins from cultured mammalian synovial cells by hydroxyapatite and calcium pyrophosphate dihydrate crystals. *Arthritis Rheum.*, **24**: 1338–1344.

Convery, F. R., Akeson, W. H., and Keown, G. H. (1972). The repair of large osteochondral defects. An experimental study in horses. *Clin. Orthop.*, **82**: 253.

Cooper, R. R. and Misel, S. (1970). Tendon and ligament insertion. *J. Bone Jt. Surg.*, **52A**: 1.

Coutts, R. D., Amiel, D., Woo, S. L.-Y., Woo, Y.-K., and Akeson, W.H. (1983). Establishment of an appropriate model for the growth of periochondrium in a rabbit joint milieu. *Trans. Orthop. Res. Soc.*, 196.

Coutts, R. D., Kaita, J., Barr, R., Mason, R., Dube, R., Amiel, D., Woo, S. L.-Y., and Nickel, V. (1982). The role of continuous passive motion in the postoperative rehabilitation of the total knee patient. *Orthop. Trans.*, **6**: 277.

Coutts, R. D., Toth, C., and Kaita, J. (1983). The role of continuous passive motion in the rehabilitation of the total knee patient. In: *Total Knee Arthroplasty—A Comprehensive Approach.* Hungerford, D., Ed., Williams & Wilkins, Baltimore.

Dahners, L. E. (1986). Ligament contraction—a correlation with cellularity and actin staining. *Trans. Orthop. Res. Soc.*, **11**: 56.

Danzig, L. A., Hargens, A. R., Gershuni, D. H., Skyhar, M. J., Sfakianos, P. N., and Akeson, W. H. (1987). Increased transsynovial transport with continuous passive motion. *J. Orthop. Res.*, **5**: 409.

Ehrlich, M. G., Mankin, H. J., Jones, H., Wright, R., Crispen, C., and Vigliani, G. (1977). Collagenase and collagenase inhibitors in osteoarthritic and normal cartilage. *J. Clin. Invest.*, **59(2)**: 226–233.

Eiken, O., Lundborg, G., and Rank, F. (1975). The role of the digital synovial sheath in tendon grafting. *Scand. J. Plast. Reconstr. Surg.*, **9**: 182.

Engkvist, O. (1979). Reconstruction of patellar articular cartilage with free autologous perichondrial grafts. An experimental study in dogs. *Scand. J. Plast. Reconstr. Surg.*, **13**: 361.

Engkvist, O. and Johansson, S. H. (1980). Perichondrial arthroplasty. A clinical study in twenty-six patients. *Scand. J. Plast. Reconstr. Surg.*, **14**: 71.

Enneking, W. E. and Horowitz, M. (1972). The intra articular effects of immobilization on the human knee. *J. Bone Jt. Surg.*, **54A**: 973.

Evans, E. B., Eggers, G. W. N., Butler, J. K., and Blumel, J. (1960). Experimental immobilization and remobilization of rat knee joints. *J. Bone Jt. Surg.*, **42A**: 737.

Fabry, G. (1982). Early biochemical and histological findings in experimental haemarthrosis in dogs. *Arch. Orthop. Traumat. Surg.*, **100**: 167.

Feagin, J. A., Abbott, H. G., and Rokous, J. A. (1972). The isolated tear of the ACL (abstr.). *J. Bone Jt. Surg.*, **54A**: 1340.

Feagin, J. A., Jr. and Curl, W. W. (1976). Isolated tear of the ACL: 5-year followup study. *Am. J. Sports Med.*, **4**: 95–100.

Fisher, R. L., Kloter, K., Bzdyra, B., and Cooper, J. A. (1985). Continuous passive motion (CPM) following total knee replacement. *Conn. Med.*, **49(8)**: 498.

Frank, C., Akeson, W. H., Woo, S. L.-Y., Amiel, D., and Coutts, R. D. (1984). Physiology and therapeutic value of passive joint motion. *Clin. Orthop. Rel. Res.*, **185**: 113.

Fronek, J., Frank, C., Amiel, D., Woo, S. L.-Y., Coutts, R. D., and Akeson, W. H. (1983). The effect of intermittent passive motion (IPM) on the healing of the medial collateral ligament. *Trans. Orthop. Res. Soc.*, 31.

Gelberman, R. H., Woo, S. L.-Y., Lothringer, K., Akeson, W. H., and Amiel, D. (1982). Effects of early intermittent passive mobilization on healing canine flexor tendons. *J. Hand Surg.*, **7**: 170.

Gillard, G. C., Reilly, H. C., Bell-Booth, P. G., and Flint, M. H. (1979). The influence of mechanical forces on the glycosaminoglycan content of the rabbit flexor digitorum profundus tendon. *Connect. Tissue Res.*, **7(1)**: 37–46.

Gospodarowicz, D., Neufeld, G., and Schweigerer, L. (1986). Cellular shape is determined by the extracellular matrix and is responsible for the control of cellular growth and function. *Mol. Cell. Endocrinol.*, **46**: 187.

Guyton, A. C., Barber, B. J., and Moffatt, D. S. (1980). Theory of interstitial pressures. In: *Tissue Fluid Pressure and Composition.* Hargens, A., Ed., Williams & Wilkins, Baltimore.

Hemler, M. E., Huang, C., and Schwartz, L. (1987). The VLA protein family. *J. Biol. Chem.*, **262**: 3300–3309.

Hohl, M. and Luck, J. V. (1956). Fractures of the tibial condyle. *J. Bone Jt. Surg.*, **38A**: 1001.

Hough, A. J., Barfield, W. O., and Sokoloff, L. (1976). Cartilage in hemophilic arthropathy; ultrastructural and microanalytical studies. *Arch. Pathol. Lab. Med.*, **100**: 91.

Ignotz, R. A. and Massague, J. (1987). Cell adhesion protein receptors as targets for transforming growth factor-β action. *Cell*, **51**: 189–197.

Inoue, M., Gomez, M. A., Hollis, J. M., Roux, R. D., Lee, E. B., Burleson, E. M., and Woo, S. L.-Y. (1986). Medial collateral ligament healing: repair vs nonrepair. *Trans. Orthop. Res. Soc.*, 78.

Ishizue, K. K., Amiel, D., Lyon, R., and Woo, S. L.-Y. (1990). Acute hemarthrosis; a histological, biochemical and biomechanical correlation of effects on the ACL in a rabbit model. *J. Orthop. Res.*, **8(4)**: 548–554.

Ishizue, K. K., Lyon, R., Amiel, D., Woo, S. L.-Y., et al. (1988). Hemarthrosis: a biochemical and mechanical evaluation of effects on the ACL and menisci. *Trans. Orthop. Res. Soc.*, **13**: 55.

Jackson, D. S. and Mechanic, G. (1974). Cross-link patterns of collagens synthesized by cultures of 3T6 and 3T3 fibroblasts and by fibroblasts of various granulation tissues. *Biochem. Biophys. Acta*, 336.

Klein, L., Dawson, M. H., and Heiple, K. G. (1977). Turnover of collagen in the adult rat after denervation. *J. Bone Jt. Surg.*, **59A**: 1065.

Kleiner, J. B., Roux, R. D., Amiel, D., Woo, S. L.-Y., and Akeson, W. H. (1986). Primary healing of the ACL. *Trans. Orthop. Res. Soc.*, **11**: 131.

Kohn, D. (1986). Arthroscopy in acute injuries of anterior cruciate-deficient knees: fresh and old intraarticular lesions. *Arthroscopy*, **2**: 98–102.

Kurkinen, M., Vaheri, A. V., Roberts, P. J., and Stenman, S. (1980). Sequential appearance of fibronectin and collagen in experimental granulation tissue. *Lab. Invest.*, **43(1)**: 47–51.

Laros, G. S., Tipton, C. M., and Cooper, R. R. (1971). Influence of physical activity on ligament insertions in the knees of dogs. *J. Bone Jt. Surg.*, **53A**: 275.

Lehto, M., Duance, V. C., and Restall, D. (1985). Collagen and fibronectin in a healing skeletal muscle injury. *Br. J. Bone Jt. Surg.*, **67(5)**: 820–828.

Limbird, R. J. and Dennis, S. C. (1987). Synovectomy and continuous passive motion (CPM) in hemophiliac patients. *Arthroscopy: J. Arthroscop. Rel. Surg.*, **3(2)**: 74.

Lindy, S., Turto, H., Sorsa, T., Halme, J., Lauhio, A., Suomalainen, K., Utto, V. J., and Wegelius, O. (1986). Increased collagenase activity in human rheumatoid meniscus. *Scand. J. Rheumatol.*, **15**: 237–242.

Lundborg, G., Myrhage, R., and Rydevik, B. (1977). Original communication: the vascularization of human flexor tendons within the digital synovial sheath region, structural and functional aspects. *J. Hand Surg.*, **2**: 417.

Lynch, A. F., Bourne, R. B., Rorabeck, C. H., Rankin, R. N., and Donald, A. (1988). Deep-vein thrombosis and continuous passive motion after total knee arthroplasty. *J. Bone Jt. Surg.*, **70(1)**: 11.

Lynch, J. A., Baker, P. L., Polly, R. E., McCoy, M. T., Sund, K., and Roudybush, D. (1984). Continuous passive motion: a prophylaxis for deep venous thrombosis following total knee replacement. *Am. Acad. Orthop. Surg.*

Lyon, R. M., Billings, E., Jr., Woo, S. L.-Y., Ishizue, K. K., Kitabayashi, L., Amiel, D., and Akeson, W. H. (1989). The ACL: a fibrocartilaginous structure. *Trans. Orthop. Res. Soc. Meet.*, **14**: 1989.

Manske, P. R., Whiteside, L. A., and Lesker, P. A. (1978). Nutrient pathways to flexor tendons using hydrogen washout techniques. *J. Hand Surg.*, **3**: 32–36.

Matthews, P. (1978). The fate of isolated segments of flexor tendons within the digital sheath—a study in synovial nutrition. *Br. J. Plast. Surg.*, **29**: 216.

McDonald, J. A., Kelley, D. G., and Broekelmann, T. J. (1982). Role of fibronectin in collagen deposition: Fab' to the gelatin-binding domain of fibronectin inhibits both fibronectin and collagen organization in fibroblast extracellular matrix. *J. Cell Biol.*, **92(2)**: 485–492.

Melzack, R. and Wall, P. D. (1970). Psychophysiology of pain. Evolution of pain theories. *Int. Anesthesiol. Clin.*, **8**: 3.

Mooney, V. and Ferguson, A. B., Jr. (1966). The influence of immobilization and motion on the formation of fibrocartilage in the repair granuloma after joint resection in the rabbit. *J. Bone Jt. Surg.*, **48**: 1145.

Mooney, V. and Stills, M. (1987). Continuous passive motion with joint fractures and infections. *Orthop. Clin. North Am.*, **18(1)**: 1.

Nagelschmidt, M., Becker, D., Bonninghoff, N., and Engelhardt, G. H. (1987). Effect of fibronectin therapy and fibronectin deficiency on wound healing: a study in rats. *J. Trauma*, **27(11)**: 1267–1271.

Neuberger A. and Slack, H. G. B. (1953). The metabolism of collagen from liver, bones, skin and tendon in the normal rat. *Biochem. J.* **53**: 47.

Nickel, V. Personal communication.

Noyes, F. R., Mangine, R. E., and Barber, S. (1987). Early knee motion after open and arthroscopic anterior cruciate ligament reconstruction. *Am. J. Sports Med.*, **15(2)**: 149.

Noyes, F. R., Torvik, P. J., Hyde, W. B., and DeLucas, J. L. (1974). Biomechanics of ligament failure. II. An analysis of immobilization, exercise and reconditioning effects in primates. *J. Bone Jt. Surg.*, **56A**: 1406.

O'Donoghue, D. H., Frank, G. R., Jeter, G. L., Johnson, W., Zeiders, J. W., and Kenyon, R. (1971). Repair and reconstruction of the anterior cruciate ligament in dogs. *J. Bone Jt. Surg.*, **53A(4)**: 710–718.

O'Donoghue, D. H., Rockwood, C. A., Jr., Frank, G. R., Jack, S. C., and Kenyon, R. (1966). Repair of the ACL in dogs. *J. Bone Jt. Surg.*, **48A**: 503.

O'Driscoll, S. W. and Salter, R. B. (1984). The induction of neochondrogenesis in free intra-articular periosteal autografts under the influence of continuous passive motion. *J. Bone Jt. Surg.*, **66A(8)**: 1248.

O'Driscoll, S. W., Kumar, A., and Salter, R. B. (1983). The effect of continuous passive motion on the clearance of a hemarthrosis. *Clin. Orthop.*, **176**: 336.

O'Driscoll, S. W., Keeley, F. W., and Salter, R. B. (1988). Durability of regenerated articular cartilage produced by free autogenous periosteal grafts in major full-thickness defects in joint surfaces under the influence of continuous passive motion. *J. Bone Jt. Surg.*, **70(4)**: 595.

Ohlsen, L. (1978). Cartilage regeneration from perichondrium. Experimental and clinical applications. *Plast. Reconstr. Surg.*, **62**: 507.

Palmer, I. (1938). On the injuries of the ligament of the knee joint: a clinical study. *Acta Chir. Scand. Suppl.*, **53**: 1–282.

Parisien, J. S. (1988). The role of arthroscopy in the treatment of postoperative fibroarthrosis of the knee joint. *Clin. Orthop. Rel. Res.*, **299**: 185.

Parker, F. and Keefer, C. S. (1935). Gross and histologic changes in the knee joint in rheumatoid arthritis. *Arch. Pathol.*, **20(4)**: 507.

Peacock, E. E. (1963). Comparison of collagenous tissue surrounding normal and immobilized joints. *Surg. Forum*, **14**: 440.

Pedowitz, R. A., Gershuni, D. H., Crenshaw, A. G., Petras, S. L., Danzig, L. A., and Hargens, A. R. (1989). Intraarticular pressure during continuous passive motion of the human knee. *J. Orthop. Res.*, **7**: 530.

Pforringer, W. (1982). Hamarthros and Kreuzbander—Biomechanische Untersuchangen Teil 1. *Unfallchirugie*, **8**: 353.

Pforringer, W. (1982). Hamarthros and Kreuzbander—Morphologische Untersuchangen Teil 2. *Unfallchirugie*, **8**: 368.

Potenza, A. D. (1963). Critical evaluation of flexor tendon healing and adhesion formation with artificial digital sheaths: an experimental study. *J. Bone Jt. Surg.*, **45A**: 1217–1233.

Potenza, A. D. (1964). The healing of autogenous tendon grafts within the flexor digital sheaths in dogs. *J. Bone Jt. Surg.*, **46A**: 1462–1484.

Poussa, M., Rubak, J., and Ritsila, V. (1981). Differentiation of the osteochondrogenic cells of the periosteum in chondrotrophic environment. *Acta Orthop. Scand.*, **52**: 235.

Ridge, S. C., Oransky, A. L., and Kerwar, S. S. (1980). Induction of the synthesis of latent collagenase and latent neutral protease in chondrocytes by a factor synthesized by activated macrophages. *Arthritis Rheum.*, **23**: 448–454.

Rippey, J. J., Hill, R. R., Lurie, A., Sweet, M., Thonar, E., and Handelsman, J. E. (1978). Articular cartilage degradation and the pathology of haemophilic arthropathy. *S. Afr. Med. J.*, **54**: 345.

Roberts, C. J., Birkenmeier, T. M., McQuillan, J. J., Akiyama, S. K., Yamada, S. S., Chen, W.-T., Yamuda, K. M., and McDonald, J. A. (1988). Transforming growth factor β stimulates the expression of fibronectin and of both subunits of the human fibronectin receptor by cultured human lung fibroblasts. *J. Biol. Chem.*, **263(10)**: 4586–4592.

Romness, D. W. and Rand, J. A. (1988). The role of continuous passive motion following total knee arthroplasty. *Clin. Orthop. Rel. Res.*, **226**: 34.

Ropes, M. W., Bennett, G. A., and Bauer, W. (1939). The origin and nature of normal synovial fluid. *J. Clin. Invest.*, **18**: 351.

Ruoslahti, E. and Pierschbacher, M. D. (1987). New perspectives in cell adhesion: RGD and integrins. *Science*, **238**: 491.

Ruoslahti, E. and Pierschbacher, M. D. (1986). Arg-Gly-Asp: a versatile cell recognition site. *Cell*, **44**: 517–518.

Salter, R. B. (1989). The biologic concept of continuous passive motion of synovial joints. *Clin. Orthop. Rel. Res.*, **242**: 12.

Salter, R. B., Bell, R. S., and Keeley, F. (1981). The protective effect of continuous passive motion on living articular cartilage in acute septic arthritis: an experimental investigation in the rabbit. *Clin. Orthop.*, **159**: 223.

Salter, R. B. and Field, P. (1960). The effects of continuous compression on living articular cartilage. *J. Bone Jt. Surg.*, **42A**: 31.

Salter, R. B., Simmonds, D. F., Malcolm, B. W., Rumble, E. J., and MacMichael, D. (1980). The biological effects of continuous passive motion on the healing of full-thickness defects in articular cartilage: an experimental investigation in the rabbit. *J. Bone Jt. Surg.*, **62**: 1232.

Schiller, S., Matthews, M. D., Cifonelli, J., and Dorfman, A. (1956). The metabolism of mucopoly saccharides in animals. Further studies on skin utilizing C14 glucose, C14 acetate, and S35 sodium sulfate. *J. Biol. Chem.*, **218**: 139.

Shimizu, T., Videman, T., Shimazaki, K., and Mooney, V. (1987). Experimental study on the repair of full thickness articular cartilage defects: effects of varying periods of continuous passive motion, cage activity, and immobilization. *J. Orthop. Res.*, **5**: 187.

Skyhar, M. J., Danzig, L. A., Hargens, A. R., and Akeson, W. H. (1985). Nutrition of the anterior cruciate ligament. Effects of continuous passive motion. *Am. J. Sports Med.*, **13(6)**: 415.

Swann, D. A., Radin, E. L., and Nazimiec, M. (1974). Role of hyaluronic acid in joint lubrication. *Ann. Rheum. Dis.*, **33**: 318.

Thaxter, T. H., Mann, R. A., and Anderson, C. E. (1965). Degeneration of immobilized knee joints in rats. *J. Bone Jt. Surg.*, **47A**: 567.

Tipton, C. M., Matthes, R. D., and Martin, R. R. (1978). Influence of age and sex on the strength of bone-ligament junctions in knee joints of rats. *J. Bone Jt. Surg.*, **60A**: 230.

Vince, K. G., Kelly, M. A., Beck, J., and Insall, J. N. (1987). Continuous passive motion after total knee arthroplasty. *J. Arthroplasty*, **2**: 281.

von Reyher, C. (1874). On the cartilage and synovial membranes of the joints. *J. Anat. Physiol.*, **8**: 261.

Warren, R. F. (1983). Primary repair of the anterior cruciate ligament. *Clin. Orthop.*, **172**: 65–70.

Weichselbaum, A. (1878). Die Feineren Verandeungen des Gelenk Knorpels bei Fungoser Synovitis und Caries der Gelenkenden. *Virch. Arch.*, **73**: 461.

Werb, Z. and Reynolds, J. J. (1974). Stimulation by endocytosis of the secretion of collagenase and neutral proteinase from rabbit synovial fibroblasts. *J. Exp. Med.*, **140**: 1482–1497.

Wessels, N. K. (1977). *Tissue Interactions and Development*, Benjamin-Cummings, Menlo Park, CA, 213–229.

Williams, I. F., McCullagh, K. G., and Silver, I. A. (1984). The distribution of types I and III collagen and fibronectin in the healing equine tendon. *Connect. Tissue Res.*, **12**: 211–227.

Woo, S. L.-Y., Ritter, M. A., Gomez, M. A., Kuei, S. C., and Akeson, W. H. (1980b). The biomechanical and structural properties of swine digital flexor tendons secondary to running exercise. *Orthop. Trans.*, **4(2)**: 165.

Woo, S. L.-Y., Gomez, M. A., Seguchi, Y., Endo, C. M., and Akeson, W. H. (1983). Measurement of mechanical properties of ligament substance from a bone-ligament-bone preparation. *J. Orthop. Res.*, **1**: 22.

Woo, S. L.-Y., Kuei, S. C., Amiel, D., Cobb, N. G., Hayes, W. C., and Akeson, W. H. (1980a). The response of cortical long bone secondary to exercise training. *Trans. 26th Annu. Meet. Orthop. Res. Soc.*, **5**: 256.

Woo, S. L.-Y., Kuei, S. C., Gomez, M. A., Winters, J. M., Amiel, D., and Akeson, W. H. (1979). Effect of immobilization and exercise on strength characteristics of bone-medial collateral ligament-bone complex. *Am. Soc. Mech. Eng. Symp.*, **32**: 62.

Woo, S. L.-Y., Matthews, J. V., Akeson, W. H., Amiel, D., and Convery, R. (1975). Connective tissue response to immobility. Correlative study of biomechanical and biochemical measurements of normal and immobilized rabbit knees. *Arthritis Rheum.*, **18(3)**: 257.

Woo, S. L.-Y., Gomez, M. A., Amiel, D., Newton, P. O., Orlando, C. A., Sites, T., and Akeson, W. H. (1987). The biomechanical and biochemical changes of the MCL following immobilization and remobilization. *J. Bone Jt. Surg.*, **69A**: 1200–1211.

Zarnett, R. and Salter, R. B. (1989). Periosteal neochondrogenesis for biologically resurfacing joints: its cellular origin. *Can. J. Surg.*, **32(3)**: 171.

3

Macromolecular Synthesis and Mechanical Stability during Fracture Repair

DOREEN E. ASHHURST
Department of Anatomy
St. George's Hospital Medical School
Tooting, London, United Kingdom

Introduction
Models for the study of fracture healing
Cellular events during the healing phase
    Healing under stable mechanical conditions
    Healing under unstable mechanical conditions
    Factors that influence the differentiation of chondrocytes in fracture
       callus
The remodeling phase of fracture repair
The types of collagen secreted during fracture healing
The proteoglycans and their associated glycosaminoglycan chains
    produced during fracture healing
Other matrix macromolecules and fracture healing
Conclusions
References

Introduction

    Healing of long bones can be divided into two phases. The initial healing phase leads to the union of the fractured cortical bone and is followed by the second, remodeling phase during which the re-united cortical bone and any callus are extensively remodeled. The realization that the first phase of fracture healing can be modified by the mechanical conditions at the fracture site came with the development of the methods for the stable fixation of fractures by the Swiss AO (Arbeitsgemeinschaft für Osteosynthesefragen) group. Their aim was to provide internal fixation sufficient to maintain a perfect anatomical reduction and to stabilize the fracture so that external splintage is unnecessary. Thus, the joints adjacent to the fracture are not immobilized and future mobility is not jeopardized by prolonged restriction of joint movement. An essential condition to maintain sufficient relative stability to achieve these aims is that the fractured surfaces are held together by a compressive force. Both histological and radiological examination of fractures treated by this method show that the amount of periosteal callus is negligible and that it consists of bone.

In contrast, when a fracture is reduced and its position maintained by a splint, plaster cast, non-compression plate, or medullary nail, relative movement occurs between the fractured surfaces; indeed there is usually a gap between them. Histological and radiological examinations reveal the development of a thick periosteal callus that contains, in the early stages of healing, a large region of cartilage, buttressed by newly formed bone, over the fracture site.

Irrespective of the method of stabilization, a fracture site in an experimental animal is surrounded by healthy mesenchymal cells 3 days after injury. It is unlikely that the mechanical conditions at the fracture site attract cells of differing differentiative potential (i.e., potential osteoblasts and chondrocytes) to unstable fractures, but only potential osteoblasts to stable fractures. It seems more logical to predict that all the mesenchymal cells that congregate around a fracture site have the same differentiative potential and that the phenotype they subsequently exhibit is determined by factors that result from the mechanical conditions at the site. Thus, in addition to the clinical importance of investigations of the cellular events during fracture healing, the ability to modulate the differentiation of the progenitor cells by altering the mechanical conditions around the fracture site provides an *in vivo* model for investigating the events leading to the differentiation of chondrocytes and osteoblasts. The identification of the extracellular matrix macromolecules and the recent development of methods for their precise localization within the cells and matrices provide tools for the investigation of the pathways of their differentiation.

Models for the Study of Fracture Healing

Fracture healing under different mechanical conditions has been investigated in dogs, rabbits, rats, and sheep. Detailed biochemical and morphological, as opposed to biomechanical, studies of all stages of healing are, for reasons of economy and ease of preparation of the material for microscopy, restricted to rodents. The rat has the advantage of greater economy, but also has disadvantages. Rat cortical bone is not Haversian and remodeling occurs primarily along the endosteal and periosteal surfaces (Kelly *et al.*, 1990). Its reaction to injury will, therefore, differ from that of human, or other Haversian bones. Second, the small size of rat bones mitigates against

A

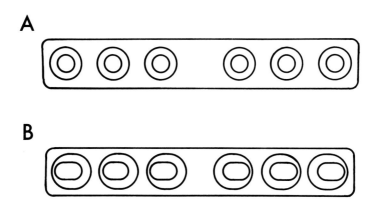

B

Fig. 1 Diagrams of the plates used to stabilize the rabbit tibia. (A) 6-hole AO/ASIF stainless steel dynamic compression plate. (B) 6-hole plastic plate. (From Ashhurst *et al.*, 1982. See reference list.)

their use as models for different methods of internal fixation. Fracture models using rat bones, such as the femur, tibia, and metatarsals, frequently rely on manual fracture and no splintage (Dunham *et al.*, 1983). More recently, Bonnarens and Einhorn (1984) developed a model in which a cerclage wire is inserted longitudinally through the femur and then the bone is fractured using a specially designed device. The resulting fractures are reproducible, while those produced by manual external force are not.

The rabbit as an experimental animal for studying fracture healing has several advantages over the rat. First, the cortical bone is Haversian and so the stimulation of remodeling after injury is more similar to that of other larger mammals. Second, the larger size of rabbit bones enables the use of several methods for the stabilization of fractures. Thus, plates of various designs, medullary nails, or external fixators have been used to stabilize osteotomies of the femur and tibia (Greiff, 1978; Slätis *et al.*, 1978; Wang *et al.*, 1981). Plaster casts have been used, but are not really successful for rabbits because they have to be replaced frequently.

A reproducible tibial fracture model in the rabbit, developed by Ashhurst *et al.* (1982) and based on the earlier model of Rahn *et al.* (1971), allows the fracture to be stabilized using plates of different materials. The fracture is made by a standard procedure. Stable mechanical conditions at the fracture site are achieved using a stainless steel, 6-hole, dynamic compression (AO-ASIF) plate (Fig. 1) that is prebent to the contours of the tibia. Unstable conditions are created with a plastic plate of similar dimensions (Fig. 1), except that the distance between the two central screws is increased to create a gap of 0.5 mm between the fractured surfaces. Both stable and unstable fractures are maintained in good alignment and there is little variability in the distribution of the tissues in the periosteal callus of fractures stabilized in the same way. In completely unstabilized, and therefore unaligned, fractures, there is great variability in the morphology of the callus because the correct relationship of the fracture fragments is not maintained.

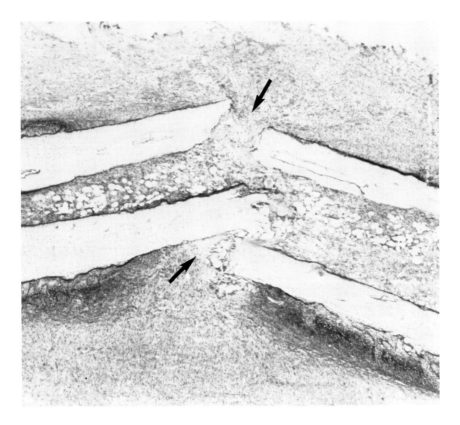

Fig. 2 Photomicrograph of a 5-day unaligned rat metatarsal fracture. Fibrous tissue surrounds the fractured surfaces of the bone (arrows). (Magnification × 31.) (Courtesy of Dr. R. Dodds, Bath Institute of Rheumatic Diseases, Bath, U. K.)

Cellular Events During the Healing Phase

A hematoma develops immediately after injury, but in experimental animals it is removed very rapidly so that by about 3 days after fracture, the periosteal surface of the fractured cortical bone is covered by a layer of fibrous tissue that extends across the fracture site, irrespective of the mechanical conditions. When the fracture gap is small, it is still filled by debris which protrudes into the external layer of fibrous tissue. If the gap is wide or the fragments are angulated, as happens frequently with unstabilized fractures, the fibrous tissue may extend around the fractured ends of the bone (Fig. 2); the reasons for this will be discussed later. The outer regions of the fibrous tissue are more compact and will form the new periosteum.

The fibrous tissue is produced by mesenchymal cells that have migrated to the fracture site and are present within it. It is usually assumed that these cells originate from the disrupted periosteum and the surrounding soft tissues (Simmons and Kahn, 1979). The involvement of blood-borne cells

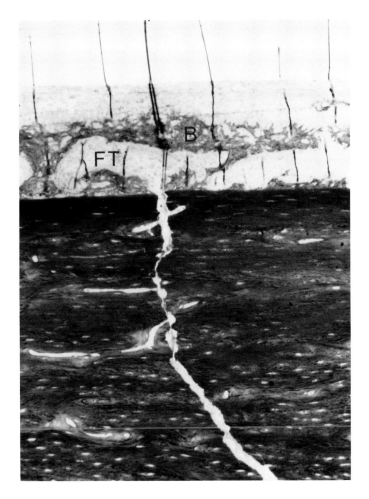

Fig. 3 Photomicrograph of the region over the fracture gap of a 4-day mechanically stable rabbit tibial fracture. Trabeculae of bone (B) are developing along the periosteal surface over the gap. The fibrous tissue (FT) between the trabeculae is well vascularized. (Magnification × 104.) (From Ashhurst, 1986. See reference list.)

and pericytes has been suggested, but not proven. Recently, Brighton and Hunt (1989) presented circumstantial evidence that endothelial cells from the marrow vessels transform into mesenchymal cells in a rabbit rib defect. This is an area which is still difficult to probe with the methods of cell labeling presently available.

Mechanical conditions at the fracture site now begin to influence cell differentiation in the callus. Close examination and comparison of the newly formed fibrous tissue associated with stable and unstable fractures reveals that whereas all the tissue associated with stable fractures is well vascularized (illustrated by the presence of bone; Fig. 3), that over the fracture site

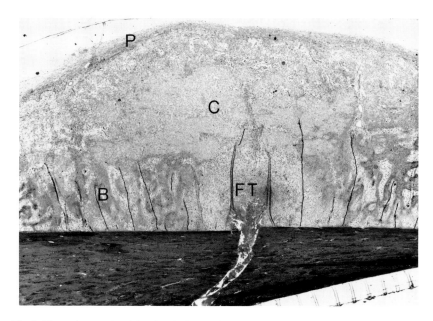

Fig. 4 Photomicrograph of the developing periosteal callus of a 6-day mechanically unstable rabbit tibial fracture. New bone (B) has formed along the periosteal surface, but it is separated from the gap by a region of avascular fibrous tissue (FT) (see Fig. 6). There is a large area over the bone and fibrous tissue in which cartilage (C) is forming. This area, too, is avascular. A new periosteum (P) has formed. (Magnification × 22.) (From Ashhurst, 1986.)

of unstable fractures contains no blood vessels (Figs. 4 and 5). The lack of blood vessels has consequences for the further development of the callus.

Regions of new bone formation are present along the surface of the cortical bone at 3 days, again, irrespective of the mechanical conditions at the fracture site. Osteoblasts are present on the surface and new bone trabeculae are being formed (Fig. 6). When the fracture is stable, bone is formed over the entire periosteal surface, including the region over the fracture site (Fig. 3), but if the fracture is unstable, new bone is not formed in the avascular area over the fracture gap (Fig. 4). In the rabbit, the distance between the new bone formation and the gap is about 0.5 mm. Further development of the periosteal callus and cortical healing are determined by the mechanical stability of the fracture until cortical union is re-established.

Healing Under Stable Mechanical Conditions

The new bone formation seen at 3 days over the entire periosteal surface continues so that by 9 days in the rabbit, a layer of cancellous bone, about 1 mm thick, has developed (Fig. 7). In man and dogs, the amount of periosteal bone formation is minimal (Schenk and Willenegger, 1967). Periosteal bone formation follows disruption of the periosteum in rabbits (Ash-

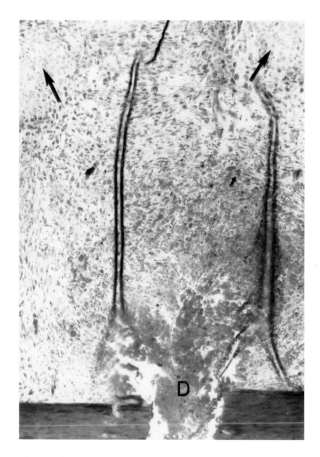

Fig. 5 Photomicrograph of the area over the fracture gap of the 6-day mechanically unstable fracture in Fig. 5. Debris (D) protrudes from the gap. The layer of cells surrounding it contains many macrophages, fibroblasts and some extravasated red cells (see Fig. 15). Cartilage (arrow) is forming away from the gap. The whole area is devoid of blood vessels. (Magnification × 80.) (From Ashhurst, 1986.)

hurst, unpublished observation) and thus it is possible that the greater amount of periosteal callus in rabbits is the result of injury to the periosteum, rather than to the bone. The periosteal tissue is well vascularized throughout and capillaries are visible over the fracture site (Fig. 8). Very small areas of cartilage are seen sporadically. They are restricted to very small areas of chondrocyte-like cells that are occasionally seen near the fracture site between 7 and 14 days after fracture. Immunohistochemistry has revealed further small regions in which chondrocyte-like cells may be present within the trabeculae of bone (Figs. 49 and 50). These are small areas of chondroid bone which are present for only a few days, and which are not removed endochondrally. The evidence for their identification will be presented later. There is no further increase in the width of the periosteal

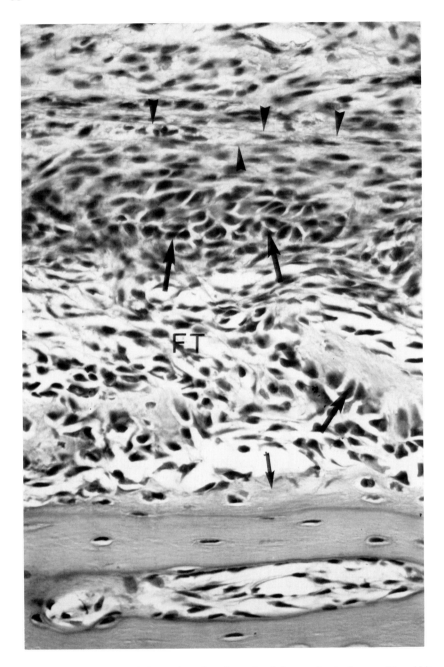

Fig. 6 Photomicrograph of the periosteal surface of a 3-day mechanically unstable rabbit tibial fracture. A new periosteum is forming and elastic fibers (arrowheads) are present. New bone is forming along the surface of the cortical bone (small arrow) and some trabeculae are extending into the fibrous tissue (FT). Osteoblasts are present on the surface of the new bone and grouped together where a developing trabeculum is seen *en face* (large arrows). (Magnification × 410.)

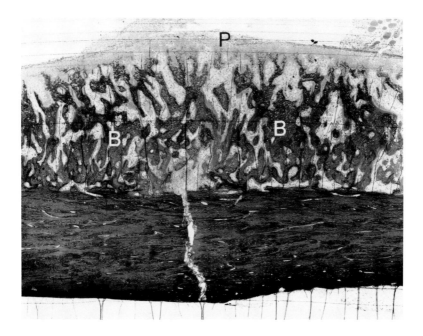

Fig. 7 Photomicrograph of a 9-day mechanically stable rabbit tibial fracture. A thin callus of new bone (B) has formed over the entire periosteal surface and is covered by a periosteum (P). (Magnification × 27.) (From Ashhurst, 1986.)

callus after about 9 days in the rabbit, but layers of new bone are laid down on the surfaces of the bone lining the spaces so that the callus becomes more compact. The periosteum is now a thick layer covering the new bone.

It is possible to examine the events leading to cortical union in different parts of the fracture gap in mechanically stable healing rabbit fractures. Because the fracture is "started" by a saw cut, 100 μm wide, in the medial cortex to which the plate is attached, this remains as a gap after the compressive force is exerted by the plate. Indeed, contact between the fractured surfaces is restricted to regions where there is perfect reduction. It has been calculated that contact is essential over only about 1% of the fractured surfaces to establish stability. The gaps are filled by debris during the first few days, but about 9 days after fracture, cells move into gaps, such as that made by the saw cut, more frequently from the periosteal than from the endosteal callus. The first cells to invade are macrophages, followed closely by fibroblasts and then by capillaries (Fig. 9). The macrophages remove the debris and a fibrous matrix is laid down by fibroblasts to support the cells and capillaries. Spindle-shaped cells line up along the fractured surfaces; these are preosteoblasts (Fig. 10). By 2 weeks, there is an epithelial layer of osteoblasts along these surfaces and layers of new bone are being secreted (Fig. 11). Further transverse layers of bone are laid down and by 3 weeks the gaps are filled to establish bony union across the fractured

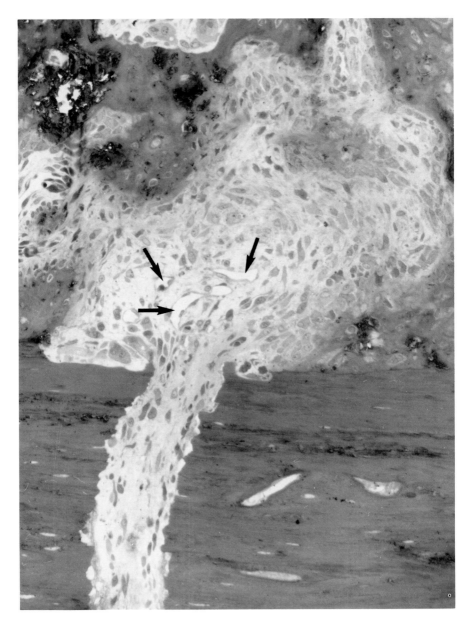

Fig. 8 Photomicrograph of the region immediately over the fracture gap of a 2-week rabbit tibial fracture. Several capillaries (arrows) are present in this fibrous tissue. (Magnification × 255.) (From Ashhurst, 1986.)

cortex (Fig. 12). It has frequently been assumed that dead bone adjacent to fractured surfaces has to be removed before new bone can be laid down on it (Ham and Harris, 1972), but this is not necessarily so (McKibbin, 1978). Very few osteoclasts are observed in the gaps. That the straight

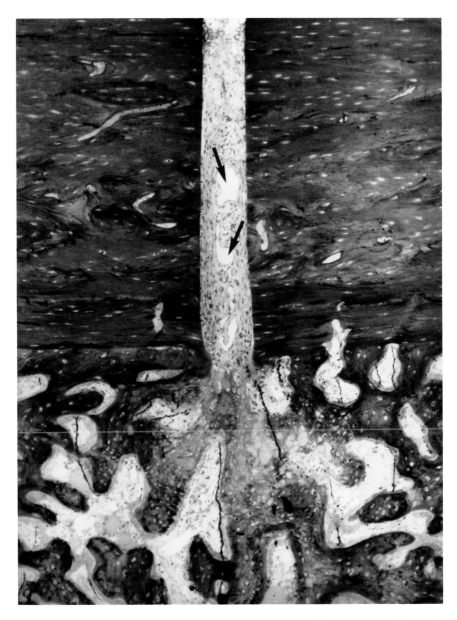

Fig. 9 Photomicrograph of the endosteal callus and fracture gap (the saw-cut region) of a 12-day mechanically stable rabbit tibial fracture. Cells and capillaries (arrows) have moved into the gap which contains fibrous tissue. This fibrous tissue is less organized away from the endosteal surface. The straight sides of the saw-cut indicate that resorption of the dead bone has not occurred. (Magnification × 100.) (From Ashhurst, 1986.)

sawcut can still be distinguished in many areas of gaps filled by new bone indicates that there are many areas in which resorption has not occurred (Fig. 12).

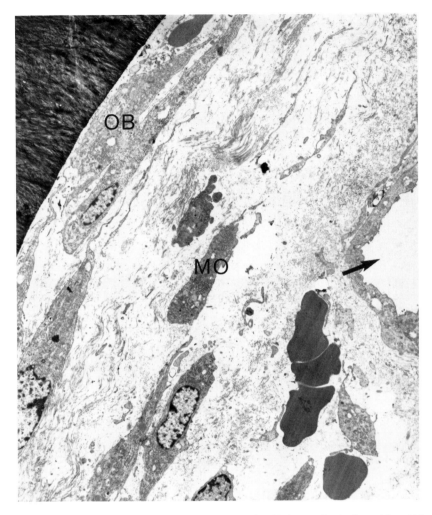

Fig. 10 Electron micrograph of part of the saw-cut of a 12-day mechanically stable rabbit tibial fracture. Spindle-shaped cells, which are probably preosteoblasts (OB), are lined up along the surface of the saw-cut. Monocytes (MO), red cells, and a capillary (arrow) are present in the fibrous tissue. (Magnification × 2900.) (From Ashhurst, 1986.)

In the regions in which there is contact, or a gap less than about 10 μm between the fractured surfaces, healing is by direct Haversian remodeling. This does not start for about 3 weeks, which is the time-lag between the stimulation of remodeling by injury and an observed increase in the number of remodeling cavities. Cavities cross the fracture (Fig. 13), which is obliterated when all the bone is remodeled. This can, however, take many weeks or months.

A third type of cortical healing is observed in stable fractures. There are some gaps of widths between 10 and 30 μm. These are too small for cells

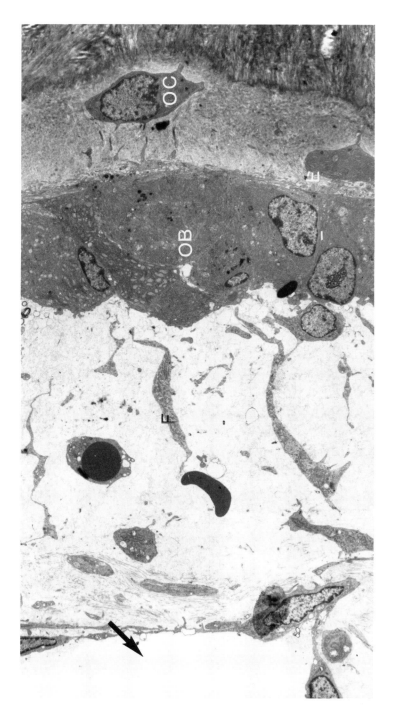

Fig. 11 Electron micrograph of part of the fracture gap of a 2-week mechanically stable rabbit tibial fracture. A layer of new bone with osteocytes (OC) has been laid down along the fractured surface. This is covered by a layer of osteoblasts (OB). The central region of the gap is filled by fibrous tissue with a capillary (arrow) and cells including fibroblasts (F). (Magnification × 2650.) (From Ashhurst, 1986.)

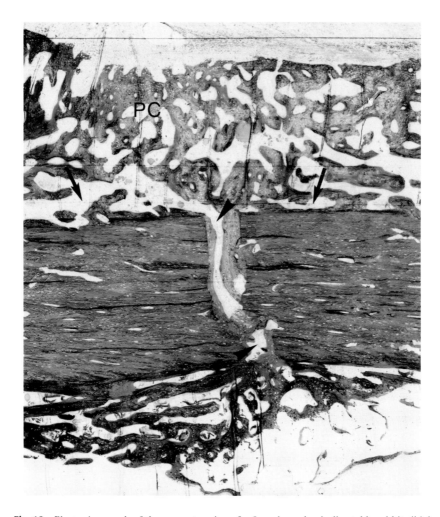

Fig. 12 Photomicrograph of the saw-cut region of a 3-week mechanically stable rabbit tibial fracture. The gap is filled by new bone to unite the cortex. The periosteal callus (PC) is compact peripherally, but along the callus-cortical boundary there are large resorption cavities (arrows). Remodeling cavities are entering the cortical bone from both the endosteal and periosteal calluses (arrowheads). (Magnification × 34.) (From Ashhurst, 1986.)

to enter, but too wide for remodeling cavities to cross. Between 3 and 4 weeks after fracture, these gaps are widened by osteoclasts. Cells and capillaries enter; some cells differentiate into osteoblasts and new bone is laid down on the fractured surfaces (Fig. 14). The spaces are gradually filled by bone to produce an irregular array of lamellae across the cortex.

Healing Under Unstable Mechanical Conditions

The new bone formation that can be seen at 3 days continues. A thick layer of cancellous bone develops along the periosteal surface, except in the

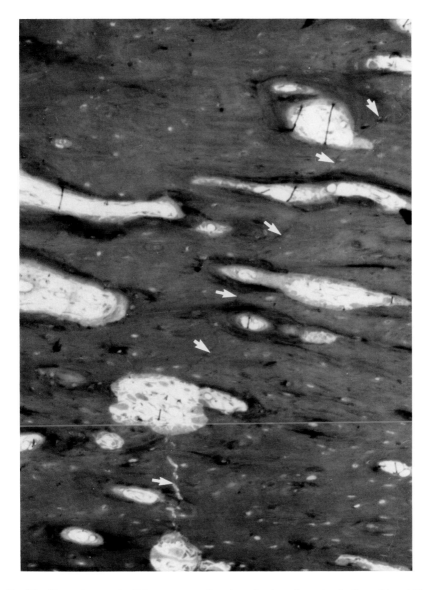

Fig. 13 Photomicrograph of the compressed region of a 4-week mechanically stable rabbit tibial fracture. Remodeling cavities are crossing the fracture line (arrows). (Magnification × 145.) (From Ashhurst, 1986.)

region above the fracture gap in which there are few, if any, blood vessels (see below). At 6 days, this avascular region associated with rabbit fractures is complex (Fig. 5). The debris protruding from the gap is covered by tissue containing macrophages and a few fibroblasts with a small amount of collagenous matrix (Fig. 15), while further from the gap some cells are begin-

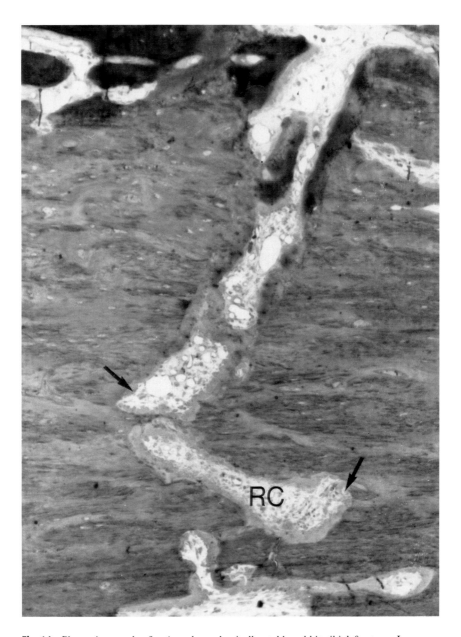

Fig. 14 Photomicrograph of a 4-week mechanically stable rabbit tibial fracture. Large re-modeling cavities (RC) cross the cortex. This is a region in which osteoclasts (arrows) have enlarged the fracture gap and so permitted its invasion by cells and capillaries. (Magnification × 130.) (From Ashhurst, 1986.)

ning to differentiate into chondroblasts and to form cartilage (Fig. 16). The region of chondrogenesis extends over the developing bone (Fig. 4). In some peripheral regions at around 7 days, the bone and cartilage matrices are

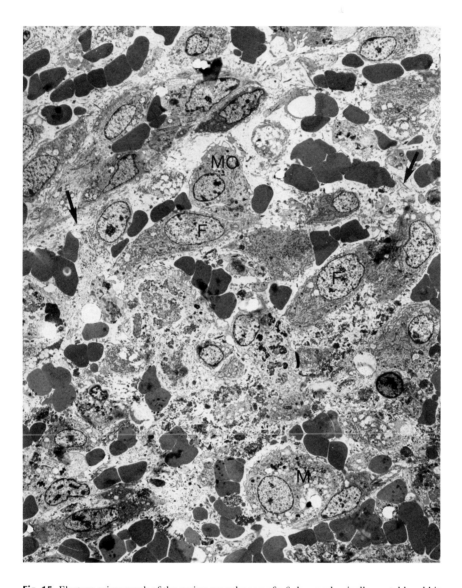

Fig. 15 Electron micrograph of the region near the gap of a 6-day mechanically unstable rabbit tibial fracture (see Fig. 4). Fibroblasts (F), macrophages (M) and monocytes (MO) are present and some collagen (arrow) has been laid down. Red cells are also scattered among the other cells. (Magnification × 1700.) (From Ashhurst, 1986.)

separated by a region of matrix that contains both types I and II collagens, i.e., an area of chondroid bone (Beresford, 1981; see below). By 10 days in the rabbit, cartilage formation is complete and is restricted to a V-shaped area over the fracture gap.

The cartilaginous matrix is heterogeneous. In some regions the cells appear healthy, in others, they are degenerating (Figs. 17 and 18). Some

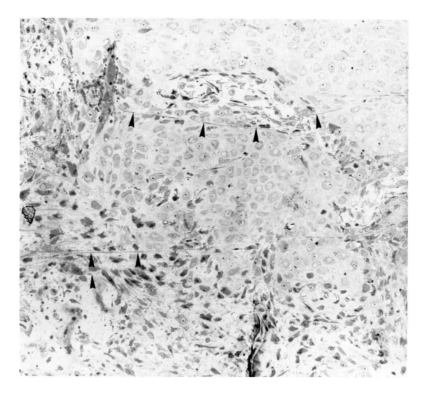

Fig. 16 Photomicrograph of an area of developing cartilage in the callus of a 6-day mechanically unstable rabbit tibial fracture. The whole area is avascular. Elastic fibers (arrowheads) pass from the fibrous tissue into the cartilage. (Magnification × 180.) (From Ashhurst, 1986.)

areas of the matrix contain only thin collagen fibrils, but in others there are bundles of thicker collagen fibrils (Fig. 18) or long elastic fibers (Fig. 17). Bone formation continues and bone grows over the cartilage from either side, to surround and separate it from the periosteum (Fig. 19). Thus, in rabbit tibial and also rib fractures (Ham, 1930, 1972) an external layer of bone bridges the fracture by 12 days.

The callus of unstable rat fractures differs in that bone does not grow over the cartilage to separate it from the periosteum. Thus, there is no subperiosteal bridging by bone external to the cartilage; instead, bone formation over the fracture is entirely endochondral (Figs. 20 and 21) (Joyce *et al.*, 1990). This has led to the term "endochondral fracture healing". The timing of the stages of healing in rats is dependent upon both the age of the rat and the strain. Endochondral ossification of the callus is almost complete in some strains, e.g., Sprague-Dawley, by 12 days (Dodds, personal communication; Urist and McLean, 1941), while in other strains, e.g., Long-Evans, it does not start until this time (Joyce *et al.*, 1990).

Immediately after cartilage formation its replacement by endochondral

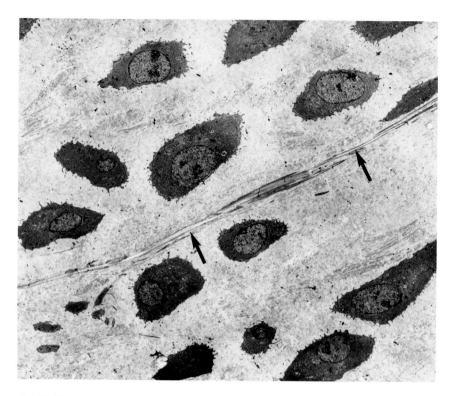

Fig. 17 Electron micrograph of part of the cartilage in the callus of a 9-day mechanically unstable rabbit tibial fracture. An elastic fiber (arrows) runs through the typical cartilaginous matrix. The chondrocytes in this area appear healthy. (Magnification × 1600.) (From Ashhurst, 1986.)

ossification starts along the lateral junctions between cartilage and bone (Fig. 22); in the rabbit it does not occur along the junction with the subperiosteal bone (Fig. 23). By 3 to 4 weeks, the cartilage is reduced to a thin central line so that the periosteal callus consists almost entirely of bone. Thus, there is now a strong external bridging callus that provides stability at the fracture site (Fig. 24). Fibrous tissue with fibroblasts and blood vessels is now present immediately over the fracture gap (Fig. 25).

The stability at the fracture gap provided by the bony callus reduces the strain and cells now enter the gap (Fig. 25). The debris in the fracture gap is removed by macrophages which invade the gap first; fibroblasts and capillaries follow. Fibrous tissue is laid down and some bone along the fractured surfaces is resorbed by osteoclasts (Fig. 26). Osteoblasts then migrate along the bone surfaces and lay down transverse lamellae, which quickly fill the gap to achieve cortical union (Fig. 27). The saw-cut regions of rabbit fractures again demonstrate that resorption of the old, dead bone is not essential before new bone is formed.

Healing that involves the endochondral replacement of a large area of

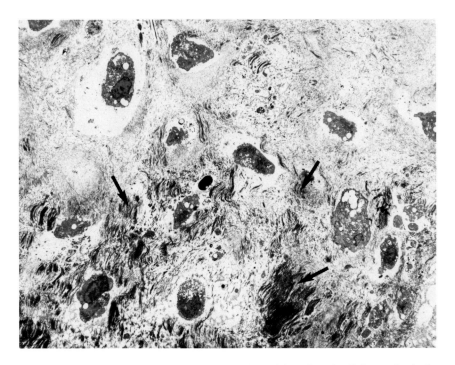

Fig. 18 Electron micrograph of a region of the cartilage of the callus of a 12-day mechanically unstable rabbit tibial fracture. The matrix is very heterogeneous; typical thin collagen fibrils are interspersed with bundles of thick collagen fibrils (arrows). The chondrocytes appear unhealthy. (Magnification × 1550.) (From Ashhurst, 1986.)

cartilage over the fracture site has recently been termed "endochondral fracture healing", though the observations leading to this nomenclature were of healing rat fractures (Joyce *et al.*, 1990; Lane *et al.*, 1986). This definition is misleading. It is pertinent here to consider what is meant by healing, or uniting, a fracture. Bony union can refer either to the continuity of bone over the fracture site in the periosteal callus, or to union of the cortical bone. As described above, in rabbit fractures, subperiosteal bone is formed to bridge the fracture by 12 to 14 days. This bone is not endochondral, but that formed to replace the underlying cartilage is. In contrast, in rat models all the bone over the fracture is formed endochondrally (see above). Thus "healing" or bony bridging by the periosteal callus may be only endochondral in part.

Factors that Influence the Differentiation of Chondrocytes in Fracture Callus

The hypothesis that cartilage forms in regions of poor blood supply and hence oxygen tension has been put forward by several groups to explain the development of the cartilaginous anlagen of the long bones during limb

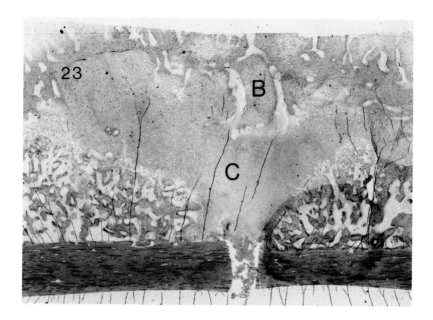

Fig. 19 Photomicrograph of a 12-day mechanically unstable rabbit tibial fracture. The cartilage (C) is now enclosed by new bone (B) that has grown over it to provide an external bridge. 23 indicates the area of Figure 23. (Magnification × 19.) (From Ashhurst, 1986.)

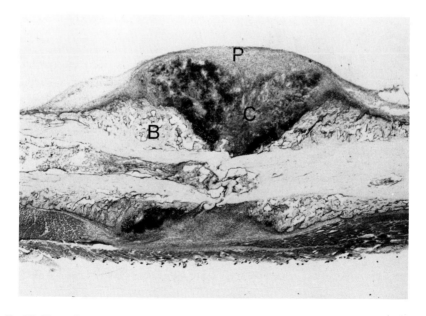

Fig. 20 Photomicrograph of an 8-day mechanically unstable rat (Sprague-Dawley) metatarsal fracture. The advancing fronts of new bone (B) recede peripherally. The central region over the fracture is filled by a large area of cartilage (C). The periosteum (P) lies directly on top of the cartilage. (Magnification × 16.) (Courtesy of Dr. R. Dodds, Bath Institute of Rheumatic Diseases, Bath, U. K.)

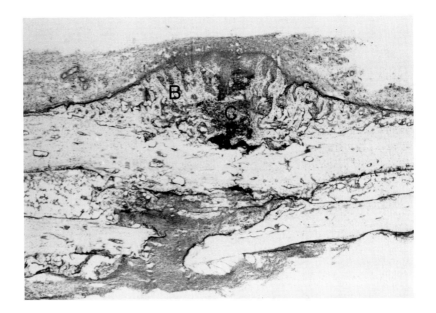

Fig. 21 Photomicrograph of a 12-day mechanically unstable rat (Sprague-Dawley) metatarsal fracture. Endochondral ossification has occurred and only a small amount of cartilage (C) remains between the advancing fronts of bone (B). (Magnification × 22.) (Courtesy of Dr. R. Dodds, Bath Institute of Rheumatic Diseases, Bath, U. K.)

development. Vascular regression from the appropriate regions of the limb bud has been observed using tracers such as India ink or fluorescently labeled low-density lipoprotein (Caplan and Koutroupas, 1973; Feinberg *et al.*, 1986; Hallmann *et al.*, 1987). It has been suggested by Wilson (1986) that condensation of the mesenchymal cells in the precartilaginous regions might produce forces that occlude the capillaries and the resulting anoxia of the area would induce chondrocytic differentiation.

That low oxygen tension influences differentiation of mesenchymal cells towards a chondrocytic phenotype was demonstrated *in vitro* by the experiments of Bassett and Herrmann (1962) and Pawelek (1969). Recent experimental evidence that the viability of chondrocytes in culture is reduced by toxic compounds physiologically derived from molecular oxygen (Tschan *et al.*, 1990), begins to explain why chondrocytes differentiate and are maintained only in regions of poor blood supply and low oxygen tension.

In the callus of mechanically unstable fractures, the region over the fracture gap will be subjected to stresses and the resulting micromovement will be important in the inhibition of angiogenesis. Carter and co-workers (Blenman *et al.*, 1989; Carter *et al.*, 1988) have constructed two- and three-dimensional finite elements models of the callus of healing fractures and have predicted the regions of high compressive dilatational stress and high intermittent stress. These correspond to the regions of cartilage formation

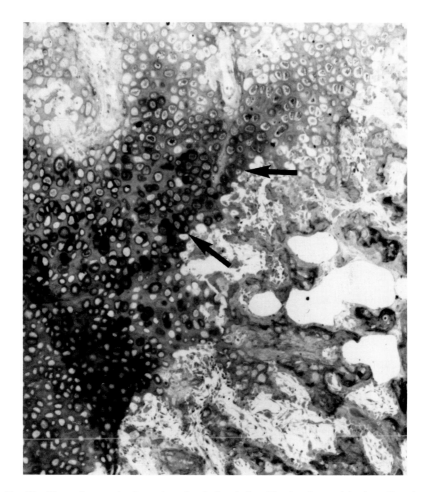

Fig. 22   Photomicrograph of a region of endochondral ossification (arrows) in the callus of a 12-day mechanically unstable rabbit tibial fracture. (Magnification × 135.) (From Ashhurst, 1986.)

and they suggest that these stresses contribute to the poor vascularity of the regions of chondrogenesis. Thus, there is strong circumstantial and theoretical evidence that the forces inherent around the fracture site of mechanically unstable fractures lead to the avascularity of the tissue and chondrogenesis. Similarly, small nodules of chondrogenesis in the callus of mechanically stable fractures are found in regions in which micromovement might occur.

The events in bony union between the cortical fragments of mechanically unstable fractures depend on the width of the gap. If it is narrow, cells do not enter until the external callus can stabilize the fracture completely. If the gap is wider (2 mm is the critical width in rabbits; Greiff, 1978), either because the fracture is displaced, or because a segment of cortical bone has

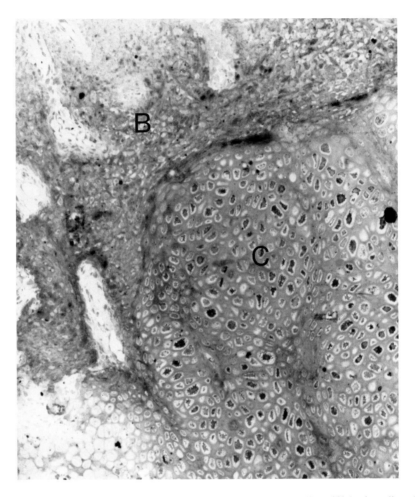

Fig. 23 Photomicrograph of the junction between bone (B) and cartilage (C) in the callus of the 12-day mechanically unstable rabbit tibial fracture in Fig. 19 (23 indicates the position of this area). Endochondral ossification is not occurring. (Magnification × 135.) (From Ashhurst, 1986.)

been lost, the relative strains are less than when the gap is narrow. Cells migrate around the fractured ends of the bone, together with capillaries to form fibrous tissue. Bone is formed on the fractured surfaces. As these growing fronts of bone approach each other, the strains in the narrowing gap become too great for the maintenance of blood vessels and cartilage is formed, which is then removed endochondrally. The events in gaps clearly support the observations that if the mechanical conditions are stable, bone formation occurs, but that if they are unstable, as in a wide gap, cartilage formation is followed by endochondral ossification.

Recently, Hulth et al. (1990) have questioned this concept that a paucity of blood vessels leads to chondrogenesis because they detected some large,

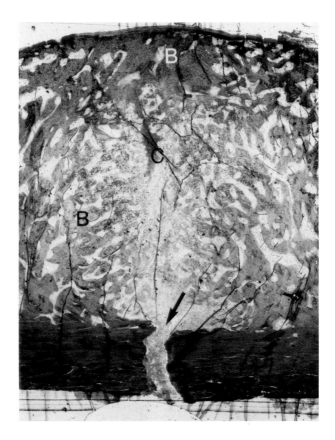

Fig. 24 Photomicrograph of a 4-week mechanically unstable rabbit tibial fracture. The cartilage (C) is reduced to a narrow central region, so that the callus consists almost entirely of bone (B). Cells and capillaries are present around the gap (arrow) — see Fig. 25. (Magnification × 20.) (From Ashhurst, 1986.)

sinusoid-like vessels in the cartilage of rat tibial fractures. Similar vessels were described in the cartilage of unstable rabbit tibial fractures by Ashhurst (1986). These vessels are not typical of the capillaries found in other parts of the periosteal callus and they are very sporadic in their occurrence. When the regions of bone and cartilage formation are compared, the sparsity of blood vessels in the presumptive cartilaginous areas compared to the abundance in areas of bone formation is obvious.

In this context it is pertinent to consider Brighton and Kreb's (1972) finding that in healing rabbit fibulae, oxygen tension is very low in the hematoma, high in fibrous tissue, but of similar lower levels in both the newly formed bone and cartilage. After remodeling, the oxygen tension in the bone increased to that of normal cortical bone. These authors consider that the low oxygen tensions in the newly formed bone and cartilage must be due to an increased oxygen consumption by the large numbers of cells

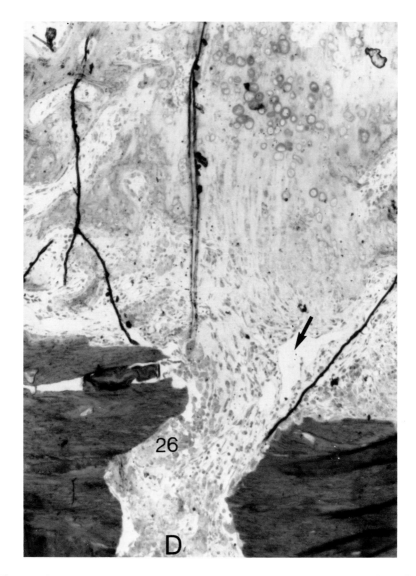

Fig. 25 Photomicrograph of the periosteal end of the fracture gap of the 4-week mechanically unstable rabbit tibial fracture in Fig. 24. Fibrous tissue with capillaries (arrow) is entering the gap. Debris (D) is still present deeper in the gap. 26 indicates the position of Fig. 26. (Magnification × 135.) (From Ashhurst, 1986.)

present, or to a decreased delivery of oxygen by the blood vessels. Certainly as mentioned previously, the lack of blood vessels in the cartilaginous regions will be an important factor. In new cancellous bone, high oxygen levels should exist in the spaces between the trabeculae. These have a rich capillary network and are lined by active osteoblasts. A plentiful supply of oxygen should, therefore, be available, but will be used rapidly by the

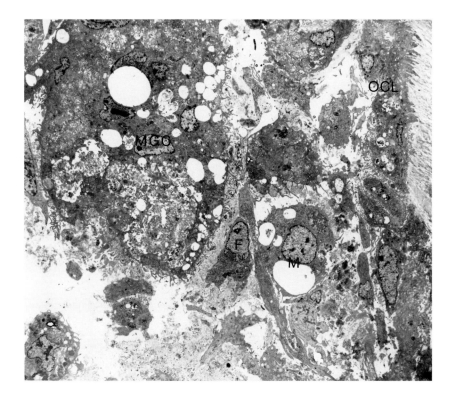

Fig. 26 Electron micrograph of the area in the fracture gap of the 4-week mechanically unstable rabbit tibial fracture in Figs. 24 and 25 and indicated by 26 on Fig. 25. The fractured surface is covered by osteoclasts (OCL). There is some debris in the gap which is being removed by macrophages (M) and a multinucleated giant cell (MGC). Fibroblasts (F) are also present. (Magnification × 1700.) (From Ashhurst, 1986.)

osteoblasts. The oxygen tension in trabeculae might be lower than in cortical bone, because the tissue is less organized and fluid flow may not be so efficient as in Haversian bone (Kelly *et al.*, 1990). The recorded oxygen tensions in the developing cancellous bone will depend on the precise location of the recording electrode, i.e., whether it is in a space, or in a trabeculum.

The Remodeling Phase of Fracture Repair

Remodeling is independent of the initial mechanical stability of the fracture. As soon as there is cortical union over even a small area of the fractured surfaces, resorption of the periosteal callus, and any endosteal callus, starts because it has fulfilled its function to stabilize the fracture. Large resorption cavities appear in the callus, particularly along its junction with the cortical bone (Fig. 28). In the rabbit this starts at 3 weeks in mechanically stable fractures and at 4 to 5 weeks in mechanically unstable fractures. Remodeling

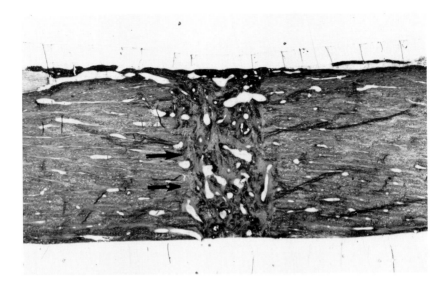

Fig. 27 Photomicrograph of the saw-cut region under the plate of a 6-week rabbit fracture that was originally mechanically unstable. The saw-cut is filled by transverse lamellae of new bone. In some regions (arrows) the straight edge of the cut is still visible. (Magnification × 29.) (From Ashhurst, 1986.)

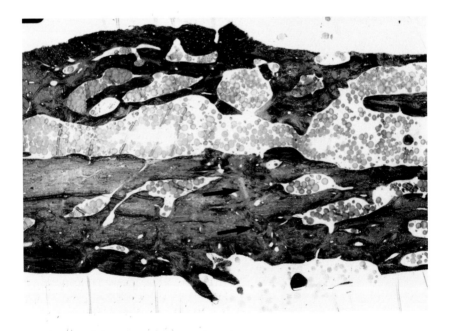

Fig. 28 Photomicrograph of a 12-week rabbit tibial fracture that was initially mechanically unstable. The periosteal callus is separated from the cortical bone by large resorption cavities. The position of the fracture can be identified by the transverse lamellae (arrows). (Magnification × 24.) (From Ashhurst, 1986.)

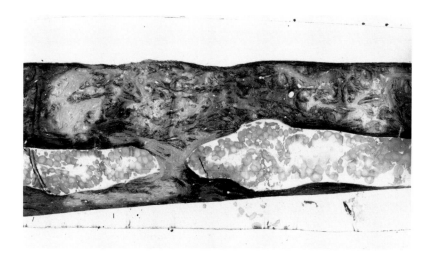

Fig. 29 Photomicrograph of the fracture region of a 26-week rabbit tibial fracture that was initially mechanically unstable. The bone is compact, but the osteons are in varying orientations. (Magnification × 27.) (From Ashhurst, 1986.)

in the cortical bone is now active (Fig. 28). The result of the extensive remodeling in the callus and in the old cortical bone is the formation of one layer (Fig. 29). The details of this process and the effects of the plates on the dimensions of, and quality of bone in, the resulting cortical bone are outside the scope of the present chapter.

The description above of the processes involved in callus formation and cortical healing is based primarily on observations of healing under different mechanical conditions in the rabbit tibia (Ashhurst, 1986). Essentially similar processes have been described in healing fractures of the rabbit rib (Ham, 1930; Ham and Harris, 1972), rat femur (Joyce et al., 1990; Urist and McLean, 1941), and dog and human long bones (Cruess and McLean, 1975; McKibbin, 1978; Schenk and Willenegger, 1967; Urist and Johnson, 1943).

The Types of Collagen Secreted During Fracture Healing

Before the development of immunological techniques for the localization of the different types of collagen during fracture healing, the problem had been approached biochemically. The incorporation of ^{3}H-proline was used to estimate the timing of collagen synthesis and it was found to be maximal in the second week in the callus of unstable rat fractures (Penttinen, 1972a). In 3-week stable rabbit tibial fractures, Paavolainen et al. (1979) found that there was no significant difference in the levels of hydroxyproline compared with intact bones, but by this time there should have been partial cortical union and callus resorption (Ashhurst, 1986). Later biochemical studies identified the three fibrous collagens. Types I and III were found to be synthesized first, followed by type II in the second week in a rabbit tibial defect model (Bruce and Dziewiatkowski, 1987), but in a similar model using the humerus of the chicken, only type I collagen was identified (Glimcher *et al.*, 1980).

Biochemical data do not give accurate information about the spatial distribution of the collagens, but this can be obtained immunohistochemically. At the present time, the only detailed immunohistochemical investigations of the collagens produced during fracture healing are those of Lane *et al.* (1986) and Page *et al.* (1986) on rabbit and rat fractures. Polyclonal antibodies to the collagens of the respective animal were made, that is to types I, II, III, and V collagens for the rabbit and types I, II, and III for the rat; details of the provenance of the antibodies is given in the papers cited and will not be discussed here. These investigations will form the basis for the following description of the distribution of the different collagens during healing under different mechanical conditions.

The first new matrix of loose fibrous tissue contains primarily of type III collagen (Fig. 30), but some type I collagen was detected in the rat. Type III collagen was identified previously in fibrous tissue of a healing fracture by Gay and Miller (1978), but the species was not given. Type V collagen is also found in the rabbit fibrous tissue (Fig. 31) and this collagen is associated particularly with the blood vessels. The periosteum reforms from the peripheral fibrous tissue and contains types III and V collagens, but no type I (Figs. 32 and 33). This finding was unexpected because the periosteum of developing chick bones contains type I collagen (Von der Mark *et al.*, 1976). Normal rabbit periosteum lacks type I collagen (Ashhurst, unpublished data).

The trabeculae of bone start to develop along the surface of the old cortical bone and grow into the fibrous tissue. Thick fibrils of type I collagen can be seen among the thin fibrils (Fig. 34). In both rabbits and rats, type I collagen is laid down among the fibrils of the original fibrous matrix, so that the newly formed bone is heterogeneous in its content of collagens. More type I collagen is produced as more trabeculae of bone develop to form a layer of thickness and distribution determined by the mechanical conditions (see above). As bone formation continues, mineralization starts in the more mature areas and the type I collagen appears to be more evenly distributed (Fig. 35). The trabeculae still contain some types III and V collagens (Figs. 36 and 37). The spaces in the bone retain the original fibrous tissue containing types III and V collagens (Figs. 36 and 37).

The same collagens are produced during the early stages of fracture healing irrespective of the mechanical conditions under which the fracture is healing. It is only from about 5 days onwards that effects of mechanical stability on collagen synthesis are seen. Thus, it is *after* new bone formation

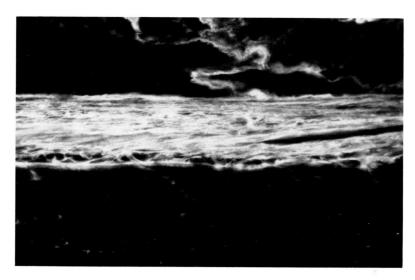

Fig. 30

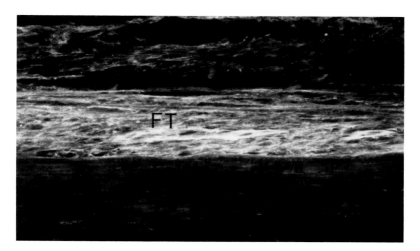

Fig. 31

Figs. 30 and 31 Photomicrographs to show the distribution of types III (Fig. 31) and V (Fig. 32) collagens in the initial fibrous tissue (FT) of a 3-day mechanically stable rabbit tibial fracture using a fluorescently (FITC) labeled second antibody. (Magnification × 300.) (From Page *et al.*, 1986. See reference list.)

is established that cartilage and, hence, type II collagen, appear in the callus of mechanically unstable fractures. The first areas in which type II collagen is laid down are along the periphery of the ingrowing regions of bone (Figs. 38 and 39), but by about 10 days, the whole area over the fracture site is filled by a matrix containing types II and IX collagens (Figs. 40 and 43) (Page *et al.*, 1986). It also contains some types III and V

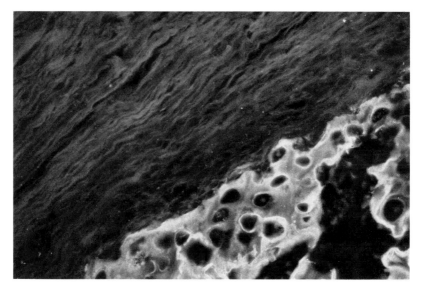

Fig. 32

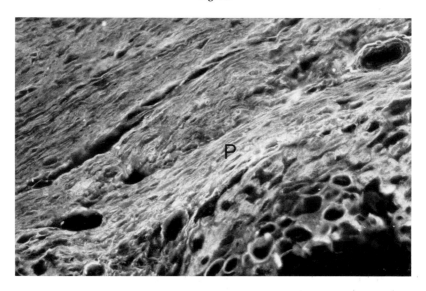

Fig. 33

Figs. 32 and 33   Photomicrographs of the regenerated periosteum (P) of a 2-week mechanically unstable rabbit tibial fracture to show the absence of type I collagen (Fig. 32) and the presence of type III collagen (Fig. 33) using a FITC-labeled second antibody. (Magnification × 300.) (From Page *et al.*, 1986.)

collagens (Figs. 41 and 42). The atypical collagens are again the remnants of the original fibrous matrix and presumably account for the heterogeneity of the collagen fibrils in the matrices seen in electron micrographs (see Fig. 18).

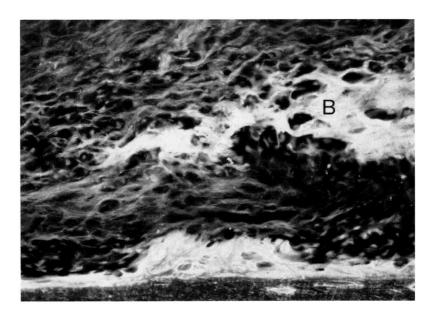

Fig. 34 Photomicrograph to show the immunofluorescence (FITC) of developing trabeculae of bone (B) containing type I collagen in the callus of a 5-day mechanically stable rabbit tibial fracture. The type I collagen fibrils are laid down among the fibrils of the initial fibrous matrix. (Magnification × 300.) (From Page *et al.*, 1986.)

The use of non-fluorescent antibody labels for the second antibody allows more precise correlation of the antigenic sites with the histology of the callus and has revealed regions of overlap of areas of matrix containing types I and II collagens; an example of this chondroid bone in a 7-day mechanically unstable rabbit fracture is shown in Figs. 38, 39, 44, and 45. The cells appear to be secreting both types of collagen into the matrix. This possibility is supported by the observation in rat fracture callus that cells along the boundary between developing bone and cartilage express the mRNAs for both types I and II collagens (Sandberg *et al.*, 1989) (see below).

Type X collagen is found in cartilage containing hypertrophic chondrocytes, i.e., in cartilage that will calcify during endochondral ossification, and also in small amounts in bone (Schmid and Linsenmayer, 1985). Its association with mineralizing regions has led to the hypothesis that it has a role in calcification (Schmid and Linsenmayer, 1985). Type X collagen is found in chicken fracture callus between 5 and 21 days after injury (Grant *et al.*, 1987). It is associated with the hypertrophic chondrocytes in regions undergoing endochondral ossification (Balian, personal communication). Its location in rabbit and rat fractures has not yet been established.

The regions of endochondral ossification are found only in the callus of unstable fractures. The mineralized cartilage is resorbed to leave spicules that bind antibodies to types I, II, III, and V collagens (Figs. 46 and 47). The appearance of type I collagen in cartilage at this time is unexpected,

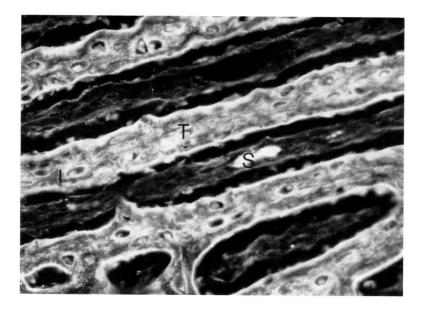

Fig. 35

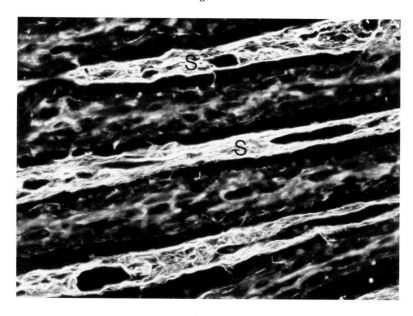

Fig. 36

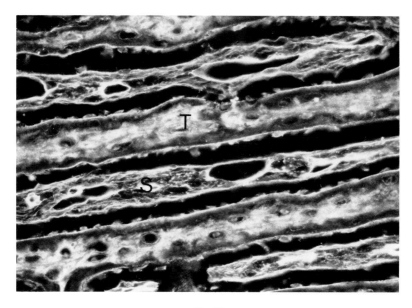

Fig. 37

Figs. 35 through 37 Photomicrographs of mineralized bone in the callus of a 4-week mechanically stable rabbit tibial fracture. The trabeculae (T) contain type I collagen (Fig. 35), but a small amount of types III (Fig. 36) and V (Fig. 37) is still present in the bone matrix. The spaces (S) contain a fibrous matrix of types III and V collagens. The second antibody is FITC-labeled. (Magnification × 300.) (From Page *et al.*, 1986.)

but it agrees with the observation of Von der Mark *et al.* (1977) that cartilage in the resorbing regions of the growth plate of chickens contains type I collagen. These authors suggest that type I collagen is laid down by osteoblasts that invade the vacated chondrocyte lacunae, but alternatively, the hypertrophic chondrocytes might produce it. This anomaly has yet to be resolved. The new bone on the spicules of cartilage contains only types I and V collagens (Fig. 48). The latter collagen is found primarily around the osteocyte lacunae and is a normal component of cortical bone (Miller, 1984 and see Volume 3, Chapter 7). The spaces in the bone contain a fibrous matrix of types III and V collagens.

The development of a large area containing type II collagen in the callus is found only in the unstable fractures. The callus of stable fractures does not normally contain any cartilage, but isolated regions consisting of about 10 cells surrounded by matrix containing type II collagen, are, however, occasionally seen in the callus of 7- to 14-day stable fractures. These regions are frequently near the fracture site, but may also be found within fully formed trabeculae of bone in the callus (Fig. 49). Type IX collagen is found in some, but not all, of these areas. Another site, in which the area of type II collagen is often greater, is along the surface of the developing bone just under the periosteum (Fig. 50). Type I collagen is also present in these areas, and indeed the matrix exhibits many features of normal bone matrix.

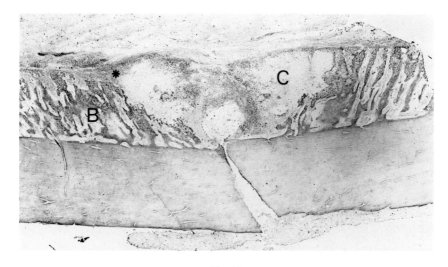

Fig. 38

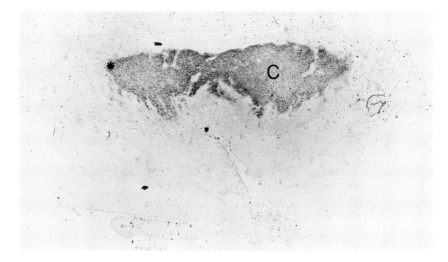

Fig. 39

Figs. 38 and 39   Photomicrographs of the whole fracture area of a 7-day mechanically unstable rabbit tibial fracture. Fig. 38 shows the distribution of type I collagen in the bone (B) and Fig. 39 that of type II collagen in the cartilage (C). A region around the periphery of the cartilage binds antibodies to both types I and II collagens. The second antibody is gold labeled; silver intensification was used. See Figs. 44 and 45 for higher magnification micrographs of the area marked *. (Magnification × 18.)

It is suggested that these regions are chondroid bone (Beresford, 1981 and see above). They disappear by 14 days, but are not removed by endochondral ossification and so it appears that the atypical collagens are removed during the normal turnover and remodeling processes in the bone. The stimulus for their initial formation is not known, but the two most common sites in which they are found correspond to regions in which there might be localized micro-motion, or shearing stresses, i.e., over the fracture site and between the hard tissue of the bone and the soft tissue of the periosteum. These areas are also characterized by their lack of blood vessels and micro-motion of the amplitude expected in regions of juxtaposition of hard and soft tissues is thought to contribute to the local inhibition of angiogenesis (see above).

A new stage of the analysis of collagen synthesis and secretion during fracture healing is developing with the availability of probes to the mRNAs for the fibrous collagens. The results of studies using Northern hybridizations (Multimäki *et al.*, 1987; Nemeth *et al.*, 1988) indicate that in the callus of rat tibial fractures immobilized with medullary nails, the mRNA for types I and III collagens are expressed first, followed by that of type II collagen towards the end of the first week. During the second week, the level of type II mRNA expression increases, but the levels of the mRNAs for both types I and II collagens decrease as new matrix production ceases. Subsequent *in situ* hybridization on sections of rat fracture callus show that osteoblasts in areas of developing new bone express the mRNA for type I collagen, but that chondrocytes along the boundaries of the cartilaginous matrix express the mRNAs for both types I and II collagens (Sandberg *et al.*, 1989). This expression of the mRNAs for both collagens is expected from the observation that both types of collagen are present in areas of chondroid bone in rabbit fracture callus. Cells that express the mRNAs for both types I and II collagens simultaneously are not confined to healing skeletal tissues. Both types I and II mRNAs are expressed by some chondrocytes during cartilage formation in developing chick limbs (Devlin *et al.*, 1988; Hayashi *et al.*, 1986). This observation led to the suggestion that type I collagen synthesis may be controlled at the transcriptional, rather than gene level (Devlin *et al.*, 1988). Leblond *et al.* (1989) presented morphological evidence for the presence of two sets of vesicles containing either type I or type II collagen within the same chondrocyte in the growing rat mandible.

The Proteoglycans and their Associated Glycosaminoglycan Chains Produced During Fracture Healing

The characterization of the proteoglycans, or rather of the glycosaminoglycans, produced during fracture healing was attempted much earlier than that of the collagens because crude biochemical and histochemical methods for polyanionic carbohydrates were available much earlier than were techniques for extracting and localizing collagens. It should be remembered that this early work preceded the detailed characterization of the proteoglycans of both bone and cartilage (see Volume 3, Chapter 8).

In an early investigation, Hudack *et al.* (1949) reported histochemical evidence for the presence of acidic polysaccharides in rabbit fracture callus,

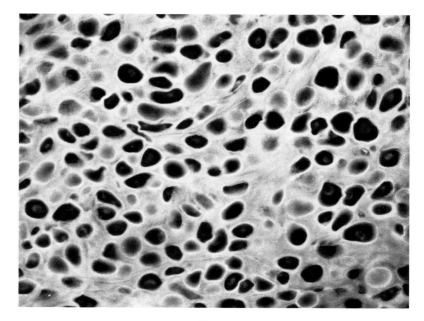

Fig. 40

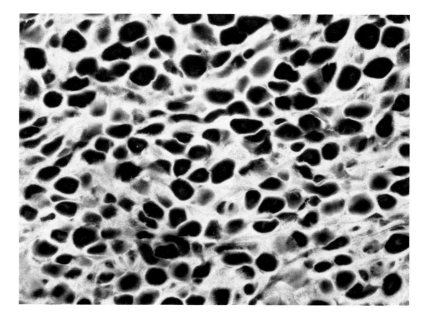

Fig. 41

Figs. 40 through 43 Photomicrographs of an area of cartilage from the callus of a 7-day mechanically unstable rabbit tibial fracture to show the binding of antibodies to types II (Fig. 40), III (Fig. 41), V (Fig. 42) and IX (Fig. 43) collagens by the matrix. The types III and V collagens are remnants of the initial fibrous matrix. The second antibody is FITC-labeled. (Magnification × 340.) (From Page *et al.*, 1986.)

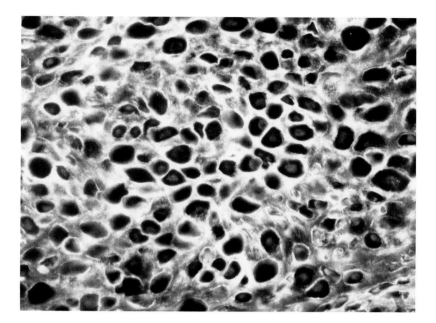

Fig. 42

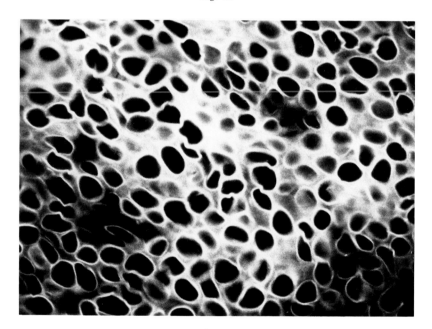

Fig. 43

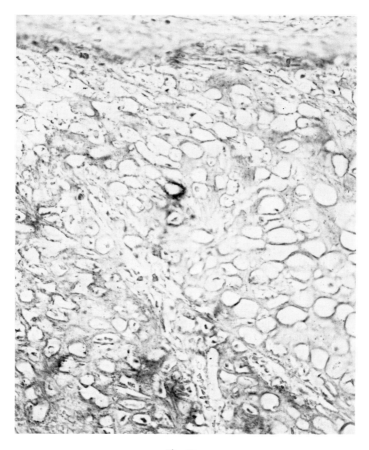

Fig. 44

but were unable to identify either hyaluronan or chondroitin sulfate after extraction. Later, Maurer and Hudack (1952) isolated a polysaccharide form 7- to 9-day unimmobilized rabbit femoral fractures which they identified as hyaluronan, because it was labile to pneumococcal hyaluronidase. The amount of sulfate extracted was very low which led them to conclude that the hyaluronan was extracted from the granulation tissue, i.e., the initial fibrous tissue and that little cartilage was present in the fracture callus. Ten years later, Zenkevich and Kasavina (1962) compared the glycosminoglycans in the bone and callus of rabbit unimmobilized foreleg fractures taken at 7, 14, 21, and 55 days after injury. They found hyaluronan and chondroitin sulfate in the callus at 7 days, but only keratan sulfate at 14 days. They also concluded that normal rabbit bone contains both chondroitin and keratan sulfates. Keratan sulfate was also identified in a rabbit tibial healing defect by Bruce and Dziewiatkowski (1987). Another study (Antonopoulos *et al.,* 1965) used callus tissue from a 1 cm rabbit radial defect from which they isolated and identified hyaluronan in the extracts at

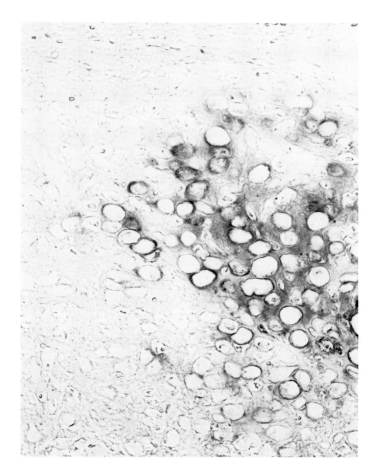

Fig. 45

Figs. 44 and 45   Photomicrographs of the area marked * in Figs. 38 and 39 to show the overlap in the distribution of types I (Fig. 44) and II (Fig. 45) collagens to form an area of "chondroid bone". The second antibody is labeled with alkaline phosphatase. (Magnification × 350.)

1, 2, and 3 weeks. Chondroitin sulfate was found in small amounts at 1 week, but in larger amounts at 2 and 3 weeks when there is much cartilage. By 4 weeks when bone predominates, the amounts are reduced. These workers did not find keratan sulfate in this or a later study (Solheim 1966).

Several biochemical studies of callus of rat humeral and tibial fractures have shown an increased content of hexosamines at 1 and 2 weeks that drops slowly as healing proceeds (Lane *et al.*, 1979, 1982; Penttinen, 1973; Udupa and Prasad, 1963). The rise and fall correlates with the formation and endochondral removal of cartilage, respectively. Penttinen (1972) identified chondroitin-4-sulfate and hyaluronan in rat callus. Lane *et al.* (1982) found that the total hexosamine content of unimmobilized tibial fractures is

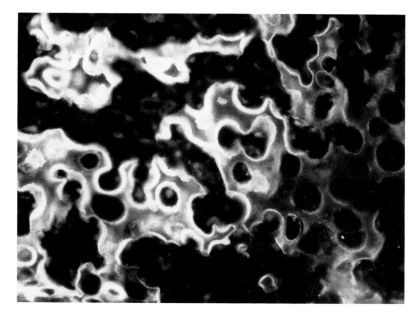

Fig. 46

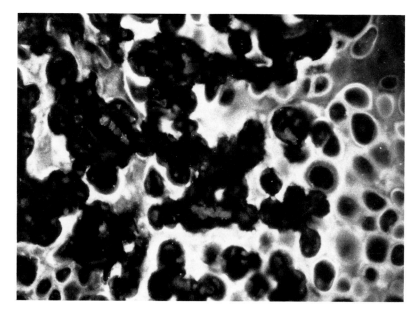

Fig. 47

Figs. 46 and 47   Photomicrographs of an area of endochondral ossification in the callus of a 2-week mechanically unstable rabbit tibial fracture. The spicules of cartilage are shown by the immunofluorescence with antibodies to type II collagen (Fig. 47). The surface of these spicules binds antibodies to type I collagen (Fig. 46). (Magnification × 340.) (From Page *et al.*, 1986.)

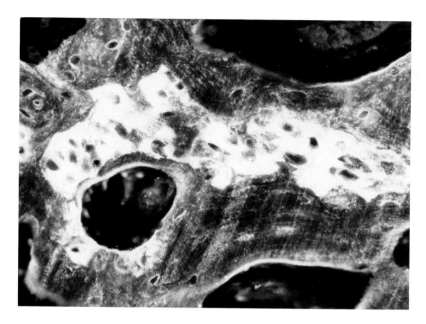

Fig. 48 Photomicrograph of a bone trabeculum in the region of endochondral ossification in the callus of a 3-week mechanically unstable rabbit tibial fracture. It contains a spicule of cartilage that binds the antibodies more strongly than the surrounding bone matrix. (Magnification × 340.) (From Page *et al.*, 1986.)

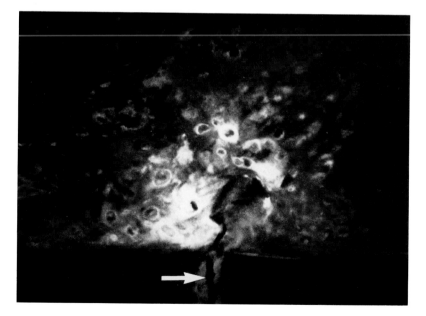

Fig. 49 Photomicrograph of the region over the fracture (arrow) of an 11-day mechanically stable rabbit tibial fracture. The immunofluorescence shows a small area in which antibodies to type II collagen are bound. (Magnification × 280.)

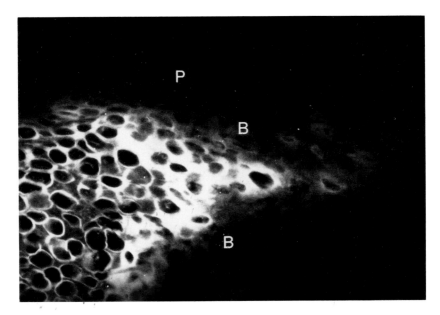

Fig. 50 Photomicrograph of an area of chondroid bone between the periosteum (P) and bone (B) of the callus of an 11-day mechanically stable rabbit tibial fracture. It is binding antibodies to type II collagen. (Magnification × 300.)

two and a half times that of fractures stabilized with an intermedullary nail (K wire). While an intermedullary nail does not provide the level of stability achieved when compression is used, this observation again illustrates that the degree of immobilization of a fracture influences the amount of cartilage and hence proteoglycans that are formed. In another investigation of the proteoglycans in rat fracture callus Yokobori *et al.* (1980) identified a "light", dermatan sulfate-containing proteoglycan and a "heavy", chondroitin sulfate-containing proteoglycan. The latter was found only when the callus contains cartilage.

The biochemical investigations reviewed above give essentially similar results, i.e., during healing under unstable mechanical conditions, proteoglycans similar to those found in cartilage can be extracted from the callus during the period in which there is a large amount of cartilage present. At the time these studies were performed, bone proteoglycans had not been characterized. It is now known from the work of Fisher *et al.* (1983), Prince *et al.* (1983), and Sato *et al.* (1985) that bone contains a large proteoglycan that is present in the soft tissues (i.e., of fibrous tissue of Haversian canals and spaces in cancellous bone) that can be extracted prior to demineralization. The core protein is similar to that of the cartilage proteoglycans, but the glycosaminoglycan side-chains are shorter. Both chondroitin-4- and -6-sulfate side chains are present. The virtual absence of this proteoglycan from cortical bone confirms its location in the soft tissues of bone. Two small proteoglycans are extracted with the mineral by EDTA. Their core proteins are of M^r around 45,000, but they are the products of different genes (Fisher et al., 1987, 1989). The chondroitin sulfate chains have a M^r of 400,000. One, known as PGI or biglycan, has two chondroitin sulfate chains, the other, PGII or decorin, has one chain. Both are present in newly formed bone and cartilaginous matrices, though their distributions differ (Bianco et al., 1990).

A distinction between rabbit and other mammalian bones, investigated to date, must now be pointed out. Rabbit bone contains keratan sulfate (Diamond et al., 1982) and the keratan sulfate chains are attached to the rabbit bone sialoprotein, which acts as the core protein (Kinne and Fisher, 1987).

The biochemical studies described so far assign the major part of the proteoglycan they characterize to the cartilage, and, of course, during healing under unstable mechanical conditions, a large area of cartilage is transiently present. Little information was obtained about the newly formed bone. Histochemical techniques have severe limitations, but provided that they are correlated with biochemical information, they can give accurate information about the precise tissue localization of the various macromolecules. The dye, Alcian Blue, used at pH 5.7 in the presence of increasing molarities of magnesium chloride, can be used to distinguish between unsulfated, and sulfated or highly sulfated glycosaminoglycans (Scott, 1980; Scott and Dorling, 1965). Using these methods, Page and Ashhurst (1987) characterized the glycosaminoglycans synthesized during healing in mechanically stable and unstable rabbit tibial fractures. The fibrous tissue binds the dye only in low magnesium chloride concentrations (Figs. 51 and 52). As this staining is labile to testicular hyaluronidase, it was concluded that the fibrous tissue contains hyaluronan and some chondroitin sulfate.

The unmineralized, newly formed bone matrix binds the dye in the presence of up to 0.8 M magnesium chloride (Figs. 53 and 54), whereas the older, mineralized matrix (Figs. 55 and 56) does not bind above 0.6 M concentrations. In addition in the mineralized matrix, the dye binding is less uniform and tends to be concentrated around the osteocyte lacunae. This observation is in agreement with that of Baylink et al. (1972) who found a reduction in staining of glycosaminoglycans on mineralization of rat tibial cortex. The identification of the glycosaminoglycans in the bone matrix as chondroitin and keratan sulfates was confirmed using specific monoclonal antibodies (Figs. 57 and 58) (Caterson et al., 1983, 1985; Page and Ashhurst, 1987). The rather low critical electrolyte concentration of the keratan sulfate suggests that it is not highly sulfated. The histochemical properties of the bone matrix are similar irrespective of the mechanical conditions under which the fracture is healing.

The large area of cartilage that develops when the fracture is unstable binds Alcian Blue in the presence of up to 0.4 M magnesium chloride at 5 days, but the concentration at which dye binding still occurs increases to

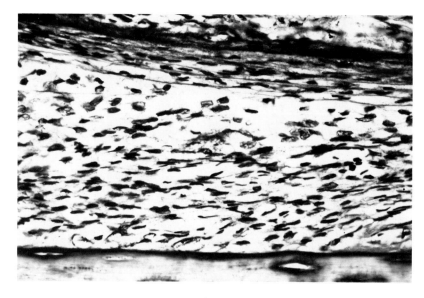

Fig. 51

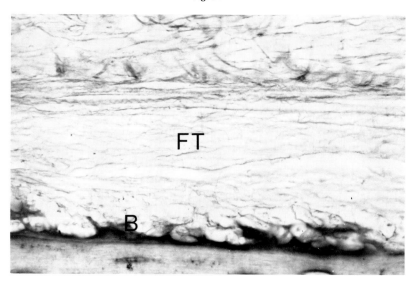

Fig. 52

Figs. 51 and 52 Photomicrograph of the fibrous tissue (FT) of a 5-day mechanically unstable rabbit tibial fracture stained with Alcian Blue, pH 5.7, in the presence of 0.1 M (Fig. 51) and 0.2 M (Fig. 52) magnesium chloride. Trabeculae of bone (B) are forming along the surface of the cortical bone. (Magnification × 340.) (From Page and Ashhurst, 1987. See reference list.)

0.8 M subsequently (Figs. 59 through 61). Dye binding is always stronger around the chondrocyte lacunae. Dye binding suggests that the cartilaginous matrix contains both chondroitin and keratan sulfates. These were identified further by the use of antibodies; chondroitin, chondroitin-4- and -6-sulfates

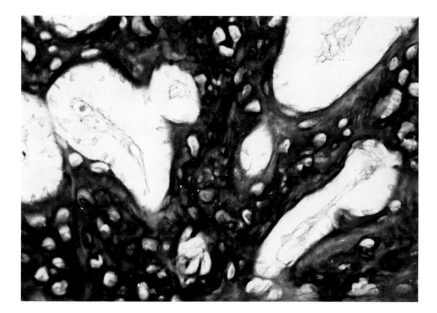

Fig. 53

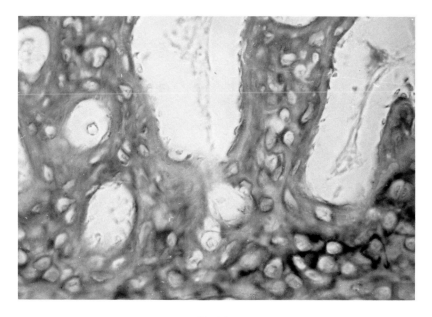

Fig. 54

Figs. 53 and 54   Photomicrographs of unmineralized, developing bone in the callus of a 5-day mechanically stable rabbit tibial fracture stained with Alcian Blue, pH 5.7, in the presence of 0.2 M (Fig. 53) and 0.6 M (Fig. 54) magnesium chloride. (Magnification × 340.) (From Page and Ashhurst, 1987.)

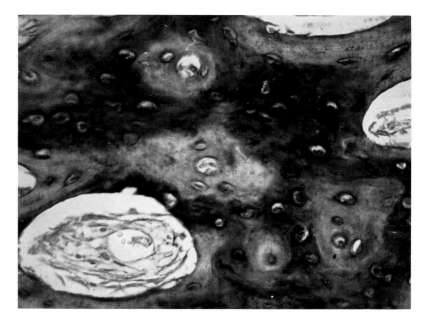

Fig. 55

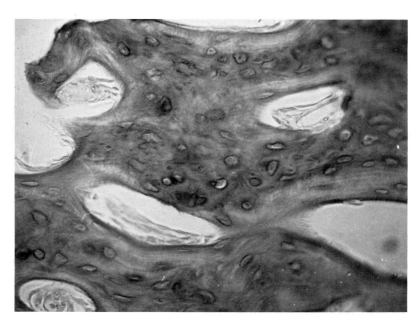

Fig. 56

Figs. 55 and 56   Photomicrographs of mineralized bone in the callus of a 21-day mechanically stable rabbit tibial fracture stained with Alcian Blue, pH 5.7, in the presence of 0.2 *M* (Fig. 55) and 0.6 *M* (Fig. 56) magnesium chloride. (Magnification × 340.) (From Page and Ashhurst, 1987.)

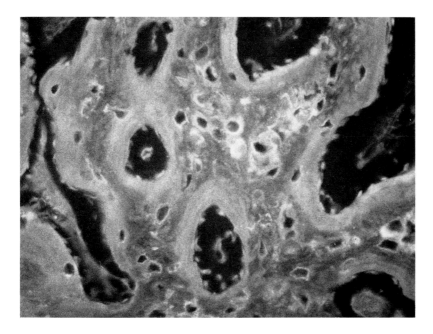

Fig. 57 Photomicrograph to show the immunofluorescent (rhodamine-label) localization of antibodies to chondroitin-4-sulfate bound by bone in the callus of a 5-day mechanically stable rabbit tibial fracture. (Magnification × 340.) (From Page and Ashhurst, 1987.)

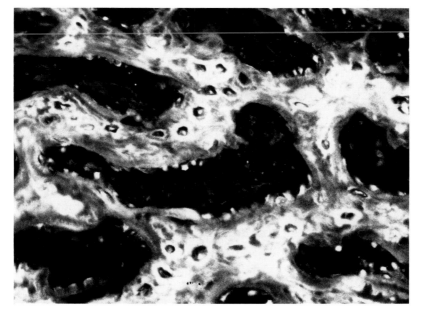

Fig. 58 Photomicrograph to show the immunofluorescent (rhodamine-label) localization of antibodies to keratan sulfate bound by bone in the callus of a 7-day mechanically unstable rabbit tibial fracture. (Magnification × 340.) (From Page and Ashhurst, 1987.)

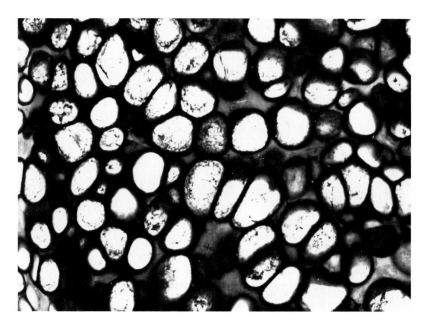

Fig. 59

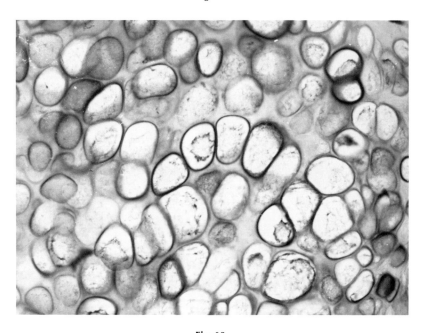

Fig. 60

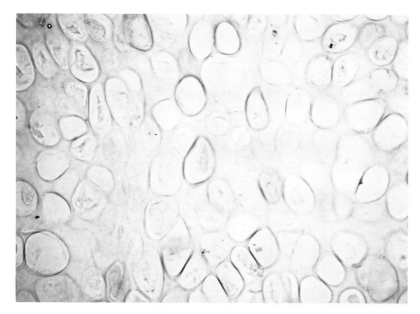

Fig. 61

Figs. 59 through 61   Photomicrographs of cartilage in the callus of a 14-day mechanically unstable rabbit tibial fracture to show the staining with Alcian Blue, pH 5.7, in the presence of 0.4 M (Fig. 59), 0.6 M (Fig. 60) and 0.8 M (Fig. 61) magnesium chloride. (Magnification × 340.) (From Page and Ashhurst, 1987.)

and keratan sulfate are present (Figs. 62 and 63). It seems reasonable to assume that the proteoglycans in the rabbit callus cartilage are similar to those in articular cartilage, except that their rather low critical electrolyte concentration compared to that of articular cartilage suggests that they may be undersulfated. Using Alcian Blue techniques, Dunham *et al.* (1983) identified large amounts of chondroitin sulfate and low levels of keratan sulfate in callus of rat unstabilized metatarsal fractures. The identification of keratan sulfate is questionable because Venn and Mason (1985) were unable to find biochemical evidence for keratan sulfate in any mouse or rat tissues. Typical cartilage proteoglycans were identified immunohistochemically in mechanically unstable rat tibial fractures by Johnell *et al.* (1988).

Small areas of cartilage in the thin callus of the mechanically stable fractures were observed only sporadically. The matrix is much less extensive than that of the cartilage in the callus of unstable fractures. At 5 days it binds Alcian Blue in the presence of up to 0.6 M concentrations of magnesium chloride, and at 1 to 2 weeks in the presence of only 0.4 M (Figs. 64 through 66). Antibodies to both chondroitin-4- and -6-sulfates and to keratan sulfate are bound (Figs. 67 and 68). Thus, the typical cartilage glycosaminoglycans are found in these nodules of cartilage, but the Alcian Blue binding suggests that they are undersulfated. It should be remembered that these areas of cartilage, or chondroid bone, are transient, persisting for only

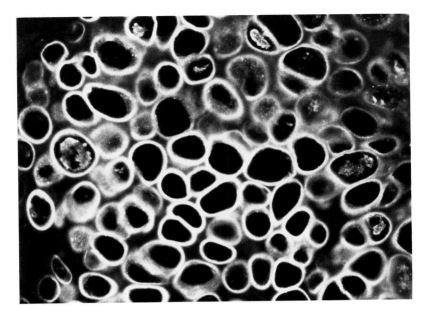

Fig. 62

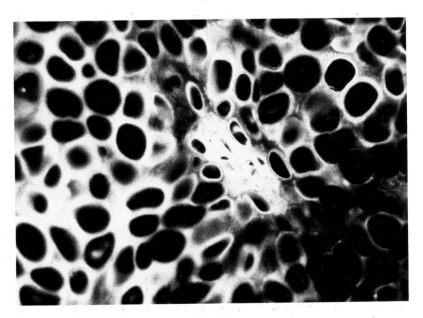

Fig. 63

Figs. 62 and 63   Photomicrograph to show the binding of antibodies to chondroitin-6-sulfate (Fig. 62) and keratan sulfate (Fig. 63) by cartilage in the callus of an 11-day mechanically unstable rabbit tibial fracture. The second antibody is rhodamine-labeled. (Magnification × 340.) (From Page and Ashhurst, 1987.)

a few days, and so the proteoglycans may not mature to achieve their normal levels of sulfation.

Other Matrix Macromolecules and Fracture Healing

While the collagens and proteoglycans comprise around 98% of the total bone mass, a number of other bone-specific proteins have recently been characterized. Osteopontin and sialoprotein have been identified (see Volume 3, Chapter 8) and in the rabbit, sialoprotein is the core protein of the keratan sulfate proteoglycan (Kinne and Fisher, 1987). Sialic acid residues bind Alcian Blue and Dunham et al. (1983) attribute some of the Alcian Blue-binding of both bone and cartilage in rat fracture callus to the presence of sialoprotein, but Page and Ashhurst (1987) were unable to detect any reduction in dye binding after treatment with neuraminidase. The very low levels of this protein make its histochemical identification somewhat doubtful. Johnell et al. (1988) were, however, able to identify a sialoprotein immunohistochemically in the new bone of the callus of rat tibial fractures.

Osteonectin, another non-collagenous protein in bone, has recently been located in newly formed endochondral bone and in some chondrocytes in the callus of a 16-day unstable rat femoral fracture using a specific monoclonal antibody (Bolander et al., 1989). Similarly, osteopontin is present in the newly formed periosteal bone of rat tibial fractures (Johnell et al., 1988). Osteocalcin has not so far been localized immunohistochemically in healing fractures.

The mRNAs of some of these molecules have been identified by Northern hybridization in extracts of rat femoral fractures by Nemeth et al. (1988). The mRNA for fibronectin is expressed early in the developing callus, followed by that of laminin on day 3 when capillaries are developing. Proteoglycan core and link protein mRNAs are found on day 6 when cartilage is developing, while that for osteocalcin appears on day 9, at the time when endochondral ossification starts.

Conclusions

Irrespective of the mechanical stability at the fracture site, bone is the major new tissue that is produced. The results of both the biochemical and immunohistochemical investigations summarized here indicate that the composition of the newly formed bone is independent of the mechanical stability of the healing fracture. A novel finding, revealed by immunohistochemistry, is that the type I collagen of the newly formed trabeculae is laid down among the types III and V collagen fibrils of the initial fibrous matrix. This means that the bone matrix is more heterogeneous in its collagen content than are other in vivo bone matrices. The proteoglycans

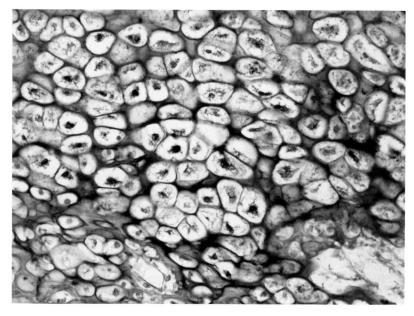

Fig. 64

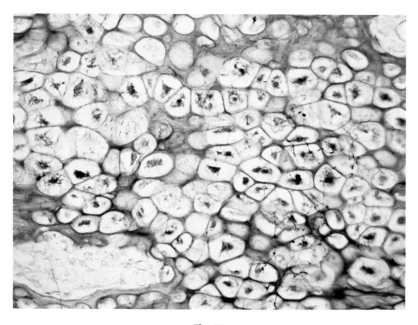

Fig. 65

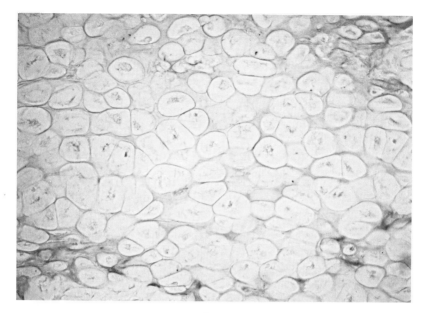

Fig. 66

Figs. 64 through 66 Photomicrographs of an area of cartilage in the callus of a 7-day mechanically stable rabbit tibial fracture to show the staining with Alcian Blue, pH 5.7, in the presence of 0.2 M (Fig. 64), 0.4 M (Fig. 65) and 0.6 M (Fig. 66) magnesium chloride. (Magnification × 340.) (From Page and Ashhurst, 1987.)

and other glycoproteins located in the bone appear to be the same as those of normal bone.

The cartilage of mechanically unstable fractures exhibits the same heterogeneity in its collagen content as the bone, again because the cartilage-specific collagens are laid down in the pre-existing fibrous matrix. The biochemical and histochemical analyses of the proteoglycans suggest that the chondroitin sulfates in the cartilage are typical of those of normal cartilage. The histochemical results do, however, suggest that the keratan sulfate is less highly sulfated than that of articular cartilage.

No biochemical analyses of proteoglycans have been performed on the callus of mechanically stable fractures. Indeed, it is unlikely that the small amounts of cartilaginous proteoglycans present would be identifiable biochemically. The histochemical tests suggest that both chondroitin and keratan sulfates are present, but that the degree of sulfation is less than that of normal cartilage. Whether the proteoglycans are more similar to cartilage than to bone proteoglycans cannot be determined histochemically.

The development of chondroid bone in the peripheral regions of the cartilage of mechanically unstable fractures, and sporadically in regions of localized micromovement in mechanically stable fractures, illustrates the lability of the osteoblastic-chondrocytic phenotype. That cells can express the mRNAs for both types I and II collagens simultaneously is further

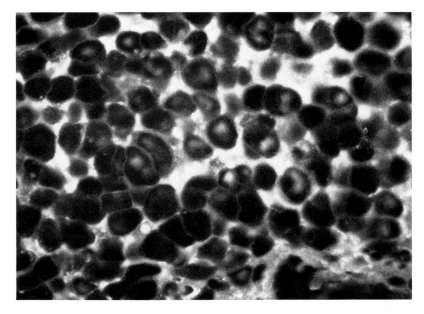

Fig. 67

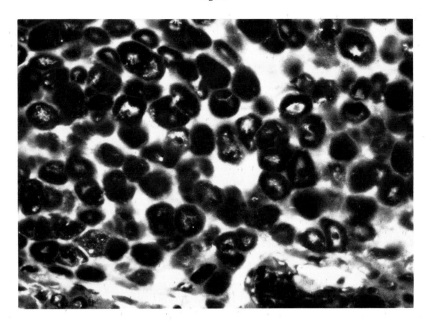

Fig. 68

Figs. 67 and 68 Photomicrographs of an area of cartilage in the callus of a 7-day mechanically stable rabbit tibial fracture to show the binding of antibodies to chondroitin-4-sulfate (Fig. 67) and keratan sulfate (Fig. 68) by the matrix. The second antibody is rhodamine-labeled. (Magnification × 340.) (From Page and Ashhurst, 1987.)

evidence that one cell can have the potential to synthesize and secrete both types of collagen (Devlin *et al.*, 1988; Hayashi *et al.*, 1986; Sandberg *et al.*, 1989).

To date the causes of delayed, or non-union, are not understood, although it is probable that there are many factors involved. Abnormalities of the macromolecules in the matrices produced during the early stages of the response to injury might contribute to the failure of healing. Non-unions are associated with the persistence of a large amount of fibrous tissue and it is, therefore, not surprising that a large amount of type III collagen was found in tissue removed at operation from a human non-union (Anderson *et al.*, 1986). In many instances this proliferation of fibrous tissue is in response to instability at the fracture site. The inherited connective tissue diseases could provide another possible cause of abnormalities in the collagens associated with healing fractures. Some of these genetic diseases cause a reduction in the amount of type III collagen synthesized by the cells, which could adversely affect the production of the fibrous tissue associated with the early stages of healing. The identification of the macromolecules synthesized during normal fracture healing discussed in this chapter will provide criteria for the recognition of abnormal tissues around a healing fracture and aid the understanding of the factors that contribute to these abnormalities.

Acknowledgments

Fig. 1 is reproduced from Ashhurst *et al.* (1982) by permission of Butterworth-Heinemann Ltd. ©. The figures from Ashhurst (1986) are reproduced with permission of the Royal Society, and those from Page and Ashhurst (1987) and Page *et al.* (1986) with permission of Chapman & Hall.

References

Anderson, A. M., Hastings, B. W., Fisher, T. R., Ross, E. R., and Shuttleworth, A. (1986). Collagen types present at human fracture sites — a preliminary report. *Injury*, **17**: 78–80.

Antonopoulos, C. A., Engfeldt, B., Gardell, S., Hjertquist, S.-O., and Solheim K. (1965). Isolation and identification of the glycosaminoglycans from fracture callus. *Biochim. Biophys. Acta*, **101**: 150–156.

Ashhurst, D. E. (1986). The influence of mechanical conditions on the healing of experimental fractures in the rabbit: a microscopical study. *Phil. Trans. R. Soc. Lond.*, **313**: 271–302.

Ashhurst, D. E., Hogg, J., and Perren, S. M. (1982). A method for making reproducible fractures of the rabbit tibia. *Injury*, **14**: 236–242.

Bassett, C. A. L. and Herrmann, I. (1961). Influence of oxygen concentration and mechanical factors on differentiation of connective tissues *in vitro*. *Nature (London)*, **190**: 460–461.

Baylink, D., Wergedal, J., and Thompson, E. (1972). Loss of proteinpolysaccharides at sites where bone mineralization is initiated. *J. Histochem. Cytochem.*, **20**: 279–292.

Beresford, W. A. (1981). *Chondroid Bone, Secondary Cartilage and Metaplasia*. Urban and Schwarzenberg, Baltimore, 454.

Bianco, P., Fisher, L. W., Young, M. F., Termine, J. D., and Gehron Robey, P. (1990). Expression and localization of the two small proteoglycans biglycan and decorin in developing human skeletal and non-skeletal tissues. *J. Histochem. Cytochem.*, **38**: 1549–1563.

Blenman, P. R., Carter, D. R., and Beaupré, G. S. (1989). Fracture healing patterns calculated from stress analyses of bone loading histories. *Trans. Orthop. Res. Soc.*, **14**: 469.

Bolander, M. E., Robey, P. G., Fisher, L. W., Conn, K. M., Prabhakar, B. S., and Termine, J. D. (1989). Monoclonal antibodies against osteonectin show conservation of epitopes across species. *Calcif. Tissue Int.*, **45**: 74–80.

Bonnarens, F. and Einhorn, T. A. (1984). Production of a standard closed fracture in a laboratory animal bone. *J. Orthop. Res.*, **2**: 97–101.

Brighton, C. T. and Hunt, R. M. (1989). Early ultrastructural changes in the intrafragmentary marrow tissue of the rib fracture. *Trans. Orthop. Res. Soc.*, **14**: 470.

Brighton, C. T. and Krebs, A. G. (1972). Oxygen tension of healing fractures in the rabbit. *J. Bone Joint Surg.*, **54A**: 323–332.

Bruce R. A. and Dziewiatkowski, D. D. (1987). Differentiation of the organic matrix in bone repair. *J. Oral Maxillofac. Surg.*, **45**: 939–944.

Caplan, A. I. and Koutroupas, S. (1973). The control of muscle and cartilage development in the chick limb: the role of differential vascularization. *J. Embryol. Exp. Morphol.*, **29**: 571–583.

Carter, D. R., Blenman, P. R., and Beaupré, G. S. (1988). Correlations between mechanical stress history and tissue differentiation in initial fracture healing. *J. Orthop. Res.*, **6**: 736–748.

Caterson, B., Christner, J. E., and Baker, J. R. (1983). Identification of a monoclonal antibody that specifically recognizes corneal and skeletal keratan sulfate. *J. Biol. Chem.*, **258**: 8848–8854.

Caterson, B., Christner, J. E., Baker, J. R., and Couchman, J. R. (1985). Production and characterization of monoclonal antibodies directed against connective tissue proteoglycans. *Fed. Proc.*, **44**: 386–393.

Cruess, R. L. and Dumont, J. (1975). Fracture healing. *Can. J. Surg.*, **18**: 403–413.

Devlin, C. J., Brickell, P. M., Taylor, E. R., Hornbruch, A., Craig, R. K., and Wolpert, L. (1988). *In situ* hybridization reveals differential spatial distribution of mRNAs for types I and II collagen in the chick limb bud. *Development*, **103**: 111–118.

Diamond, A. G., Triffitt, J. T., and Herring, G. M. (1982). The acidic macromolecules in rabbit cortical bone tissue. *Arch. Oral Biol.*, **27**: 337–345.

Dunham, J., Catterall, A., Bitensky, L., and Chayen, J. (1983). Metabolic changes in the cells of the callus during healing in the rat. *Calcif. Tissue Int.*, **35**: 56–61.

Feinberg, R. N., Latker, C. H., and Beebe, D. C. (1986). Localized vascular regression during limb morphogenesis in the chicken embryo. I. Spatial and temporal changes in the vascular pattern. *Anat. Rec.*, **214**: 405–409.

Fisher, L. W., Hawkins, G. R., Tuross, N., and Termine, J. D. (1987). Purification and partial characterization of small proteoglycans I and II, bone sialoproteins I and II, and osteonectin from the mineral compartment of developing human bone. *J. Biol. Chem.*, **262**: 9702–9708.

Fisher, L. W., Termine, J. D., Dejter, S. W., Whitson, S. W., Yanagishita, M., Kimura, J. H., Hascall, V. C., Kleinman, H. K., Hassell, J. R., and Nilsson, B. (1983). Proteoglycans of developing bone. *J. Biol. Chem.*, **258**: 6588–6594.

Fisher, L. W., Termine, J. D., and Young, M. F. (1989). Deduced sequence of bone small proteoglycan I (biglycan) shows homology with proteoglycan II (decorin) and several nonconnective tissue proteins in a variety of species. *J. Biol. Chem.*, **264**: 4571–4576.

Gay, S. and Miller, E. J. (1978). *Collagen in the Physiology and Pathology of Connective Tissue*. G. Fischer, Stuttgart, New York, 109.

Glimcher, M. J., Shapiro, F., Ellis, R. D., and Eyre, D. R. (1980). Changes in tissue morphology and collagen composition during the repair of cortical bone in the adult chicken. *J. Bone Joint Surg.*, **62A**: 964–973.

Grant, W. T., Wang, G.-J., and Balian, G. (1987). Type X collagen synthesis during endo-chondral ossification in fracture repair. *J. Biol. Chem.*, **262**: 9844–9849.

Greiff, J. (1978). Bone healing in rabbits after compression osteosynthesis: a comparative study between the radiological and histological findings. *Injury*, **10**: 257–267.

Hallman, R., Feinberg, R. N., Latker, C. H., Sasse, J., and Risau, W. (1987). Regression of blood vessels procedes cartilage differentiation during chick limb development. *Differentia-tion*, **34**: 98–105.

Ham, A. W. (1930). A histological study of the early phases of bone repair. *J. Bone Joint Surg.*, **12**: 827–844.

Ham, A. W. and Harris, W. R. (1972). Repair and transplantation of bone. In: *The Biochemistry and Physiology of Bone*, Vol. III, 2nd ed. Bourne, G. H., Ed., Academic Press, New York, 337–399.

Hayashi, M., Ninomiya, Y., Parsons, J., Hayashi, K., Olsen, B. R., and Trelstad, R. L. (1986). Differential localization of mRNAs of collagen types I and II in chick fibroblasts, chon-drocytes, and corneal cells by *in situ* hybridization using cDNA probes. *J. Cell Biol.*, **102**: 2302–2309.

Hudack, S. S., Blunt, J. W., Higbee, P., and Kearin, G. M. (1949). A probable acid muco-polysaccharide present in granulation tissue. *Proc. Soc. Exp. Biol. Med.*, **72**: 526–528.

Hulth, A., Johnell, O., Lindberg, L., Paulsson, M., and Heinegård, D. (1990). Demonstration of blood-vessel like structures in cartilaginous callus by anti-laminin and anti-heparan sulfate proteoglycan antibodies. *Clin. Orthop.*, **254**: 289–293.

Johnell, O., Hulth, A., Heinegård, D., and Franzen, A. (1988). Immunolocalization of bone and cartilage specific proteins and proteoglycans in experimental fracture healing. *Calcif. Tissue Int.*, **42 (Suppl.)**: A32.

Joyce, M. E., Jingushi, A., and Bolander, M. E. (1990). Transforming growth factor-β in the regulation of fracture repair. *Orthop. Clin. North Am.*, **21**: 199–209.

Kasavina, B. S. and Zenkevich, G. D. (1960). Mucopolysaccharides of the chondral and bone tissue in the course of osteogenesis and regeneration. *Biokhimiya*, **25**: 669–674.

Kelly, P. J., Montgomery, R. J., and Bronk, J. T. (1990). Reaction of the circulatory system to injury and regeneration. *Clin. Orthop.*, **254**: 275–288.

Kinne, R. W. and Fisher, L. W. (1987). Keratan sulfate proteoglycan in rabbit compact bone is bone sialoprotein II. *J. Biol. Chem.*, **262**: 10206–10211.

Lane, J. M., Boskey, A. L., Li, W. K. P., Eaton, B., and Posner, A. S. (1979). A temporal study of collagen, proteoglycan, lipid and mineral constituents in a model of endochondral osseous repair. *Metab. Bone Dis. Rel. Res.*, **1**: 319–324.

Lane, J. M., Golembiewski, G., Boskey, A. L., and Posner, A. S. (1982). Comparative bio-chemical studies of the callus matrix in immobilized and non-immobilized fractures. *Metab. Bone Dis. Rel. Res.*, **4**: 61–68.

Lane, J. M., Suda, M., Von der Mark, K., and Timpl, R. (1986). Immunofluorescent locali-zation of structural collagen types in endochondral fracture repair. *J. Orthop. Res.*, **4**: 381–329.

Leblond, C. P., Marchi, P., and Luder, H. (1989). Evolution of cartilage cell and matrix in the growing rat mandibular condyle. *Proc. 11th Annu. Meet. Am. Soc. Bone Mineral Res.*, Montreal, S406.

Maurer, P. H. and Hudack, S. S. (1952). The isolation of hyaluronic acid from callus tissue of early healing. *Arch. Biochem.*, **38**: 49–53.

McKibbin, B. (1978). The biology of fracture healing in long bones. *J. Bone Joint Surg.*, **60B**: 150–162.

Miller, E. J. (1985). Recent information on the chemistry of the collagens. *Proc. 2nd Int. Conf. Chem. Biol. Mineralized Tissues*. W. T. Butler, Birmingham, 80–93.

Multimäki, P., Aro, H., and Vuorio, E. (1987). Differential expression of fibrillar collagen genes during callus formation. *Biochem. Biophys. Res. Commun.*, **142**: 536–541.

Nemeth, G. G., Heydemann, A., Guterman, S., Smith, L. S. W., Martin, G. R., and Bolander, M. E. (1988). Gene expression in fracture healing. *Trans. Orthop. Res. Soc.*, **13**: 505.

Paavolainen, P., Penttinen, R., Slätis, P., and Karaharju, E. (1979). The healing of experimental fractures by compression osteosynthesis. II. Morphometric and chemical analysis. *Acta Orthop. Scand.*, **50**: 375–383.

Page, M. and Ashhurst, D. E. (1987). The effects of mechanical stability on the macromolecules of the connective tissue matrices produced during fracture healing. II. The glycosaminoglcyans. *Histochem. J.*, **19**: 39–61.

Page, M., Hogg, J., and Ashhurst, D. E. (1986). The effects of mechanical stability on the macromolecules of the connective tissue matrices produced during fracture healing. I. The collagens. *Histochem. J.*, **18**: 251–265.

Pawelek, J. M. (1969). Effects of thyroxine and low oxygen tension on chondrogenic expression in cell culture. *Dev. Biol.*, **19**: 52–72.

Penttinen, R. (1972). Carbohydrate components of fracture callus in rats. *Ann. Med. Exp. Biol. Fenn.*, **50**: 163–167.

Penttinen, R. (1973). Metabolism of fracture callus of rat in vitro. II. Incorporation of ^{35}S-sulphate, ^{3}H-proline and ^{32}P-phosphate. *Acta Physiol. Scand.*, **87**: 208–212.

Prince, C. W., Rahemtulla, F., and Butler, W. T. (1983). Metabolism of rat bone proteoglycans *in vivo*. *Biochem. J.*, **216**: 589–596.

Rahn, B. A., Gallinaro, P., Baltensperger, A., and Perren, S. M. (1971). Primary bone healing. An experimental study in the rabbit. *J. Bone Joint Surg.*, **53A**: 783–786.

Sandberg, M., Aro, H., Multimäki, P., Aho, H., and Vuorio, E. (1989). *In situ* localization of collagen production by chondrocytes and osteoblasts in fracture callus. *J. Bone Joint Surg.*, **71A**: 69–77.

Sato, S., Rahemtulla, F., Prince, C. W., Tomana, M., and Butler, W. T. (1985). Proteoglycans of adult bovine compact bone. *Connect. Tissue Res.*, **14**: 65–75.

Schenk, R. and Willenegger, H. (1967). Morphological findings in primary fracture healing. *Symp. Biol. Hung.*, **7**: 75–86.

Schmid, T. M. and Linsenmayer, T. F. (1985). Immunohistochemical localization of short chain cartilage collagen (Type X) in avian tissues. *J. Cell Biol.*, **100**: 598–605.

Scott, J. E. (1980). The molecular biology of histochemical staining by cationic phthalocyanin dyes: the design of replacements for Alcian Blue. *J. Microsc.*, **119**: 373–381.

Scott, J. E. and Dorling, J. (1965). Differential staining of acid glycosaminoglycans (mucopolysaccharides) by Alcian Blue in salt solutions. *Histochemie*, **5**: 221–233.

Simmons, D. J. and Kahn, A. J. (1979). Cell lineage in fracture healing in chimeric bone grafts. *Calcif. Tissue Int.*, **27**: 247–253.

Slätis, P., Karaharju, E., Holmström, T., Ahonen, J., and Paavolainen, P. (1978). Structural changes in intact tubular bone after application of rigid plates with and without compression. *J. Bone Joint Surg.*, **60A**: 516–522.

Solheim, K. (1966). Distribution of glycosaminoglycans, hydroxyproline and calcium in healing fractures. *Acta Soc. Med. Upsal.*, **71**: 1–13.

Tschan, T., Höerler, I., Houze, V., Winterhalter, K. H., Richter, C., and Bruckner, P. (1990). Resting chondrocytes in culture survive without growth factors, but are sensitive to toxic oxygen metabolites. *J. Cell Biol.*, **111**: 257–260.

Udupa, K. N. and Prasad, G. C. (1963). Chemical and histochemical studies on the organic constituents in fracture repair in rats. *J. Bone Joint Surg.*, **45B**: 770–779.

Urist, M. R. and Johnson, R. W. (1943). Calcification and ossification. IV. The healing of fractures in man under clinical conditions. *J. Bone Joint Surg.*, **25**: 375–426.

Urist, M. R. and McLean, F. C. (1941). Calcification and ossification. I. Calcification in the callus in healing fractures in normal rats. *J. Bone Joint Surg.*, **23**: 1–16.

Venn, G. and Mason, R. M. (1985). Absence of keratan sulphate from skeletal tissues of mouse and rat. *Biochem. J.*, **228**: 443–450.

Von der Mark, K. and Von der Mark, H. (1977). The role of three genetically distinct collagen types in endochondral ossification and calcification of cartilage. *J. Bone J. Surg.*, **59B**: 458–464.

Von der Mark, K., Von der Mark, H., and Gay, S. (1976). Study of differential collagen synthesis during development of the chick embryo by immunofluorescence. II. Localization of type I and type II collagen during long bone development. *Dev. Biol.*, **53**: 153–170.

Wang, G.-J., Dunstan, J. C., Reger, S. I., Hubbard, S., Dillich, J., and Stamp, W. G. (1981). Experimental femoral fracture immobilized by rigid and flexible rods (a rabbit model). *Clin. Orthop.*, **154**: 286–290.

Wilson, D. J. (1986). Development of avascularity during cartilage differentiation in the embryonic limb. *Differentiation*, **30**: 183–187.

Yokobori, T., Oohira, A., and Nogami, H. (1980). Proteoglycans synthesized in calluses at various stages of fracture healing in rats. *Biochim. Biophys. Acta*, **628**: 174–181.

Zenkevich, G. D. and Kasavina, B. S. (1962). The composition of acid mucopolysaccharides of bone and bone callus tissues in the regeneration process. *Biokhimiya*, **27**: 279–285.

4

The Use of Grafts Composed of Cultured Cells for Repair and Regeneration of Cartilage and Bone

Z. NEVO, D. ROBINSON, and N. HALPERIN
Department of Chemical Pathology
Sackler School of Medicine
Tel Aviv University
Ramat Aviv, Tel Aviv
and
Department of Orthopaedic Surgery
Assaf Harofeh Medical Center
Zeriffin, Israel

Introduction

The biological approach to solve the problematic repair of cartilage and bone defects is undergoing a revolution. Its benefits over artificial devices like prostheses are self evident, either for massive bone loss or for joint resurfacing. The latter causes bone-stock loss and becomes loose with time.

More and more, new uses for a variety of human tissues have brought tissue banking as a biological solution to the clinical problems. Although implants of skeletal tissues have been in use for many years, the employment of grafts composed of cultured cells to reconstruct joints with cartilage and bone is a relatively new experimental orthopedic tool. The current chapter deals with implants composed of various cultured cells and the prospectives for such implants becoming a routine clinical orthopedic treatment.

Historical Background

The possibility of replacing damaged tissues of the body by donor tissues has fascinated humankind since primordial times. Homer mentions the legendary chimera created by the gods. This creature had the body of a goat, the head of a lion, the tail of a serpent, and a goat's head at the back (Homer). This amusing deed of xenogeneic transplantation remains beyond the capabilities and dreams of modern science (the limited experience in xenogeneic transplantation will be described later). The ancients were also well aware of the limited regenerative potential of musculoskeletal tissues, and hence the potential benefit which could be derived from transplantation of parts. This is well attested to by the legend of Cosmas and Damian (Gordon, 1960). These saints were famous for their miraculous healing feats until their martyrdom. However, their most impressive deed was performed posthumously. A parishioner's gangrenous and cancerous leg was amputated by them, and a new leg taken from a dead moor was implanted. The parishioner reportedly could walk on his new leg. Already during the Renaissance period, Tagliacozzi described the main obstacle to successful transplantation between individuals, i.e., the recognition of non-self (Tagliacozzi, 1597). Despite the great advances made by medical science in the 400 years since his time, allogeneic transplantation is still experimental for most tissues of the body.

Self Repair of Articular Cartilage

Articular cartilage has a limited ability to self repair. The essential component of wound healing in any tissue is an inflammatory reaction dependent on vasomotor changes as well as migration of leukocytes. This reaction cannot take place in articular cartilage which is normally avascular. Thus, injuries to cartilage could be divided into superficial ones which do not traverse the subchondral bone plate and deep ones which do transverse the bone plate and render the wound vascular.

Several authors have demonstrated the lack of autogenous repair of cartilage lesions superficial to the bone plate (Ghadially, 1983a; DePalma, 1966; Mankin, 1974). Defects in the articular surface which extend into spongy bone lead to exposure of blood vessels, allowing migration of fibroblasts and endothelial cells. The final result is a vascularized granulation tissue (Ghadially, 1983b; Mankin, 1974). This chain of events depends on several factors including the species and age of the animal, as well as the size of the defect.

Defects in dogs appear to heal with the formation of fibrocartilage after 4 weeks. The tissue later undergoes metaplasia and transforms into hyaline cartilage after 3 months (Shands, 1931). Similar results were reported in rabbits, with the formation of hyaline cartilage after 8 weeks (Hjertquist and Lemperg, 1971). The repair tissue appeared to consist of hyaline cartilage in one third of the cases and of fibrocartilage in the rest. Other authors have reported similar results in the rabbit (Meachim and Roberts, 1971; Shimizu et al., 1987; Mitchell and Shepard, 1976), although some of them reported much lower rates of self healing of about 10% (Bentley, 1988).

We did not observe any self healing in chickens in a series of over 100 animals (Itay et al., 1987; Robinson et al., 1989; Robinson et al., 1990). Abrasion arthroplasty in humans has unpredictable results. Fibrocartilage might form after abrasion to bleeding subchondral bone (Johnson, 1986). However, other authors encountered cases without any significant repair reaction (Milgram, 1985).

Age has a major influence on the rate of cartilage wound healing. Older rabbits tend to react to chondral injury by degenerative changes with a decrease in chondroitin sulfate synthesis, cluster formation, cell necrosis, a diminution in the number of cells, and lack of mitosis. On the other hand, young rabbits seem to mount a vigorous reparative reaction with the formation of fibrocartilage, in which some of the cells undergo metaplasia to hyaline cartilage (Dustmann and Puhl, 1976). This might explain the different rates of self healing observed by various authors.

The size of the defects is also of great importance. A matrix flow phenomenon takes place in cartilage wounds. This phenomenon tends to decrease wound size (Ghadially, 1983b). Because of this phenomenon any experiments in cartilage repair need to be controlled for cartilage flow, i.e., large enough defects have to be created.

The repair tissue is never completely similar to hyaline cartilage biochemically, though it might appear similar microscopically. The collagen in the tissue is mainly type I early in the repair stage and type I still comprises 20% of the total collagen in the tissue 1 year after injury. Furthermore, the repair tissue tends to lose hexosamine and thus becomes more fibrous in nature (Furakawa et al., 1980). These biochemical changes seem to seal the repair tissue fate. Longer term follow-ups demonstrate loss of glycosaminoglycans and gradual deterioration of the tissue. The final result seems to be an osteoarthrotic joint surface composed of fibrous tissue and eburnated bone (Wedge et al., 1986; Hjertquist and Lemperg, 1971).

The unpredictability of self-repair of cartilage as well as the frequency of cartilage damage in the population has encouraged research into cartilage transplantation.

Transplantation of Cartilage Fragments and Osteochondral Grafts

The obvious approach to biological resurfacing of joints would be with cartilage fragments. This method has been used both clinically and experimentally. Silver (1969) has transplanted autogeneic and allogeneic cartilage fragments from the radial head of domestic fowls. The grafts were initially successful with most chondrocytes surviving the transplantation. However, most grafts were eventually replaced by fibrous tissue. Somewhat better results were reported in sheep using fragments both autogeneic and allogeneic in origin, which were fixed to the site of implantation by fibrinogen-based tissue adhesive (Passl *et al.*, 1976a,b). The addition of a sliver of bone to the implant facilitates fixation of the implant. Such osteochondral grafts have been employed quite extensively. However, despite early success with survival of the cells and sometimes union of the hosts bone to the grafted bone sliver, later results are unpredictable; the bone generates a vigorous immune response. Furthermore, the transplanted cartilage slowly degenerates (Hesse and Hesse, 1976), a degeneration that is particularly prominent in arthritic joints (Paccola *et al.*, 1979).

A critical factor in the success of such grafts is the achievement of complete joint congruity which serves to dampen the immunological reaction as well as to prevent secondary osteoarthrosis (Tanaka *et al.*, 1980; Aichroth, 1969).

The use of autogenous grafts would of course obviate the problems of cartilage immunogenicity. (Benum, 1975; Gibson, 1965; Hjertquist and Lemperg, 1970; Stover *et al.*, 1989). However, as little tissue is available for autogenous transplantation, this method does not solve the problem of repair of major weight bearing joints. The problems of graft fixation still remain even with autogenous grafts. Because of these unsolved problems osteochondral grafting is not a commonly performed procedure.

Implants Composed of Cultured Chondrocytes

Already at the initial attempts of isolating chondrocytes and establishing procedures for their culturing, the idea of putting the cells back to work *in vivo* has evolved. The earliest reports of growing chondrocytes cultures appeared in the 1960s (Holtzer *et al.*, 1960; Kawiak *et al.*, 1965; Chan *et al.*, 1967; Manning and Bonner, 1967). The procedure became feasible mainly due to the availability of powerful degrading enzymes such as trypsin, collagenase, and hyaluronidase which disintegrate the complexed cartilage territorial matrix, releasing single chondrocytes (Horwitz and Dorfman, 1970; Green, 1971). Special attention should be paid to maintenance of the proper growth conditions, e.g., substrata (Bates *et al.*, 1987) and reduced oxygen atmosphere (Nevo *et al.*, 1988) of such cultures, as the stability of the cartilaginous phenotype is labile and easily lost *in vitro*, giving rise to dedifferentiated cells (Holtzer *et al.*, 1960; Coon, 1966; Chacko *et al.*, 1969). These dedifferentiated cells express non-cartilaginous characteristic traits in shape, amounts, and composition of metabolic synthetic products. However, it was shown that such dedifferentiated cells are shifted back to typical homogeneous cultures of chondrocytes upon changing their growth conditions to those better supporting chondroid expression (Holtzer and Abbott, 1968; Benya and Shaffer, 1982; Nevo *et al.*, 1972; Solursh and Meier, 1974). Examples are transferring cells from monolayers to either pure suspension, or suspensions over hydrated-gel-coated plates (e.g., collagens; agar; agarose) (Srivastava *et al.*, 1974; Bates *et al.*, 1987).

In summary, one should ensure, prior to implantation, that the chondrocytes cultures, even those derived from a single chondrocytic cell, preserve their cartilaginous nature during culturing, subculturing, and at the storage period within the delivery substances (for details see below).

The development of decent tissue culture techniques for chondrocytes paved the way to a new approach for repairing cartilaginous tissues employing transplants composed of cultured cartilage cells. The isolated cells cultured *in vitro* increase their mass up to 30 times (Bentley, 1988). Long term cultures can serve also as a storage system for such cells.

An important advantage of cultured cells, as compared to tissue grafts, is the ability to form their implant into any needed shape, thus allowing accurate joint congruity (its importance has been mentioned before) with diminished rejection reaction.

However, the greatest advantage of transplanting cultured cells, in contrast to tissue fragments, has been their ability to better survive the transplanting procedure. The survival of articular cartilage depends on diffusion of nutrients from the synovial cavity. The vessels of the subchondral bone are not very important for the survival of normal articular cartilage (Sengupta, 1974). The number of chondrocytes which can survive under a given area of articular surface is constant. It is related to the thickness of the cartilage layer and is approximately 25,000 cells/mm^2 of articular surface (Stockwell, 1979). In any case, immediately after transplantation the grafted tissue depends solely on diffusion for its nutrients. This dependence of the grafted tissues on nutrient diffusion leads to necrosis of the grafts. This is especially true for the central areas of thick osteochondral grafts (Sengupta, 1974; Paccola, 1989), as well as for the bone forming capacity of transplanted periosteum (Poussa, 1980). The transplantation of single cells is advantageous, as synovial circulation through the graft is facilitated and in fact is probably immediately established.

The first experiments of such kind were performed by Chesterman and Smith (1965) who used suspensions of adult chondrocytes, immediately after isolation, without prior culturing. When these cells were implanted into cancellous bone of the iliac crest they proliferated rapidly and induced bone formation. No signs of a rejection reaction were found. The cells eventually underwent hypertrophy and later induced ossification. Thus, after about 6 months the chondrocytes were difficult to locate among the newly formed bone. In contrast to the results with live implanted chondrocytes, cartilage cells frozen without the cryopreservative dimethyl-sulfoxide, most probably non-vital cells, disappeared rapidly and failed to induce the formation of new bone.

The same group also attempted the repair of mechanically induced lesions in the articular surface with isolated chondrocytes. They placed the chondrocyte suspension into full thickness defects of rabbits humeral heads. The final results were cartilage nodules embedded in fibrous tissue. This was attributed by them to overgrowth of tissue from the marrow spaces.

Other experiments were performed by Bentley and his group (Bentley and Greer, 1971; Bentley et al., 1978; Aston and Bentley, 1986; Bentley, 1988). These authors observed that cells isolated from the epiphyses of young rabbits could be successfully transplanted into defects in the joint of adult rabbits. On the other hand, cells isolated from the articular cartilage of young rabbits barely survived and were surrounded by fibrous tissue as well as inflammatory cells. Another phenomenon observed by these authors was the reconstitution by the isolated cells of the typical layers of articular cartilage. The success rates achieved by those authors were less than 50% which may be mainly related to the desertion of the lesion sites by the implanted cells. The highest rates of success were achieved by a mild enzymatic digestion, as a pretreatment to the tissue serving as a source for the chondrocytic cells to be implanted. This treatment left intact a part of the chondroid matrix surrounding the individual cells. This advantage could be attributed to the immunoprotective effect of the matrix. However, such failure rates would of course not be suitable for human trials. In fact the success rates are higher using fragments of articular cartilage rather than isolated or cultured cells (Bentley, 1988).

A method attempting to improve the results of such grafts made of cultured cells has been described by Green (1977) who used cells isolated from immature rabbits and grown for 10 days *in vitro* on decalcified bone in culture. The cells formed a chondroid tissue which was later transplanted onto 5 mm defects in the articular surface of mature rabbits. The success rate was only 25%. However, conceptually it should be considered as a landmark paper, as it is first to use a delivery substance in which the cells are embedded. Use of such a substance is critical, as it allows anchoring of the cells to the implantation site.

Others reported the employment of a periosteal cover which is sutured to the cartilage surrounding the defect (Grande et al., 1987; Brittberg et al., 1989). This periosteum serves as a lid holding the cells in place. Furthermore, periosteum and perichondrium themselves have a certain chondrogenic quality (Jaroma and Ritsila, 1987; Niedermann et al., 1985; Rubak et al., 1982a; Rubak et al., 1982b; Rubak, 1982; O'Driscoll and Salter, 1984; O'Driscoll and Salter, 1986; O'Driscoll et al., 1989; Engkvist, 1979; Engkvist et al., 1980) even after freezing (Moran et al., 1989). The results are variable and quite unpredictable (Upton et al., 1981), this being perhaps related to the site of origin of the graft material (Vachon et al., 1989).

The approach employing cells covered by periosteum had a much higher rate of success than previous ones, over 80% (Grande et al., 1987). However, this approach is technically very demanding and has the basic fault of the sutures damaging the surrounding cartilage. In fact, it is difficult to visualize how a whole condyle could be resurfaced, not to mention a whole joint.

Establishing reliable procedures for isolation and culturing chondrocytes together with the discovery of naturally occurring biodegradable adhesive substances, such as those based on fibrin (Passl et al., 1976a,b; Helbing et al., 1979; Helbing et al., 1980; Helbing, 1981), paved the way for the utilization of implants composed of cultured cells. These kind of glues were termed biological resorbable immobilizing vehicles (BRIV) (Itay et al., 1987). At the beginning of the 1980s the whole concept of grafting cultured chondrocytes embedded in an adhesive delivery substance underwent reconsideration and reevaluation as to each of the components composing these kinds of implants.

The following points were examined:

(1) The cell source: including immunological considerations
(2) The culturing conditions of chondrocytes
(3) The delivery substance(s), the application procedure, and the fate of the implant

The Cell Source

Theoretically, three types of donor cells could be envisioned: autogeneic, allogeneic, and xenogeneic.

The use of autogeneic cells would be the best, as no immunological problems should be encountered. Unfortunately, cartilage is not an abundant tissue in the body, and few areas are functionally unimportant and could be sacrificed. Though sternal or rib cartilages could be sacrificed, these tissues in adult humans are relatively acellular. In addition, the few cells present are hardly proliferating; upon attempts in culture to "force" them to proliferate employing various growth factors, they undergo a characteristic shift exerting traits of dedifferentiated cells (Nevo et al., unpublished observations). The greatly limited ability of adult cartilage to proliferate has been well documented in the literature. The marked decrease in cellularity of human cartilage is also well documented, taking place particularly during the first post-natal years (Stockwell, 1979). Furthermore, when cells of various aged donors are compared, the quality of the reconstituted cartilage differs significantly. Cells taken from 1- to 2-month-old rabbits reconstituted an abnormal appearing tissue after transplantation intramuscularly; in contrast, cells from younger rabbits reconstituted normal appearing cartilage (Moskalewski and Rybicka, 1977).

Callus tissues developing as a response to long bone fractures, in both

normal chick neonates (2- to 4-weeks old) and in vitamin D deficient counterpart, were examined as potential sources for non-embryonal proliferating
chondrocytes. Epiphyseal growth plates of ricketic chick neonates which
have large epiphyses as a result of the delayed ossification were also used
for cell isolation. All the above cell preparations were basically isolated
according to the procedure described for chick embryonal chondrocytes
(Nevo et al., 1972). These cultured cells used for the implants were grown
either as high density monolayer cultures (Lidor et al., 1987a,b) or as
suspension over soft agar coated plates (Nevo et al., 1972). However, these
cells do not reconstitute articular cartilage when transplanted into defects
in joint surfaces. Instead, a rather dense fibrous tissue is formed.

The limited potential of adult or even adolescent cartilage cells to proliferate led us to abandon both autogenous tissue and cadaver allogeneic
tissue, as a source of cells.

Therefore, the obvious promising source for proliferating chondrocytes is
allogeneic embryonal chondrocytes. Embryonal cells have a high rate of
proliferation that allows culturing masses of cells.

A detailed description of experimentation of our group with allogeneic
embryonal chondrocytes to correct defects in cartilage and bone in chick
will be provided in the next pages.

However, in the case of human allogeneic embryonal chondrocytes, both
the limited amounts of healthy sterile samples (of aborted fetuses) as well
as moral considerations, might raise difficulties employing this potential
source. This brings us to consider the implantation of xenogeneic cells.
Therefore, a short discussion of the immunology of cartilage graft is
unavoidable.

Allogeneic transplantation of visceral organs demands immunosuppression. However, at least one of the musculoskeletal tissues, cartilage, seems
to possess a certain degree of immunoprivilege. Cartilage is unique among
body tissues as the cells are surrounded by a thick coat of matrix, and the
tissue as a whole is relatively avascular. The relatively low antigenicity of
cartilage fragments is attested to by the lack of lymph node reaction to a
single subcutaneous transplant of cartilage in rabbits. A repeat transplantation does lead to a moderate degree of hyperplasia of the local lymph
nodes (Craigmyle, 1958). Cartilage allografts can survive for prolonged
periods (Craigmyle, 1955).

The intensity of the rejection reaction evoked depends on the site of
transplantation as well as on the form of the cartilage. The importance of
the transplantation site to the chances for cartilage graft survival in lambs
has been delineated by McKibbin and Ralis (1978). Even grafts into pre-
sensitized animals survive when implanted orthotopically, i.e., intra-arti-
cularly. On the other hand, similar grafts implanted intramuscularly are
rejected. Similar results have been observed by us in chickens.

The form of cartilage transplanted is also very important. The invasion
of the transplanted tissue appears to affect mainly the cut surface of the

cartilage. Immune cells seem to be hindered by the perichondrium. Transplantation of isolated cartilage cells evokes an intense immune reaction when allogeneic cells are used (Moskalewski and Kawiak, 1965; Moskalewski et al., 1966). This immune reaction seems to sensitize the animals against cartilage fragments as well. Thus co-transplantation of cartilage fragments and cells leads to invasion of the fragments.

As cartilage enjoys a certain amount of immunoprivilege, this might allow it to survive a xenogeneic transplantation. Relatively few experiments were conducted in which xenogeneic cartilage cells were implanted. Implantation of guinea pig cartilage into rabbits induced a massive rejection reaction. Weight of regional lymph nodes increased 400% (Craigmyle, 1958). In this paper the histological changes in the cartilage are not detailed. Implants of isolated chondrocytes derived from rats and implanted into hamster's cheek pouch survived reasonably well. The tissue was reconstituted and the chondrocytes underwent hypertrophy, despite a dense cellular infiltrate. However, their osteogenic capacity was lost (Thyberg and Moskalewski, 1979).

This led us to attempt to transplant xenogeneic cultured cartilage cells. We attempted to transplant across a particularly large immunologic barrier, i.e., avian embryonal chondrocytes into adult guinea pigs. The animals were observed for 6 months after transplantation. The chondrocytes in the implant proliferated and reconstituted the joint surface (Fig. 1). This contrasted sharply with the appearance of control defects which appeared either empty or filled with granulation tissue. The chondrocytes in the reparative tissue of the experimental group were of avian origin as attested to by the obviously different cellular morphology. No signs of round cell infiltrates were evident, but a synovial hypertrophy was seen after 3 months, as well as after longer observation periods. The repair tissue slowly degenerated. However, the arthrosis caused in the control animals by the creation of large untreated defects in the articular surface was retarded in the experimental group. The animals did not favor the legs which underwent chondrocytes' transplantation. Moreover, the range of movement in operated joints of the animals transplanted with chondrocytes was better than in the untreated controls.

In order to substantiate the alien donor origin of chondrocytes in reparative tissues we have implanted embryonal Japanese quail chondrocytes into chicks. The quail cells have a prominent nucleolus which can be readily identified (Jotreau and LeDouarin, 1978). The repair tissue in grafted defects contained cartilage cells which were obviously of quail origin. Implantation of rabbit chondrocytes into nude mice led to the formation of mouse-derived bone spicules (Wright et al., 1985). Survival of both allogeneic (Malejczyk et al., 1988) and xenogeneic cartilage (Ostrowski et al., 1970) has been reported to be improved by use of immunosuppressive agents. However, immunosuppression is not a likely adjunct for treatment of orthopedic pathologies which are not life threatening.

One can conclude from this series of xenogeneic transplantation that

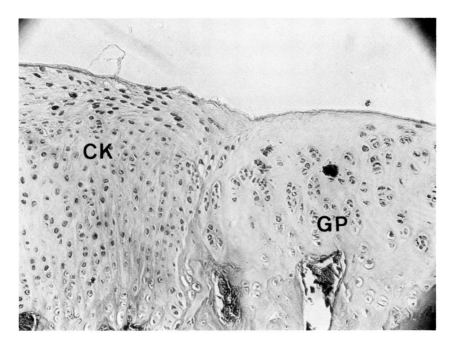

Fig. 1 Xenogeneic embryonal chick chondrocytes reconstitute a cartilaginous reparative tissue (CK). The adjoining guinea pig cartilage (GP) shows early osteoarthrotic changes. (H & E, magnification × 100.)

chondrocytes can survive for prolonged periods without evoking a classical rejection reaction without the employment of immunosuppression agents.

Further studies are necessary in order to conclude whether such transplants could and should be attempted in humans, and second, which species should prove to be the best donor. An even more important conclusion is that restoring the articular surface, and by that the joint congruity can actually delay the course of secondary osteoarthrosis and improve joint function.

The Culturing Conditions of Chondrocytes

The method of culturing of the cells is of the utmost importance. The chondrocytic phenotype is known to be unstable under *in vitro* conditions (Holtzer *et al.*, 1960). This is especially true for chondrocytes grown on monolayer cultures. The phenotype can be stabilized by the use of suspension cultures (Yasumoto *et al.*, 1980; Coon, 1966). Dedifferentiated cells can re-express their chondrocytic phenotype when transferred to agarose gels (Benya and Shaffer, 1982; Srivastava *et al.*, 1974).

The initial concentration of cells in monolayers should be kept high, i.e., in the range of 3 to 5 × 10^6 cells per 35 mm Petri dishes. This also tends to prevent dedifferentiation. Culturing under low oxygen tension (8% O_2) was found to further preserve the chondrocytic phenotype (Nevo *et al.*, 1988). Furthermore, culturing under such conditions also serves to delay the known accelerated aging of chondrocytes in culture.

The integrity of the matrix surrounding the cultured chondrocytes is crucial for successful transplantation. This is probably the most important single factor which determines the chances of survival of such grafts. The cells in Chesterman and Smith experiments (1965) were isolated using trypsin and collagenase solution. They were transplanted immediately following their isolation. The trypsin and collagenase solutions at least partially removed the surrounding matrix. This exposed the cell membrane and its transplantation antigens. Chondrocytes whose surrounding matrix has been removed are as antigenic as lymphocytes (Elves, 1974; Heyner, 1969). The chondrocytes have to be given time to synthesize and restore their matrix coat. This can be done *in vitro* by allowing a minimal restoration period of about 48 h after isolation, or, alternatively, by using a delivery substance to temporarily shield the cells from the immune reaction. Keeping an intact surrounding matrix is also essential for another reason. The chondrocytic phenotype is not a stable one; cartilage cells tend to lose their phenotypic expression and to dedifferentiate (Coon, 1966; Holtzer *et al.*, 1960). The proper natural matrix environment tends to prevent such a transition.

Delivery Substance(s), Application Procedure, and the Fate of the Implant

Assuming an appropriate source of proliferating chondrocytes has been found and a phenotypically stable homologous culture of chondrocytes established, transfer of cells from the culture to the lesion sites is needed. Therefore, a multipurpose substance(s) to store, deliver, and fix the cells into the defect sites must be found. A proper milieu for supporting the cells during shipment outside the incubator at varying temperatures and in an air atmosphere is being sought.

An ideal delivery substance should have several unique properties. It should be simple to sterilize and be stable enough to be suitable for shipping. Its viscosity should be easily controllable, thus allowing an even distribution of cells, as well as introduction through narrow gauge arthroscopic cannulae on the one hand, but be viscous and adhesive enough to secure fixation of the cells to the implantation sites on the other. Needless to say, it has to be biocompatible and biodegradable and offer a permissive milieu for cell proliferation and matrix production. The material has to be shapable into any form, thus conforming exactly to the three-dimensional shape of the shallow areas of eburnated bone in osteoarthrosis. Optimally it should inhibit fibroblast proliferation and prevent invasion of immune cells as well as diffusion of immunoglobulins. However, it must be permeable to nutrients from the synovial fluid.

We began our studies using a fibrin based glue in which the cells were mixed prior to implantation (Itay et al., 1987). The success rate was about 75%. However, this delivery substance had several drawbacks. It is in itself cytotoxic to chondrocytes, the majority of cells undergo lysis when cultured in it, and upon in vivo implantation the residual surviving cell fraction rapidly proliferates. Another problem with the fibrin based system was the difficulty of achieving an even distribution of the cells in the semisolidified mixture. Frequently, islands of acellular mixture were formed. Using such acellular regions for implantation is risking the repair outcome. Furthermore, the viscosity of the fibrin based delivery substance is too high and cannot be manipulated, sometimes leading to dislodgement of the implant as a whole. On the other hand, its viscosity is not high enough to serve as an intact cover for totally eburnated articular surface. Fibrinogen is also a well-known promoter of vascular invasion and fibroblast proliferation.

Screening for new suitable delivery substance(s) has yielded interesting information. A recent report in the literature described the use of mussel adhesive protein as a delivery substance for chondrocytes (Grande and Pitman, 1988). This material has higher bonding strength than fibrinogen based compounds and appears promising. However, it is a foreign protein which could lead to severe immunologic reactions.

As chondrocytes can be successfully grown in and on various hydrated gels, such as agar, agarose, and collagen (Yasui et al., 1982), can these substances serve as delivery agents? The locally condensed environment, as well as the three-dimensional nature of such cultures, seem to promote chondrocyte differentiation and the preservation of the chondrogenic phenotype. Cells cultured under these conditions with a heavy intact matrix coat can be successfully transplanted allogeneically. They reconstitute a tissue containing mostly type II collagen (Wakitani, 1989). Collagen certainly seems promising, especially if collagen type II could be used. However, collagen has two possible drawbacks. Collagen is mildly antigenic and the risk of adverse reactions exists. Collagen is also an excellent promoter of fibroblast growth and vascularization. These properties of collagen are, theoretically at least, detrimental to cartilage regeneration.

The material of choice currently investigated in our laboratory (Robinson et al., 1989a,b) is hyaluronic acid. Sodium hyaluronate (NaHa) was obtained from Biotechnology General (BTG) Ltd., Kiryat Weizmann, Rehovot, Israel and conformed with the following specifications:

NaHa by assay (%)	90
Molecular weight (MDa)	2.01
Protein (mg/g)	0.2
Absorbance at 257 nm (1% solution)	0.02
Endotoxin (1% solution) (EU/mg)	0.125
Inflammation	non-inflammatory

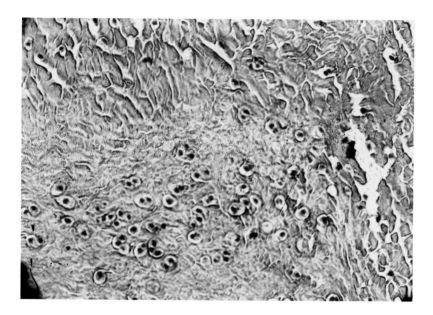

Fig. 2 Allogeneic transplanted embryonal chick chondrocytes thrive in the hyaluronic acid gel as a delivery substance. Note numorous mitoses. (H & E, magnification × 200.)

Only the high molecular weight, i.e., over 2,000,000 Da, was found suitable. Hyaluronic acid is not antigenic. The high molecular weight variety stimulates chondrogenesis *in vitro* (Knudson and Toole, 1987; Kujawa and Caplan, 1986). Hyaluronic acid, particularly the high molecular weight form, reduced scar formation and vascular invasion (Weiss *et al.*, 1989a,b; Matsubara *et al.*, 1989). This material also protects both mechanically and biochemically, by reducing free radicals which damage chondrocytes (Larsen *et al.*, 1989). The viscosity of the chondrocyte hyaluronic-acid mixture is easily controlled and manipulated. The cells thrive in the hyaluran gel and rapidly divide while maintaining their phenotype and synthesizing new matrix (Fig. 2). The material undergoes degradation and resorption *in vivo* after 2 weeks. A cartilaginous tissue is reconstituted which resembles hyaline cartilage morphologically, histologically, and histochemically and has a similar elasticity (Figs. 3, 4 and 5). Furthermore, cells left accidentally in hyaluran for 1 week on a laboratory bench, at room temperature in air, have survived, and were capable of incorporating massive amounts of radioactive sulfate. Therefore, it appears that hyaluran might serve as a convenient short- and long-term (days) storage milieu of chondrocytes destined for transplantation.

The main difficulty which the hyaluronic acid does not solve is transplanting whole joints. As long as one attempts to resurface areas within the joint, the need for a form retaining implant is not great. However, in order to replace a whole surface, a shape-retaining implant is necessary. It should

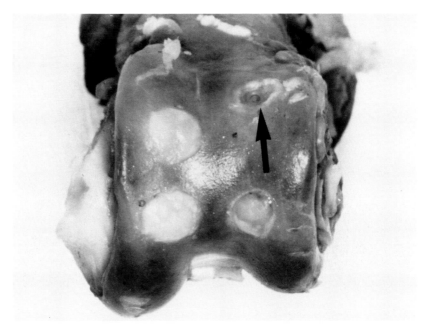

Fig. 3 Six weeks after implantation of embryonal chondrocytes into four mechanically created defects in the articular surface of the lower tibia. Note complete healing of three of the defects with restoration of the articular surface. The fourth one (arrow) is only partially filled. (Magnification × 8.)

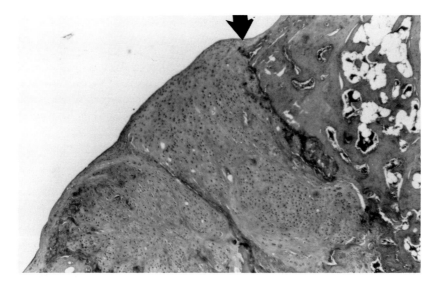

Fig. 4 Low power micrograph of chondrocytes in hyaluronic acid implanted defect 2 months postoperatively. The defect area is filled completely by newly formed cartilage. Note the lobular arrangement of the chondrocytes and the excellent integration of original and new cartilage surface (arrow). No trace of the delivery substance can be seen. (H & E, magnification × 40.)

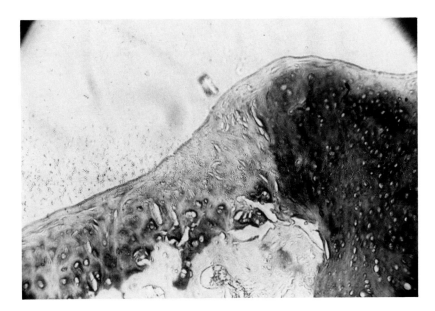

Fig. 5 The cartilaginous reparative tissue, which formed in the defect, stains intensively with a specific dye for sulfated glycosaminoglycans. (Alcian Blue, magnification × 200.)

be rigid enough to allow early continuous passive motion. The latter method has been conclusively shown to improve cartilage repair and joint function (Dhert *et al.*, 1987; Moran *et al.*, 1989; Shimizu, 1987; Salter, 1984).

Joint defects have a tendency to heal in a dimple-like fashion. This creates a conical crater and is true for both grafted defects and defects under going self-repair. Implantation of hydroxyapatite has been shown to prevent the central pitting in ungrafted osteochondral defects (Bucholz, 1989). A search for a solid framework to impregnate it with the implant composition of hyaluronic acid-containing chondrocytes was conducted. Recent attempts by our group to graft a porous hydroxyapatite implant saturated with cells did not achieve very good results. The implant tended to remain exposed and to lead to osteoarthrosis of the joint.

A further attempt in this direction was the employment of decalcified bone matrix prepared according to previously described methods (Nimni *et al.*, 1988; Syftestad and Urist, 1982). Cylinders of such decalcified bone were perforated by a small diameter high speed dental burr. They were later saturated with hyaluronic acid based mixture containing 5 to 10 × 10^6 cells/ml. Such cylinders were fitted into defects of the articular surface covering over 90% of the joint surface. The implants were fixed in place by crossed k-wires. After 4 to 6 weeks good healing of the defects with accurate restoration of joint congruity was observed in all joints (Fig. 6). This was in contrast to the findings in control joints (Robinson *et al.*, in preparation).

To date, the combined use of hyaluronic acid and decalcified bone matrix seems the most promising method of repairing whole joint surfaces. By use

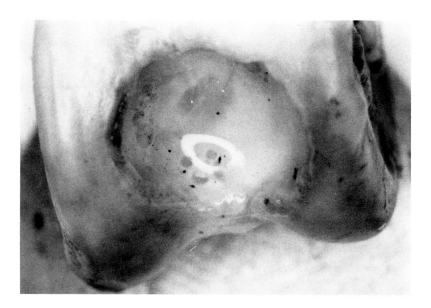

Fig. 6 A micrograph of a transplanted defect, one month post operation, with a combination of chondrocytes embedded in hyaluronic acid and impregnated into demineralized chick bone matrix. (Magnification × 10.)

of this combination (cells + delivery substance + scaffold) the success rate can be improved from 25% for decalcified bone alone (Green, 1977) and 80% for hyaluronic acid alone (Robinson et al., 1990) to close to 100%. The decalcified bone is only mildly immunogenic and allografts of freeze-dried bone do not evoke an immune response in humans and animals (Friedlander, 1983).

Decalcified bone is also a potent source of bone morphogenetic protein (Nimni, 1988). This helps to maintain the phenotype of the implanted cells (Green, 1977) as well as promoting chondrogenesis (Friedenberg et al., 1989).

We have already discussed the immunogenicity of cartilage and chondrocytes used to repair joint surfaces. Here it is worthwhile to note that the immune reaction is dependent on the site of implantation (McKibbin and Ralis, 1978). The joint surface appears to be a privileged site. Immune reaction to allogeneic chondrocytes implanted in collagen matrix was assessed according to the blast-formation of peripheral blood lymphocytes (Wakitani et al., 1989). No significant sensitization was observed. On the other hand, Kawabe et al. (1987) found a severe immunological reaction. The latter authors assessed the parameters of passive hemagglutination testing, chromium release assay, and immunofluorescence. A specific cell mediated reaction was observed; moreover, evidence of humeral immunity was observed. Cell survival 3 weeks after implantation was only 26%. The rate of synovitis was similar in control and grafted defects in rabbits (Grande *et al.*, 1987). Our experience has been different. We did not observe any round cell infiltrates, and no round cells were present in the synovial fluid.

Cell survival rates using the hyaluran as a glue exceed 90% (Robinson *et al.*, 1989, 1990). The method of cell culturing in the work published by Kawabe *et al.* (1987) is not described in detail. However, monolayer cultures of chondrocytes contain relatively little matrix. This exposes cellular surface antigens and sensitizes the immune system. The fibrinogen glue used was probably also responsible for decreased cell survival.

The quality of the repair tissue has crucial importance for the success of this method of cultured cells to joint repair. The repair tissue stains intensively by dyes specific for sulfated glycosaminoglycans (Bentley and Greer, 1971; Itay *et al.*, 1987; Robinson *et al.*, 1990). The repair tissue synthesizes almost exclusively type II collagen (Wakitani *et al.*, 1989; Yoshihashi, 1983). These findings contrast with the situation in ungrafted defects. The repair tissue incorporates radioactive sulfate ten times more than that of the granulation tissue, 4 weeks after implantation. This rate is four times higher than that of normal cartilage. This high rate of synthesis decreases 6 months after transplantation. The rate of radioactive calcium incorporation increased in grafted defects from 2 months after implantation and continued to increase through the 6 months of observation (Itay *et al.*, 1987). This correlated with the formation of a tide mark by the repair tissue and hypertrophy of the cells. Eventually a large portion of the defect underwent ossification leaving only a layer of cartilage of similar thickness to the normal articular cartilage. At present the longest observation period available after chondrocyte grafts is 18 months (Robinson *et al.*, 1989, 1990). The repair tissue shows no signs of deterioration, neither does the joint become osteoarthrotic nor lose range of motion. This is in contrast to the control joint (untreated defects) which deteriorate over time with the formation of osteophytes (Riddle *et al.*, 1970) at least in some species.

The implantation of embryonal cells into recipients of various ages offers an interesting opportunity for studying the effect of the environment on the pace and rate of aging.

A skeletally immature recipient tolerated the grafts less well than adult rabbits, as demonstrated by a lower success rate though not by a more intense infiltration (Bentley, 1978) when cells were grafted. We have compared the repair achieved by 4-month-old chicks to that in 3-year-old chickens. Embryonal chondrocytes implanted in older chickens underwent an accelerated aging process. The defects filled up completely after 1 month as compared to 3 months in young chicks. Endochondral ossification began after 2 months in the older group, while it commenced only after 6 months in the young. Another unique response observed only in the old group was the accumulation of hematopoietic centers (Robinson, 1989). This influence of the recipient on the rate of aging is of interest though not enough data are available for any valid conclusions regarding the environmental mechanism.

Other Applications of Transplants Composed of Cultured Chondrocytes

Cultured chondrocyte implants can be used for many other applications besides the repair of articular cartilage and bone defects in joints. Applications in maxillofacial surgery and tracheal surgery are quite obvious, but are outside the scope of this chapter, and will not be dealt with any further. Other applications in the field of orthopedic surgery are discussed one by one in the coming pages.

Growth Plate Reconstruction

Repair and regeneration of growth plate in general is discussed in details in Chapters 7 and 8 of this volume. Shortly, the physis is responsible for longitudinal growth of the skeleton. Injuries of up to 25% of the physis do not retard growth, unless a bony bridge is formed. Grafts of inert tissue (Bright, 1981) as well as fat tissue (Langeskiold et al., 1987; Langeskiold, 1988) can prevent the reformation of the osseous bridge after its resection. Autogenous transplants, whether vascularized or nonvascularized, have also been reported as successful transplants; however, they have little clinical relevance as there are few if any growth plates which can be sacrificed (Brown, 1988; Zaleske et al., 1982; Nettelblad et al., 1984).

Allogeneic transplants of cartilage fragments and whole unvascularized physis was not successful. The failure was attributed to an immune reaction occurring in the reserve zone, which is partially vascularized (Ring, 1955; Harris et al., 1965). Nevertheless, more recent works stress the importance of the lack of vascularization within the implants. Thus, others reported that allogeneic vascularized physes have been successfully transplanted (Drzewiecki et al., 1989). Growth continued though at a slower rate and the physis closed prematurely. It appears that grafts of isolated and cultured allogeneic cells could survive better than tissue fragments in the early devascularized period, immediately after transplantation.

Such studies performed by Kawabe et al. (1987) demonstrated survival and matrix production by cultured allogeneic chondrocytes. The physis continued to grow at a reduced rate in most animals. In contrast, implantated dead cells were absorbed and did not prevent the formation of a bone bridge with deformity. Much more work is needed before a firm conclusion regarding the potential use of cultured cells in reconstruction of growth plates can be reached.

Bone Growth Augmentation and Replacement

Another field in which cartilage cells have proved of some use is in bone growth augmentation. This approach might be important in two areas, i.e., (a) fractures, and (b) bone stock loss and osteoporosis. Transplants of allogeneic chondrocytes have been shown to stimulate bone formation in adult and old-aged hosts, by induction of the process of endochondral ossification (Shimomura *et al.*, 1975; Ksiazek and Moskalewski, 1983; Miki and Yamamuro, 1987; Thyberg and Moskalewski, 1979). This property was not found in xenogeneic transplants (Thyberg and Moskalewski, 1979).

Embryonal bone consisting mainly of cartilage has been reported to induce endochondral ossification in drill holes in long bones of rabbits. On the other hand, neither dead embryonal bone nor adult bone can induce endochondral ossification (Steinman, 1947). Other studies refuted this claim (Cleland and Sevastikoglou, 1962).

Embryonal bone can also be used to bridge massive segmental defects in rats (Nevo *et al.*, 1983; Nevo *et al.*, 1977; Siegal *et al.*, 1972; Siegal *et al.*, 1977). The embryonal bone survives in contrast to adult bone, most probably because of protective anti Ia-alloantibodies (Segal *et al.*, 1979). Any system involving bone induction has to be compared to the activity of bone morphogenetic protein alone or in combination with autogeneic bone marrow. Very little research of this kind has been published to date. Nimni *et al.* (1988) have reported the transplantation of embryonal calvaria cells in conjunction with demineralized bone matrix implanted subcutaneously in old rats. The amount of bone induced was higher in implants containing embryonal cells than in implants to which autogenous bone marrow was added. This activity could not be equaled by embryonal muscle cells or fibroblasts. The bone cylinders by themselves did not induce any new bone formation at all. These authors suggested that the mechanism of bone induction by embryonal calvarial cells was different than the mechanism of action of bone morphogenetic protein. This subject has not yet been sufficiently explored. Chondrocytes have also been grafted into fractures. The cells from the growth plate enhanced fracture repair while cells derived from articular cartilage delayed the repair process (Laurence and Smith, 1968). Once again this subject has not been adequately explored. Any future work will have to consider the beneficial effect of cartilage matrix on general wound healing, as for example, skin lacerations (Prudden and Allen, 1965; Paulette and Prudden, 1959). Thus, any specific enhancement of fracture healing by implantation of cultured cells might be related solely to the matrix.

Osteoporosis

An additional area in which cartilage cells have been used is the augmentation of density of osteoporotic bone. The basic pathology in senile osteoporosis is a constant deficit incurred in the process of skeletal remodeling. This deficit leads first to thinning of the trabeculae; however, the pathology at this stage is potentially reversible. Later on, the trabeculae disappear completely. This stage is not reversible with any of the currently used treatment modalities such as exercise, calcitonin, vitamin D metabolites, or female hormones (Frost, 1985; Recker, 1981). The implantation of

bone morphogenetic protein induces bone formation in the rabbit metaphysis (Nilsson and Urist, 1985). This reaction is quantitatively greater
than that which could be ascribed solely to the osteogenic response to
trauma of the bone marrow (Bab *et al.*, 1985).

In addition, it was suggested that removal of bone marrow from long
bones increases the overall formation of bone and cartilage in the body (Bab
et al., 1985). Recently, the mechanism for the above phenomenon was elucidated, pointing to an elevation of a potent osteogenic growth peptide
(OGP) as the response to bone marrow aspiration (Bab *et al.*, 1988). Here
is the place to note that the future of bone and cartilage repair lies in the
combination of cartilaginous and osteogenic growth factors (for details see
Chapter 10 of this volume) with or without implants of cultured cells. In
addition to cultured chondrocytes, one should consider osteogenic cells from
various sources. Again, the best sources are embryonal tissues (e.g., calvaria), though osteoprogenitor cells for establishing bone cells in culture
may be derived from adult tissues such as the deep layers of resting periosteum, from the marrow cavity and external and internal callus (Fell, 1932;
Peck *et al.*, 1964; Dziak and Brand, 1974; Binderman *et al.*, 1974; Aubin *et
al.*, 1982).

Upon implanting embryonal chondrocytes into full thickness articular
defects transversing the subchondral bone in chickens, we observed massive
bone formation in the subchondral areas in the vicinity of the cartilaginous
implants (unpublished data, Robinson *et al.*). This led us to examine the
effect of implantation of such a cell composition (chondrocytes in 2% hyaluronic acid) on increasing bone density of the metaphysis of old osteoporotic chickens. We drilled a tunnel 3 cm long and 3 mm in diameter
beginning in the middle of the intercondylar notch of the distal tibia (Figs.
7 through 10). In this defect we installed 0.2 ml of a mixture of hyaluronic
acid and embryonal cartilage cells (5×10^6 cells/ml). We observed an
increased bone density in the metaphysis of the implanted bones up to 15
months after the operation. This increase in bone mass was greater than
that which could be ascribed solely to the effect of trauma to the bone
marrow (the control group was sham operated). We are currently conduct-
ing detailed histomorphometric, biochemical, and biomechanical analyses
of this model.

Summary and Discussion of Future Research Avenues

It seems that now we are on the verge of adding cell therapy to the
armamentarium of the orthopedic surgeon. This line of therapy offers the
exciting possibility of healing skeletal lesions caused by pathological states.
Furthermore, rejuvenation of parts of the skeletal system by tissue and cells
of young donors could be contemplated.

In order that such therapy be a practical alternative to the currently used

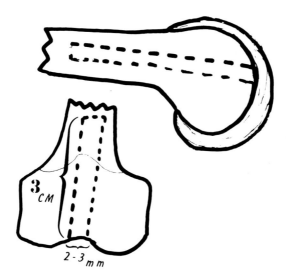

Fig. 7 A diagram showing the operation approach of the cell implants into the metaphysis (broken line ---- the tunnel drilled).

metallic and ceramic prostheses, a convenient and reliable method of isolating, growing, maintaining, and storing cells has to be developed. Currently, the only method available for cartilage storage is freezing of the tissue in the presence of a cryopreservative such as glycerol or dimethyl sulfoxide (Tomford and Mankin, 1989). This method is far from perfect, especially due to the low survival rates of the chondrocytes. However, it was previously shown that embryonal skeletal tissues of bone and cartilage so stored can later be successfully transplanted (Nevo *et al.*, 1983). Alternatively, cartilage cells can be kept in long-term cultures, at least up to 60 days (Brighton *et al.*, 1979). This method is probably not cost efficient and also is limited in duration. On the other hand, a 30-fold increase in cell number can be achieved (Bentley, 1988). Hyaluronic acid, as has already been mentioned, was found in our experimentation to be the best storage milieu of viable cells for a week outside an incubator. Thus, deep frozen cells could be thawed, grown for a short restoration period embedded in hyaluronic acid, and be available for surgery for a couple of days.

However, the origin of cartilage cells for human trials is a most vexing problem. Embryonal cells are advantageous both from the point of proliferation and because of their relative immunoprivilege. However, use of embryonal tissue is currently not only a pure scientific problem but rather a moral one. The use of adult cadaver cartilage is possible but with great limitations in amounts; the mitotic potential of adult cells is very low.

An alternative source of cells would preferably be autogenous. The most promising candidates are the so-called chondrogenic and osteogenic stem cells. As to the osteogenic cells, two types are known at present. The first

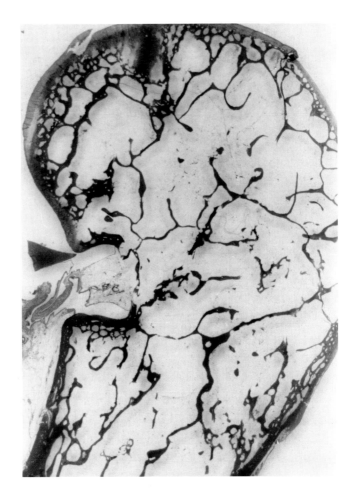

Fig. 8 A typical osteopenic bone of a 3-year-old chicken. Note sparsity of bony trabeculae. (H & E, magnification × 40.)

type are the cells induced by bone morphogenetic protein in soft tissues. The other type are bone marrow stromal fibroblasts (Beresford, 1989). These cells can be induced to express a cartilaginous phenotype by incubation *in vivo* in the presence of bone morphogenetic protein, especially if combined with electrical current (Friendenberg *et al.*, 1989). The potential of such cells in regenerating both articular and growth plate cartilage as well as in inducing bone formation is currently our main interest. A possible improvement in the application procedure is the introducing of a biodegradable scaffold substance to hold the cells and the delivery substance in the defect site.

In the future, more complicated experiments employing specific growth factors have to be carried out to explore the possibility of inducing mitosis

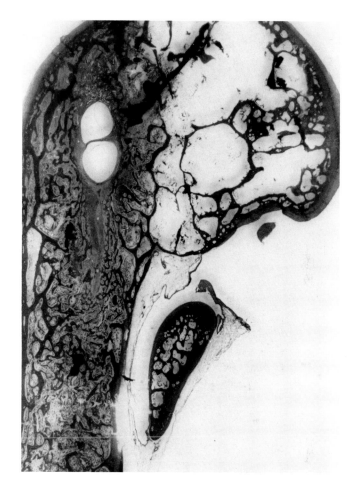

Fig. 9 A bone of a 3-year-old chicken similar to the one in Fig. 7, 6 weeks after transplantation of embryonal chondrocytes embedded in hyaluronic acid. Note the dense newly formed trabeculae along the line of injection. (H & E, magnification × 40.)

in adult chondrocytes. Such techniques might allow the removal of a cartilage slice from the patient, isolating cells, and incubating them with growth factors. After a sufficient mass of cells has been obtained, the cells could be transplanted back into the same patient and used to repair bone and cartilage defects of the joints. The most promising and recommended combination of growth factors to date is a combination of insulin-like growth factor TGF-β and acidic fibroblast growth factor used in concert. These agents can cause a 40-fold increase in thymidine incorporation of adult bovine chondrocytes in organ culture (Osborn *et al.*, 1989). Inductive molecules for repair and regeneration of bone and cartilage are discussed elsewhere in this volume (Chapter 6).

In conclusion, many scientific achievements have broadened our knowl-

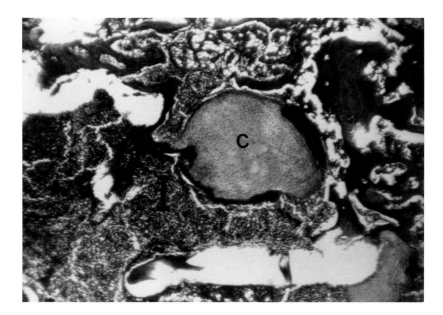

Fig. 10 At a larger magnification an island of implanted chondrocytes (c) that survived 6 weeks after operation, surrounded by a dense cellular infiltrate (I). Note formation of bony trabeculae around the implant. (H & E, magnification × 200.)

edge regarding the acceleration and manipulation of bone and cartilage repair and regeneration. Currently, attempts are being made to introduce cell culturing techniques for the benefit of preparing implants containing cultured cells for repairing defective bone and cartilage tissues. It is still a long way to the fulfillment of the prophet's vision on the revival of the dried bones in the valley (see the *Book of Ezechiel*, Chapter 37).

Acknowledgments

Data in this chapter originated from research projects of the authors which were supported in part by grants from the U.S.-Israel Binational Science Foundation Nos. 84-00365 & 88-00428 and Chief Scientist Office, Ministry of Industry and Chamber.

References

Aichroth, P. M. (1969). Transplantation of joint surfaces by cartilage grafts. *Br. J. Surg.*, **56**: 855.
Aston, J. E. and Bentley, G. (1986). Repair of articular surfaces by allografts of articular and growth plate cartilage. *J. Bone J. Surg.*, **68B**: 29–35.

Aubin, J. E., Heersche, J. N., Merrilees, M. J., and Sodek, J. (1982). Isolation of bone cell clones with differences in growth, hormone responses, and extracellular matrix production. *J. Cell Biol.*, **92**: 542–461.

Bab, I., Gazit, D., Massarawa, A., and Sela, J. (1985). Removal of tibial marrow induces increased formation of bone and cartilage in rat mandibular condyle. *Calcif. Tissue Int.*, **37**: 551–555.

Bab, I., Gazit, D., Muhlrad, A., and Shteyer, A. (1988). Regenerating bone marrow produces a potent growth factor activity to osteogenic cells. *Endocrinology*, **123**: 345–362.

Bates, G. P., Schor, S. L., and Grant, M. E. (1987). A comparison of the effects of different substrata on chondrocyte morphology and the synthesis of collagen types IX and X. *In Vitro Cell. Dev. Biol.*, **23**: 374–380.

Bentley, G. (1988). Transplant potential of the growth plate. In: *Behavior of the Growth Plate*, Uhthoff, H. K. and Wiley, J. J. Eds., Raven Press, New York, 65–71.

Bentley, G. and Greer, R. B. (1971). Homotransplantation of isolated epiphyseal and articular cartilage chondrocytes into joint surfaces of rabbits, *Nature*, **230**: 385–388.

Bentley, G., Smith, A. U., and Mukerjhee, R. (1978). Isolated epiphyseal chondrocyte allografts into joint surfaces. *Ann. Rheumat. Dis.*, **37**: 449–458.

Benum, P. (1975). Autogenous transplantation of apophyseal cartilage to osteochondral defects of joints. *Acta Orthop. Scand.*, **46**: 11–24.

Benya, P. D. and Shaffer, J. D. (1982). Dedifferentiated chondrocytes re-express the differentiated collagen phenotype when cultured in agarose gels. *Cell*, **30**: 215–224.

Beresford, J. N. (1989). Osteogenic stem cells and the stromal system of bone and marrow. *Clin. Orthop.*, **240**: 270–279.

Binderman, I., Duksin, D., Harell, A., Sacks, L., and Katchalsky, E. (1974). Formation of bone tissue in culture from isolated bone cells. *J. Cell Biol.*, **61**: 427–439.

Bright, R. W. (1981). Further canine studies with medical elastomer X7-2320 after osseous bridge resection for partial physeal plate closure. *Trans. Orthop. Res. Soc.*, **6**: 108.

Brighton, C. T., Shadle, C. A., Jimanez, S. A., Irwin, J. T., Lane, J. M., and Upton, M. (1979). Articular cartilage preservation and storage. *Arthritis Rheum.*, **22**: 1093–1101.

Brittberg, M., Nilsson, A., Peterson, L., Lindahl, A., and Isaksson, O. (1989). Healing of injured rabbit articular cartilage after transplantation of autologous cultivated chondrocytes. The Bat Sheva Seminar on Methods Used in Research on Cartilaginous Tissues, Israel. March 16-26, 1989.

Brown, K. L. B. (1988). Vascularized epiphyseal grafts. In: *Behavior of the Growth Plate*. Uhthoff, H. K. and Wiley, J. J., Eds., Raven Press, New York.

Bucholz, R. W., Holmes, R., and Mooney, V. (1981). Regeneration of articular cartilage over coralline hydroxyapatite. *Orthop. Trans.*, **5**: 322.

Chacko, S., Abbott, J., Holtzer, S., and Holtzer, H. (1969). The loss of phenotype traits of differentiated cells. VI. Behavior of the progeny of a single chondrocyte. *J. Exp. Med.*, **130**: 417–442.

Chan, R. D., Coon, H. G., and Chan. M. B. (1967). Cell culturing and cloning techniques. In: *Methods in Developmental Biology*. Wilt F. H. and Wessells, N. K., Eds., Thomas Y. Crowell, New York, 413–450.

Chesterman, P. J. and Smith, A. U. (1965). Homotransplantation of articular cartilage and isolated chondrocytes. An experimental study in rabbits. *J. Bone J. Surg.*, **50B**: 184–197.

Cleland, H. N. and Sevastikoglou, J. A. (1962). Experimental studies of embryonic bone transplantation. *Acta Orthop. Scand.*, **32**: 1–26.

Coon, H. G. (1966). Clone stability and phenotypic expression of chick cartilage cells in vitro. *Proc. Natl. Acad. Sci. U.S.A.*, **55**: 66–73.

Craigmyle, M. B. L. (1955). Studies of cartilage autografts and homografts in the rabbit. *Br. J. Plast. Surg.*, **8**: 93–100.

Craigmyle, M. B. L. (1958). Regional lymph nodes changes induced by cartilage homo- and heterografts in the rabbit. *J. Anat.*, **92**: 74–83.

DePalma, A. F., McKeever, C. D., and Subin, D. K. (1966). Process of repair of articular cartilage demonstrated by histology and autoradiography with tritiated thymidine. *Clin. Orthop.*, **48**: 229–242.

Dhert, W. J. A., O'Driscoll, S., Van Royen, B. J., and Salter, R. B. (1987). Effects of immobilization and continuous passive motion on postoperative muscle atrophy in mature rabbits. *Can. J. Surg.*, **31**: 185–188.

Drzewiecki, A. E., Randolph, M. A., and Weiland, A. J. (1989). Vascularized growth plate transplantation. *Trans. Orthop. Res. Soc.*, **14**: 465.

Dustmann, H. O. and Puhl, W. (1976). Altersabhangige Heilungs Moglich-Keiten von Knorpelwunden. *Z. Orthop.*, **114**: 749–764.

Dziak, R. and Brand, J. S. (1974). Calcium transport in isolated bone cells. I. Bone cell isolation procedures. *J. Cell Physiol.*, **84**: 75–83.

Elves, M. W. (1974). A study of the transplantation antigens on chondrocytes from articular cartilage. *J. Bone J. Surg.*, **56B**: 178–185.

Engkvist, O. (1979). Reconstruction of patellar articular cartilage with free autologous perichondrial grafts, *Scand. J. Plast. Reconstr. Surg.*, **13**: 361–369.

Engkvist, O. and Johansson, S. J. (1980). Perichondral arthroplasty. *Scand. J. Plast. Reconstr. Surg.*, **14**: 71–87.

Fell, H. B. (1932). The osteogenic capacity in vitro of periosteum and endosteum isolated from limb skeleton of fowl embryos and young chicks. *J. Anat.*, **66**: 157–180.

Friedenberg, Z. B., Brighton, C. T., Michelson, J. D., Bednar, J., Schmidt, R., and Brockmeyer, T. (1989). The effects of demineralized bone matrix and direct current on an "in vivo" culture of bone marrow cells. *J. Orthop. Res.*, **7**: 22–27.

Friedlander, G. E. (1983). Immune responses to osteochondral allografts. *Clin. Orthop.*, **174**: 58–68.

Frost, H. M. (1985). The pathomechanics of osteoporosis. *Clin. Orthop.*, **200**: 198–225.

Furakawa, T., Eyre, D. R., Koide, S., and Glimcher, M. J. (1980). Biomechanical studies on repair cartilage resurfacing experimental defects in the rabbit knee, *J. Bone J. Surg.*, **62A**: 79–89.

Ghadially, F. N. (1983a). In: *Fine Structure of Synovial Joints.* Butterworths, London, 261–279.

Ghadially, F. N. (1983b). In: *Fine Structure of Synovial Joints.* Butterworths, London, 280–306.

Gibson, T. (1965). Cartilage grafts. *Br. Med. Bull.*, **21**: 153–156.

Gordon, B. L. (1960). *Medieval and Renaissance Medicine.* P. Owen, London, 38.

Grande, D. A. and Pitman, M. I. (1988). The use of adhesives in chondrocyte transplantation surgery preliminary studies. *Bull. Hosp. J. Dis. Orthop. Inst.*, **48**: 140–148.

Grande, D. A., Singh, I. J., and Pugh, J. (1987). Healing of experimentally produced lesions in articular cartilage following chondrocyte transplantation. *Anat. Rec.*, **218**: 142–148.

Green, W. T. (1971). Behavior of articular chondrocytes in cell culture. *Clin. Orthop.*, **75**: 248–260.

Green, W. T. (1977). Articular cartilage repair. *Clin. Orthop.*, **124**: 237–250.

Harris, W. R., Martin, R., and Tile, M. (1965). Transplantation of epiphyseal plates. *J. Bone J. Surg.*, **47A**: 897–914.

Helbing, G. (1981). Transplantation Isolierter Chondrozyten in Gelenkknorpel Defekte. *Med. Habilit.*, 3355–3359.

Helbing, G., Burri, C., Heit, W., Neugebauer, R., and Ruter, A. (1980). In vivo synthesis of cartilage after transplantation of chondrocytes in animal experiments. *Chir. Forum Exp. Klin. Forsch.*, 47–51.

Helbing, G., Neugebauer, R., and Mohr, W. (1979). In vitro cultured chondrocytes as homologous cartilage transplant. *Hefte Unfallheilkd.*, **138**: 319–322.

Hesse, W. and Hesse, I. (1976). Umbauvorgange bei autologen gelenkknorpeltransplantaten, *Langzeit Ergebnisse. Vehr. Anat. Ges.*, **70S**: 685–690.

Heyner, S. (1969). The significance of the intercellular matrix in the survival of cartilage allografts. *Transplantation*, **8**: 666–676.

Hjertquist, S. O. and Lemperg, R. (1970). Microchemical studies on glycosaminoglycans and calcium in autologous costal cartilage transplanted to an osteochondral defect on the femoral head of adult rabbits. *Calcif. Tissue Res.*, **5**: 153–169.

Hjertquist, S. O. and Lemperg, R. (1971). Histological, autoradiographic and microchemical studies of spontaneously healing osteochondral articular defects in adult rabbits. *Calcif. Tissue Res.*, **8**: 54–72.

Holtzer, H. and Abbott, J. (1968). Oscillations of the chondrogenic phenotype in vitro. In: *Results and Problems in Cell Differentiation*, Vol. 1. Ursprung, H., Ed., Springer-Verlag, New York, 1–16.

Holtzer, H., Abbott, J., Lash, J., and Holtzer, S. (1960). The loss of phenotypic traits by differentiated cells in vitro. I. Dedifferentiation of cartilage cells. *Proc. Natl. Acad. Sci. U.S.A.*, **49**: 643–647.

Homer, *Iliad*, Book 6, 189f. Hessiod, Theog. 319ff.

Horwitz, A. L. and Dorfman, A. (1970). The growth of cartilage cells in soft agar and liquid suspension. *J. Cell Biol.*, **45**: 434–438.

Itay, S., Abramovici, A., and Nevo, Z. (1987). Use of cultured embryonal chick epiphyseal chondrocytes as grafts for defects in chick articular cartilage. *Clin. Orthop.*, **220**: 284–303.

Jaroma, H. J. and Ritsila, V. A. (1987). Reconstruction of patellar cartilage defects with free periosteal grafts, *Scand. J. Plast. Reconstr. Surg.*, **21**: 175–181.

Johnson, L. L. (1986). *Arthroscopic Surgery, Principles and Practice*, 3rd ed., C. V. Mosby, St. Louis.

Jotreau, F. V. and LeDouarin, N. M. (1978). The developmental relationship between osteocytes and osteoclasts: a study using the quail-chick nuclear marker in endochondral ossification. *Dev. Biol.*, **63**: 253–265.

Kawabe, N., Ehrlich, M. G., and Mankin, H. J. (1987). Growth plate reconstruction using chondrocytes allograft transplants. *J. Pediatr. Orthop.*, **7**: 381–388.

Kawabe, N., Yoshinao, M., and Hirotani, H. (1989). The repair of full thickness articular cartilage defects. Immune responses to reparative tissue by growth plate chondrocytes implants. *Trans. Orthop. Res. Soc.*, **14**: 143.

Kawiak, J., Moskalewski, S., and Darzynkiewicz, Z. (1965). Isolation of chondrocytes from calf cartilage. *Exp. Cell Res.*, **39**: 59–68.

Knudson, C. B. and Toole, B. P. (1987). Hyanluronate-cell interactions during differentiation of chick embryo limb mesoderm. *Dev. Biol.*, **124**: 82–90.

Ksiazek, T. and Moskalewski, S. (1983). Studies on bone formation by cartilage reconstructed by isolated epiphyseal chondrocytes, transplanted syngeneically or across known histocompatibility barriers in mice. *Clin. Orthop.*, **172**: 233–250.

Kujawa, M. J. and Caplan, A. I. (1986). Hyaluronic acid bonded to cell-culture surfaces stimulates chondrogenesis in stage 24 limb mesenchyme cell cultures. *Dev. Biol.*, **114**: 504–518.

Langeskiold, A. (1988). Growth plate regeneration. In: *Behavior of the Growth Plate*. Uhthoff, H. K. and Wiley, J. J., Eds., Raven Press, New York, 47–50.

Langeskiold, A., Osterman, K., and Valle, M. (1987). Growth of fat grafts after operation for partial bone growth arrest: demonstration by computerized tomography scanning. *J. Pediatr. Orthop.*, **7**: 389–394.

Larsen, N. E., Lombard, K. M., and Balasz, E. A. (1989). The effect of hyaluronan on cartilage and chondrocyte response to mechanical and biochemical perturbation. *Trans. Orthop. Res. Soc.*, **14**: 151.

Laurence, M. and Smith, A. U. (1968). Experiments in chondrocyte homografting in the rabbit. *J. Bone J. Surg.*, **50B**: 226.

Lidor, C., Dekel, S., and Edelstein, S. (1987b). The metabolism of vitamin D_3 during fracture healing in chicks. *Endocrinology*, **120**: 389–393.

Lidor, C., Dekel, S., Hallel, T., and Edelstein, S. (1987a). Levels of active metabolites of vitamin D_3 in the callus of fracture repair in chicks. *J. Bone J. Surg.*, **69B**: 132–136.

Malejczyk, J. and Moskalewski, S. (1988). Effect of immunosuppression on survival and growth of cartilage produced by transplanted allogeneic epiphyseal chondrocytes, *Clin. Orthop.*, **232**: 292–303.

Mankin, H. J. (1974). The reaction of articular cartilage to injury and osteoarthritis. *N. Engl. J. Med.*, **291**: 1285–1292, 1335–1340.

Manning, W. K. and Bonner, W. (1967). Isolation and culture of chondrocytes from human adult articular cartilage. *Arthritis Rheum.*, **10**: 235–239.

Matsubara, T., Hirata, S., Saegusa, Y., and Hirohata, K. (1989). Inhibition of vascular endothelial cell proliferation by hyaluronic acid but not by proteoglycans. *Trans. Orthop. Res. Soc.*, **14**: 424.

McKibbin, B. and Ralis, Z. A. (1978). The site dependence of the articular cartilage transplant reaction. *J. Bone J. Surg.*, **60B**: 561–566.

Meachim, G. and Roberts, C. (1971). Repair of the joint surface from sub-articular tissue in the rabbit knee. *J. Anat.*, **109**: 317–327.

Miki, T. and Yamamuro, T. (1987). The fate of hypertrophic chondrocytes in growth plates transplanted intramuscularly in the rabbit. *Clin. Orthop.*, **218**: 276–282.

Milgram, J. W. (1985). Injury to articular cartilage joint surfaces, *Clin. Orthop.*, **192**: 168–173.

Mitchell, N. and Shepard, N. (1976). The resurfacing of adult rabbit articular cartilage by multiple perforations through the sub-chondral bone. *J. Bone J. Surg.*, **58A**: 230–233.

Moran, M. E., Kreder, H. J., Salter, R. B., and Keeley, F. N. (1989). Biological resurfacing of major full thickness defects in joint surfaces by neochondrogenesis with cryopreserved allogeneic periosteum stimulated by continuous passive motion. *Trans. Orthop. Res. Soc.*, **14**: 542.

Moskalewski, S. and Kawiak, J. (1965). J. Cartilage formation after homotransplantation of isolated chondrocytes. *Transplantation*, **3**: 737–742.

Moskalewski, S., Kawiak, J., and Rymaszewska, T. (1966). Local cellular response evoked by cartilage formed after auto- and allogeneic transplantation of isolated chondrocytes. *Transplantation*, **4**: 572–581.

Moskalewski, S. and Rybicka, E. (1977). The influence of the degree of maturation of donor tissue on the reconstruction of elastic cartilage by isolated chondrocytes. *Acta Anat.*, **97**: 231–240.

Nettelblad, H., Randolph, M. A., and Wieland, A. J. (1984). Free microvascular epiphyseal plate transplantation. *J. Bone J. Surg.*, **66A**: 1421–1430.

Nevo, Z., Beit-Or, A., and Eilam, Y. (1988). Slowing down aging of cultured embryonal chick chondrocytes by maintenance under lowered oxygen tension. *Mech. Ageing Devel.*, **45**: 157–165.

Nevo, Z., Horwitz, A. L., and Dorfman, A. (1972). Synthesis of chondromucoprotein by chondrocytes in suspension. *Dev. Biol.*, **28**: 219–228.

Nevo, Z., Lev El, A., Siegal, T., Altaraz, C., Segal, S., Dolev, S., and Nebel, L. (1983). Fresh and cryopreserved fetal bones replacing massive bone loss in rats. *Calcif. Tissue Int.*, **35**: 62–69.

Nevo, Z., Lev El, A., Siegal, T., Segal, S., Altaraz, C., and Dolev, S. (1977). ^{35}S, ^{45}Ca incorporation and matrix integrity: valuable parameters for transplantation. *Isr. J. Med. Sci.*, **12**: 975–976.

Niedermann, B. Boe, S., Lauritzen, J., and Rubak, J. M. (1985). Glued periosteal grafts in the knee, *Acta Orthop. Scand.*, **56**: 457–460.

Nilsson, O. and Urist, M. R. (1985). Response of the rabbit metaphysis to implants of bovine bone morphogenetic protein. *Clin. Orthop.*, **195**: 275–281.

Nimni, M. E., Bernick, S., Ertl, D., Nishimoto, S. K., Paule, W., Strates, B. S., and Villaneuva, J. (1988). Ectopic bone formation is enhanced in senescent animals implanted with embryonal cells. *Clin. Orthop.*, **234**: 255–267.

O'Driscoll, S. W., Delaney, J. P., and Salter, R. B. (1989). Experimental patellar resurfacing using periosteal autografts: reasons for failure. *Trans. of the 35th Annu. Meet. Orthopaedic Res. Soc.*, **14**: 145.

O'Driscoll, S. W. and Salter, R. B. (1984). The induction of neochondrogenesis in free intra-articular periosteal autografts under the influence of continuous passive motion. *J. Bone J. Surg.*, **66A**: 1248–1257.

O'Driscoll, S. W. and Salter, R. B. (1986). The repair of major osteochondral defects in joint surfaces by neochondrogenesis with autogenous osteoperiosteal grafts stimulated by continuous passive motion. *Clin. Orthop.*, **208**: 131–140.

Osborn, K. D., Trippel, S. B., and Mankin, H. J. (1989). Growth factor stimulation of adult articular cartilage. *J. Orthop. Res.*, **7**: 35–42.

Ostrowski, K., Wlodarski, K., Skarzinska, S., and Poltorak, A. (1970). Immunodepressive treatments allowing formation of cartilage and bone induced by xenogeneic transplantations. *Coll. R. Soc. Biol. (Paris)*, **164**: 2258–2262.

Paccola, C. A. J., Xavier, C. A. M., and Goncalves, R. P. (1979). Fresh immature articular cartilage allografts. *Arch. Orthop. Traumatol. Surg.*, **93**: 253–259.

Passl, R., Plenk, H., Radaskiewicz, T., Sauer, G., Holle, J., and Spangler, H. P. (1976a). Zum Problem der Reinen Homologen Gelenksknorpel Transplantation. *Verh. Anat. Ges.*, **70S**: 675–678.

Passl, R., Plenk, H., Sauer, G., Spangler, H. P., Radaskiewicz, T., and Holle, J. (1976b). Die Homologe Reine Gelenksknorpeltransplantation im Teirexperiment. *Arch. Orthop. Unfall Chir.*, **86**: 243–256.

Paulette, R. E. and Prudden, J. F. (1959). Studies on the acceleration of wound healing with cartilage. *Surg. Gynecol. Obstet.*, **108**: 408–410.

Peck, W. A., Birge, S. J., and Fedak, S. A. (1964). Bone cells: biochemical and biological studies after enzymatic isolation. *Science*, **146**: 1476–1477.

Poussa, M., Rubak, J., and Ritsila, V. (1980). The effect of the thickness of the cortical bone on bone formation by osteoperiosteal grafts. *Acta Orthop. Scand.*, **51**: 29–35.

Prudden, J. F. and Allen, J. (1965). The clinical acceleration of healing with a cartilage preparation. *JAMA*, **192**: 352–356.

Recker, R. R. (1981). Continuous treatment of osteoporosis. *Orthop.Clin. North Am.*, **12**: 611–627.

Riddle, W. E. (1970). Healing of articular cartilage in the horse. *J. Am. Vet. Med. Assoc.*, **157**: 1471–1479.

Ring, P. A. (1955). Transplantation of epiphyseal cartilage. *J. Bone J. Surg.*, **37B**: 642–657.

Robinson, D., Halperin, N., and Nevo, Z. (1989). Fate of allogeneic embryonal chick chondrocytes implanted orthotopically, as determined by the host's age. *Mech. Ageing Dev.* **50**: 71–80.

Robinson, D., Halperin, N., and Nevo, Z. (1990). Regenerating hyaline cartilage in articular defects of old chickens using implants of embryonal chick chondrocytes embedded in a new natural delivery substance. *Calcif. Tissue Int.*, **46**: 246–253.

Rubak, J. M. (1982). Reconstruction of articular cartilage defects with free periosteal grafts. *Acta Orthop. Scand.*, **53**: 175–180.

Rubak, J. M., Poussa, M., and Ritsila, V. (1982a). Effects of joint motion on the repair of articular cartilage with free periosteal grafts. *Acta Orthop. Scand.*, **53**: 187–191.

Rubak, J. M., Poussa, M., and Ritsila, V. (1982b). Chondrogenesis in repair of articular cartilage defects by free periosteal grafts in rabbits. *Acta Orthop. Scand.*, **53**: 181–186.

Salter, R. B., Hamilton, H. W., Wedge, J. H., Tile, M., Torode, I. P., O'Driscoll, S. W., Murnaghan, J. J., and Saringer, J. H. (1984). Clinical application of basic research on continuous passive motion for disorders and injuries of synovial joints. *J. Orthop. Res.*, **1**: 325–342.

Segal, S., Siegal, T., Altaraz, H., Lev-El, A., Nevo, Z., Nebel, L., Katznelson, A., and Feldman, M. (1979). Fetal bone grafts do not elicit allograft rejection because of protecting anti-Ia alloantibodies, *Transplantation*, **28**: 88–95.

Sengupta, S. (1974). The fate of transplants of articular cartilage in the rabbit. *J. Bone J. Surg.*, **56B**: 167–177.

Shands, A. R. (1931). The regeneration of hyaline cartilage in joints, *Arch. Surg.*, **22**: 137–178.

Shimizu, T., Videman, T., Shimazaki, K., and Mooney, V. (1987). Experimental study on the repair of full thickness articular cartilage defects: effects of varying periods of continuous passive motion, cage activity and immobilization. *J. Orthop. Res.*, **5**: 187–197.

Shimomura, Y., Yoneda, T., and Suzuki, F. (1975). Osteogenesis by chondrocytes from growth cartilage of rat rib. *Calcif. Tissue Res.*, **19**: 179–187.

Siegal, T. and Marcus, Z. H. (1972). Studies on orthotopic homografts and allografts of rat fetal bones. *Proc. XII SICOT Congr. Exc. Med. ISC*, **291**: 142–167.

Siegal, T., Segal, S., Nevo, Z., Lev-El, A., Altaraz, C., Katznelson, A., and Nebel, L. (1977). Replacement of massive bone loss by massive fetal bone transplantation. *Transpl. Proc.*, **9**: 351–353.

Silver, W. A. (1969). Transplantation of articular cartilage in fowls. *Br. J. Surg.*, **56**: 700.

Solursh, M. and Meier, S. (1974). Effects of cell density on the expression of differentiation by chick and embryo chondrocytes. *J. Exp. Zool.*, **187**: 311–322.

Srivastava, V. M. L., Malemud, C. J., and Sokoloff, L. (1974). Chondroid expression by lapine articular chondrocytes in spinner culture following monolayers growth. *Connect. Tissue Res.*, **2**: 127–136.

Steinman, C. (1947). The healing of drill-hole defects in the long bones of adult rabbits especially following the use of embryonic bone transplants. *Anat. Rec.*, **99**: 427–441.

Stockwell, R. A. (1979). *Biology of Cartilage Cells*. Cambridge University Press, Cambridge.

Stover, S. M., Pool, R. R., and Lloyd, K. C. K. (1989). Repair of surgically created osteochondral defects with autogenous sternal osteochondral grafts. *Trans. Orthop. Res. Soc.*, **14**: 543.

Syftestad, G. T. and Urist, M. R. (1982). Bone aging. *Clin. Orthop.*, **162**: 288–297.

Tagliacozzi, G. (1597). De curtorum chirurgia per insitioneum, Venice.

Tanaka, H., Inoue, M., Suzuki, M., and Nojima, M. (1980). A study on experimental homocartilage transplantation. *Arch. Orthop. Traumatol. Surg.*, **96**: 165–169.

Thyberg, J. and Moskalewski, S. (1979). Bone formation in cartilage produced by transplanted epiphyseal chondrocytes. *Cell Tissue Res.*, **204**: 77–94.

Tomford, W. W., Hang, H. H., and Mankin, H. J. (1989). Cryopreservation of articular cartilage slices. *Trans. Orthop. Res. Soc.*, **14**: 146.

Upton, J., Sohn, S. A., and Glowacki, J. (1981). Neocartilage derived from transplanted perichondrium: what is it?. *Plast. Reconstr. Surg.*, **68**: 166–172.

Vachon, A. M., McIlwraith, C. W., Trotter, G. W., Norddin, R. W., and Powers, B. E. (1989). Neochondrogenesis in free intra-articular, periosteal and perichondrial autografts in the horse. *Trans. Orthop. Res. Soc.*, **14**: 541.

Wakitani, S., Kimura, T., Hirooka, A., Ochi, T., Yoneda, M., Yasui, N., Owaki, H., and Ono, K. (1989). Repair of rabbit articular surfaces with allograft chondrocytes embedded in collagen gel. *J. Bone J. Surg.*, **71B**: 74–80.

Wedge, J. H., Powell, J. N., Ulmer, B. G., and Reynolds, R. (1986). Biodegradable resurfacing of the hip in dogs. *Clin. Orthop.*, **208**: 76–80.

Weiss, C., Dennis, J., Suros, J. M., Delinger, J., Badia, A., and Gross, J. (1989a). Sodium hylan for the prevention of post laminectomy scar formation. *Trans. Orthop. Res. Soc.*, **14**: 44.

Weiss, C., Suros, J. M., Dennis, J., Delinger, J., Badia, A., Gross, J., and Ermenco, S. (1989b). Effect of Na-Hylan on articular cartilage. *Trans. Orthop. Res. Soc.*, **14**: 539.

Wright, G. C., Miller, K., and Sokoloff, L. (1985). Induction of bone xenografts of rabbit growth plate chondrocytes in the nude mouse. *Calcif. Tissue Int.*, **37**: 250–256.

Yasui, N., Osawa, S., Ochi, T., Nakashima, H., and Ono, K. (1982). Primary culture of chondrocytes embedded in collagen gels. *Exp. Cell Biol.*, **50**: 92–100.

Yasumoto, S., Kato, Y., Oguri, K., Yamagata, S., and Yamagata, T. (1980). Maintenance and phenotypic properties by chondrocytes cultured in suspension. *Dev. Growth Differ.*, **22**: 445–459.

Yoshihashi, Y. (1983). Tissue reconstitution by isolated articular chondrocytes in vitro. *Nippon Seikeigekagakkai Zasshi*, **57**: 629–641.

Zaleske, D. J., Ehrlich, M. G., Piliero, C., May, J. W., and Mankin, H. J. (1982). Growth plate behavior in whole joint replantation in the rabbit. *J. Bone J. Surg.*, **64A**: 249–258.

5

The Reactions of Bone to Non-Cemented Implants

TOMAS ALBREKTSSON
Biomaterials Group
Department of Handicap Research
University of Gothenburg
Gothenburg, Sweden

Introduction

What will happen if an implant (or a transplant) is introduced to the body? If, hypothetically, the implant material is inert, the healing of it will follow the same principles that govern fracture healing. There is an inevitable trauma at the insertion of the implant, a trauma that in one way or the other will trigger a healing response. This is identical to what happens in the fracture zone. Cells undifferentiated at the time of implant insertion will undergo mitosis and start to form new tissue after proper induction. In the case of a fracture the proper main direction for the induction is towards bone forming cells. In the case of an inserted joint implant the present author is of the opinion that the ideal goal is the same: cellular differentiation to osteoblasts. If the cellular differentiation is disturbed in the case of a fracture, for instance, because of continuous movements of the fracture ends, soft tissue differentiation will ensue. The end result is a pseudarthrosis. If the implant moves in its site a similar series of events will follow with the end result an implant pseudarthrosis — a fibrous capsule. However, an implant (like a large segmental bone graft that seldom is replaced to any greater degree with new bone) may still function provided it is not overloaded. In fact, this is the situation with most currently used cemented or non-cemented orthopedic reconstructions in this the first generation of such clinically used implants. The fibrous embedment of the devices is stable enough to guarantee some function provided a careful loading. In today's clinical practice of implant reconstructions, however, the observation of more and more failures with increasing time of implantation indicate that the interfacial situation is far from ideal. This is very different from the endpoint of fracture healing — bone ideally heals with new bone without any scar formation. The properly healed fracture is not prone to new breakage. In fact, a similar situation is also clinically achievable with implants. There is evidence of a continuous undisturbed anchorage of consecutively inserted, directly bone-anchored, load-bearing mandibular fixtures over follow-up times of at least 15 years (Albrektsson and Lekholm, 1989). Fig. 1a demonstrates the outcome of one type of currently used non-cemented implants (but is in principle valid for any type of orthopedic joint replacements of today) whereas Fig. 1b demonstrates the more ideal failure curve seen if bone is allowed to heal as bone around the foreign device.

The aim of the present paper is to summarize current knowledge on non-cemented implants and to critically analyze such implants with respect to the theoretically ideal end-point which to the author is represented by the implant that is directly anchored to bone. In the first part of this paper I will try to briefly summarize cemented and non-cemented implants with some historical data. I will then present a literature review with special emphasis on hip and knee joint anchorage elements. Conditions that may indirectly influence the anchorage function such as revision arthroplasties, wear products from adjacent joints, infections, or other disorders will be only briefly commented on. Besides, there is an excellent recently published overview on the influence of prosthesis design on wear and loosening phenomena (Mittlmeier and Walter, 1987). Thereafter, the current knowledge of how to achieve bone incorporation of implanted devices will be evaluated with comparisons to the clinical situation of today's orthopedic treatment routines. One major point here is to present the multifaceted aspects of bone implant anchorage that surely does not only depend on the materials and presence or absence of micromotion.

Cemented and Non-Cemented Implants

At the closing of a meeting on the Bone Implant Interface arranged by the American Academy of Orthopaedic Surgeons in Chicago in September of 1983 (Lewis and Galante, 1985) the participants were asked whether bone cement was going to remain one way to anchor joint implants in the future or whether it was to be regarded as a biological parenthesis. Everyone

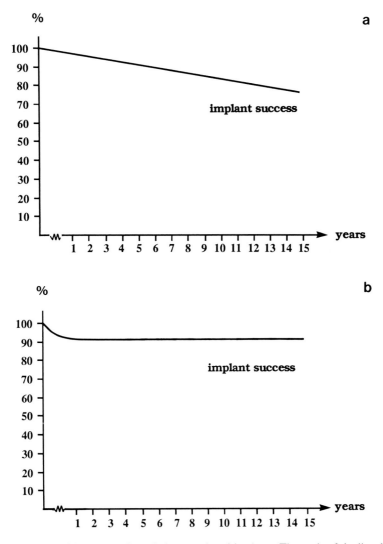

Fig. 1 **(a)** Typical failure curve for soft tissue anchored implants. The angle of the line does, of course, depend on factors such as used success criteria, but the main point is that more and more implants are being lost with increasing time. **(b)** Typical failure curve for directly bone-anchored implants. There is an initial loss of implants depending on failures to achieve the desired bone anchorage. Thereafter, however, there are hardly any failures.

who commented on this question was convinced that bone cement was to be part of the orthopedic world "forever". Personally, I am convinced of the opposite. The cemented interface is constantly in the risk of failure even at loadings generally looked upon as being in the physiological range. Bone cement does age and the need for revision surgery increases with time. In addition, the obvious environmental problems of toxic bone cement products (short-term monomer as well as long-term dimethylparatoluidin, (Linder, 1982; Lintner, 1983; Albrektsson, 1984; Albrektsson and Linder, 1984) will alone constitute a reason for abandoning methylmethacrylates as soon as we have realistic alternatives. Bone cement works in conflict to the cells of the body whereas the aim for a biomaterial is to have it co-operating with the organism. Having said this, however, we must realize that we are far from reaching this ideal state with currently used non-cemented implants. Therefore, in spite of its shortcomings, bone cement remains the most logical alternative in many clinical situations today, at the same time an intensive research effort must be devoted to replace it in the future.

Early Endoprosthetic Attempts to Repair the Hip and Knee Joint

The first endoprosthetic replacements for major joints were non-cemented ones. One of the first attempts to use a foreign material in hip joint arthroplasty was a glass cup inserted by Smith-Petersen in 1923 to cover a re-shaped head of the femur (Amstutz 1985). Hey-Groves replaced the femoral head with an ivory implant in 1922 and the first total hip endoprosthesis was implanted by Wiles in 1938 (Refior et al., 1988), the same year as a cast Cr-Co-Mo femoral cup was described (Smith-Petersen, 1939). The Judet acrylic hip was introduced in 1946 (Judet and Judet, 1950). The clinical outcome of these initially used hip hemiarthroplasties was not very encouraging, but the experience gathered has served as an important step in the development of present day hip reconstructions.

The first operated endoprosthesis of the knee seems to be the vitallium femoral condyle mold inserted by Campbell (1940) and tried in four cases, however, with poor clinical results (Walldius, 1957). Inspired by the work with plexiglass hip prostheses performed by the Judet brothers, Walldius, in 1951, constructed a knee prosthesis of the same material (Walldius, 1957). The Walldius acrylic knee was a hinge prosthesis jointed together by a stainless steel rod and, at least initially, reinforced by central stainless steel cores. Thirty-two artificial knees were inserted in many severely crippled patients who often had been totally unable to walk for years before surgery. Two patients died, two cases needed a later knee amputation, and four other devices failed. The remaining 24 knees were reported to have an excellent result after a follow-up of 1 to 6 years (Walldius, 1957).

Early studies on retrieved acrylic implants revealed a fibrous tissue coat a few millimeters in thickness around hip (Judet et al., 1954) as well as around knee implants (Walldius, 1957). This soft tissue coat was regarded as a positive shock absorber by Walldius; he even recommended the preservation of it, should a reoperation be necessary. In addition, wear products from plexiglass hip joints resulting in fibrosis and foreign body reactions were already described by Mittelmeier and Singer (1956). It is, thus, obvious that various tissue reactions to joint replacement materials actively debated in the 1990s were observed and discussed 30 to 40 years ago.

Tissue Response to Hip Prostheses

From a design and surface point of view non-cemented hip prostheses have been divided into many different categories. For instance, Schatzker *et al.* (1989) separated ingrowth and press-fit stem prostheses. Naturally, however, an ingrowth prosthesis may also be a press-fit one and this differentiation may, therefore, be slightly unclear in some cases. Oh (1987) refers to non-cemented stem implants as macroporous and microporous, the latter as a rule having an average pore size of 250 μm (Engh *et al.*, 1987), yet Zweymüller *et al.* (1988) discuss microirregularities in the 3 to 5 μm range. Brånemark and afEkenstam (1979) have even patented an implant surface with irregularities of the nanometer size, even if there seems to be a lack of biological evidence that such a microporous surface is advantageous compared to, for instance, a surface with irregularities in the 1 to 10 μm size (Fig. 2a,b).

One type of ingrowth prostheses is the fenestrated one such as the Mittelmeier design (Mittelmeier, 1983). However, several other prosthetic designs may have major fenestrations as well as some other means for bone anchorage such as the Zweymüller original hip design (Zweymüller, 1983). In this review I regard major fenestrations as an additional mode for implant fixation and will not treat them separately. In the following discussion I will use a classification of hip joints presented in Table 1. This classification distinguishes between surface replacement hips and press-fitted ones, the latter category being subdivided into ingrowth, granulated, super press-fitted, and threaded ones.

Surface Replacement

Acetabular Cup

Experimental Studies.   In an experimental series, Jasty and Harris (1988) used a Chrome-Cobalt-Molybden cup with a porous surface and implanted this device into 15 dogs. They found that these cement-free cups did not show any evidence of the development of radiolucent lines at radiography. Histologically they observed a uniform bone ingrowth over follow-ups of 3 weeks to 3 months. At the latter time the bone was organized and it was reported that the ingrown trabeculae had penetrated the depths of the porous region to the solid substrate. If, on the other hand, a surgical technique that resulted in a central gap between the acetabular component and bone was used, this lead to persistent radiolucencies and a poor and patchy bone ingrowth was observed over the same follow-up period. Changing the design of the cup to a hemispherical type with a fiber mesh of commercially pure titanium resulted in a significant increase of bone compared to the porous-coated design. Calcium phosphate coatings on the

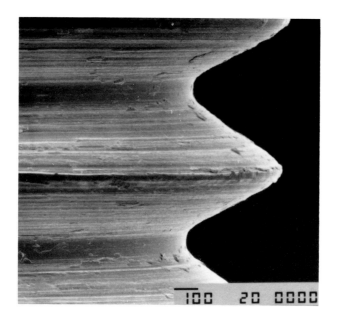

a

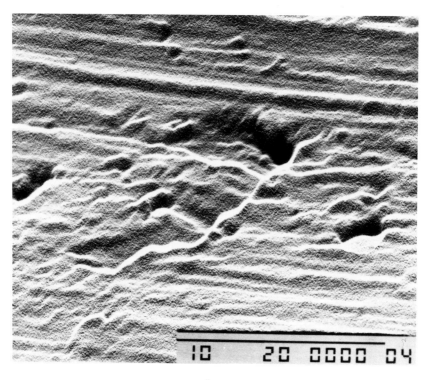

b

Table 1.
Design-Based Classification of Hip Prostheses

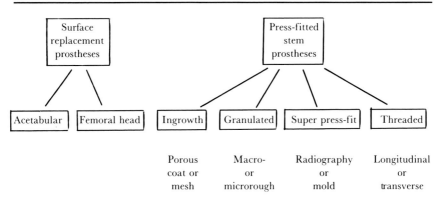

meshwork resulted in a significantly increased bone ingrowth at 3 weeks but not at 6 weeks or 3 months. Tooke *et al.* (1988) presented an experimental investigation of threaded and porous coated (pore size 75 μm) Ti-6A1-4V acetabular cups inserted in canines. At 2 and 6 months after surgery the authors found no bone in direct contact with the threaded cups and in three of the porous-coated cups, whereas the other porous-coated cups showed bone ingrowth. A mechanical test revealed greater movement with the threaded design compared to the porous-coated one at 6 months of follow-up. Huiskes (1987) presented a finite element analysis suggesting an explanation for the regular reports of loosened threaded acetabular cups.

Clinical Development and Retrieval Analyses. Charnley (1979) reported an increasing failure rate with time with cemented cups. Jasty and Harris (1988) concluded that as many as 25% or more of cemented acetabular components were loose over clinical follow-ups of 4 to 12 years.

Current clinical development seems to result in a rapid increase of the use of cement-free acetabular cups. Morscher (1983) referred to five main types of cement-free acetabular cups introduced in Europe; the cylindric socket (Griss and Heimke, 1981), the square socket (Griss *et al.*, 1978), the conic cup (Endler and Endler, 1982), the ellipsoid threaded ring (Lord and Bancel, 1983), and the hemispheric cup (Boutin, 1974; Engelhardt, 1983). Clinical reports from the use of similar types of fiber mesh titanium to those

Fig. 2 (a) Even if bone tissue cannot invade pores of much smaller size than 100 μm there is experimental evidence that surface micro-irregularities in the 1–100 μm size are advantageous for the stability of directly bone anchored implants. **(b)** Some investigators have even suggested that so-called micropits of a size between 10 and 1000 nm are important for the bone response although, to the knowledge of the present authors, there is no experimental backing up of this hypothesis.

used in the canine work by Jasty and Harris (1988) seem to indicate a good clinical outcome with respect to function and absence of radiolucent lines on radiographic examinations (Sumner *et al.*, 1987; Haddad *et al.*, 1987).

Collier and co-workers have presented an extensive overview of the fate of 226 retrieved uncemented porous-coated hip prostheses of which 162 were subjected to a detailed macroscopic and microscopic examination. Only 16% of the acetabular components showed evidence of bone ingrowth. However, in this material clinically loose components were also included. The authors summarized that the tissue in the retrieved cups ranged from loose, thin-fibrous tissue to highly organized fibers to bone ingrowth. In no case was more than 50% of the surface of the cup invaded by bone.

Femoral Cups

Surface replacement prostheses have been attractive as these designs call for a minimal removal of bone. Should the clinical results of such replacements be favorable, the procedure would be ideal. This is due, not in the least, to the fact that if a long-term failure would occur another conventional type of prosthesis could be easily inserted as the bone stock remains. However, to date, the clinical outcome of surface replacement prostheses has not been very positive and the procedure has been abandoned by most clinicians. Nevertheless, it should be remembered that many of the clinically introduced types of surface replacement hips have been cemented such as the Wagner cup (Wagner, 1978; Head, 1981) and the ICLH-prosthesis (Fig. 3a, b) (Freeman and Bradley, 1982; Herberts *et al.*, 1983) and that this may be part of the reason for the relatively poor results that have been achieved. Gerard (1978) developed a non-cemented double cup total hip arthroplasty.

Gerard *et al.* (1985) reported the clinical results of 145 cases followed for 5 to 8 years with a failure rate of some 20%. Willems *et al.* (1988) reported the histopathologic results of 15 failed Gerard double cup arthroplasties. It was observed that 9 of the 15 failures showed a clear resorption of the femoral head. There was a fibrous membrane between the foreign material and the bone. The fibers were directed parallel to the metal surface. The membrane contained a few lymphocytes and macrophages. Willems *et al.* (1988) blamed the osteonecrosis of the femoral head on injury to the retinacular vessels at the dorsal side of the neck. Schreiber and Jacob (1984), although referring to the ICLH-prosthesis, suggested that the bone resorption observed under the cup is explained by stress protection. Irrespective of the failure mechanism, similar problems with femoral head resorption have been reported by many investigators of cup arthroplasties (Bell *et al.*, 1985; D'Ambrosia *et al.*, 1972). Campbell *et al.* (1989), who investigated ten femoral components retrieved after an average clinical function time of 29 months, indicated another failure mechanism relating to wear of titanium alloy. The authors demonstrated that titanium alloy debris-filled histiocytes may cause a rapid and marked bone destruction within the femoral head and lead to failure despite an excellent ingrowth fixation.

The team around Amstutz has published several in-depth papers on the outcome of double cup arthroplasties (Amstutz, 1985; Amstutz *et al.*, 1987; Amstutz *et al.*, 1988) that have been used experimentally and clinically at the author's clinic since 1977. When evaluated in canines, there was primary bone ingrowth in all cases where initial stability was achieved at surgery (Amstutz, 1985). Between 18 and 24 months after surgery, however, cysts that were metallic-laden were observed in one third of the animals. The metallic debris originated primarily from loosened beads from the porous replacements (Amstutz *et al.*, 1987). Kim *et al.* (1986) presented results from a canine series where a short metal stem had been used in conjunction with the femoral surface replacement. Again, bone ingrowth was sufficient in the prosthesis, but there were other problems in the form of femoral neck resorption.

The clinical results of femoral hip replacements without stems were evaluated as so far promising at a follow-up time of 1 to 2.5 years. One retrieved clinical specimen showed excellent bone ingrowth (Amstutz *et al.*, 1987). In another retrieval analysis of nine femoral components (Campbell *et al.*, 1989) bone ingrowth was seen in seven of those cases and in five patients there were similar types of large cysts as those described by Amstutz *et al.* (1987). With a clinical experience of some 100 patients the authors concluded that their initial results were promising, but that the clinical use of porous surface replacements should proceed with caution (Amstutz *et al.*, 1988).

Press-Fit Prostheses

Ingrowth

Various Types of Soft Tissue Attachment.   Pilliar and colleagues in Toronto are the most well-known researchers behind the introduction of *porous-coated implants* (Welsh *et al.*, 1971; Cameron *et al.*, 1973; Pilliar *et al.*, 1975; Pilliar *et al.*, 1981; Pilliar, 1987). In their contribution of 1981, the authors described two types of soft tissue attachment to canine femoral porous stainless steel implants followed for 6 months. Apart from the previously often described fibrous capsule type of soft tissue embedment, the authors also found evidence of oblique fibers that anchored to the bone in a Sharpey's fiber-like fashion. The authors regarded this soft tissue as acting in one way or the other as an adequate implant-supportive membrane in contrast to "ordinary" fibrous capsules that have a fiber orientation parallel to the surface of the implanted device. Interestingly, Pilliar *et al.* (1981) were unable to detect any bone ingrowth in their porous devices, a fact they attributed to interfacial micromovements.

Experimental Investigations on Pore Size and Pore Distribution.   Bobyn *et al.* (1980) investigated the optimal pore size for bone fixation of ingrowth

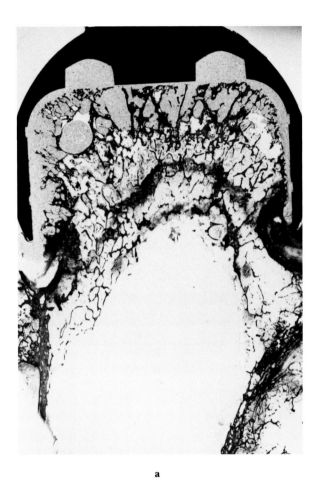

a

Fig. 3 (a) Many originally used femoral surface replacement cups were cemented. The clinical outcome of such devices was, generally, not favorable. (b) However, non-cemented cups often showed a soft tissue interface.

implants. The earlier experiments by Welsh *et al.* (1971) and Cameron *et al.* (1973) had used a chrome-cobalt alloy implant with a pore size of 50 to 100 μm. Chrome-cobalt implants with pore sizes varying from 20 to 800 μm and a porous coating of at least three particles thickness were inserted in the femur of dogs. Instron mechanical tests revealed that implants with a pore size of 20 to 50 μm were significantly less stable in bone than were implants with greater pore sizes. The maximal shear strength of fixation was of the order of 17 MPa. The authors suggested that the most appropriate pore size for their porous implants would be between 50 and 400 μm. In fact, Hulbert *et al.* (1969) showed that a pore size of 100 μm was necessary for bone ingrowth whereas a minimal of 150 μm seemed necessary for osteon formation. The data by Hulbert *et al.* (1969) were verified by

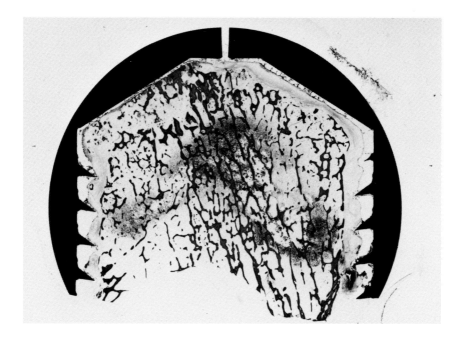

Fig. 3b

Albrektsson (1979). The latter author used a commercially pure titanium implant with a built-in optical system so that actual bone ingrowth could be studied in the live animal by the use of vital microscopy. The implant was manufactured in such a way that bone could invade one single macropore, the size of which was altered between 25 and 400 μm. Occasionally bone ingrowth was observed in pores of a size of only 70 μm, but in such cases the bone never matured properly. Actual Haversian canals were seen with pore sizes of 150 μm or more (Albrektsson, 1979; 1986) (Fig. 4).

Clemow *et al.* (1981) addressed the different question of optimal shear strength and stiffness of porous implants and came to the conclusion that the implant stability in the bone bed increased with decreasing pore size in the range of 325 to 175 μm. Bobyn (1977) compared interfacial shear strengths between a single and a multiple particle layer and came to the conclusion that the multiple particle layer resulted in an increase of 12% in shear strength, everything else being equal. These findings were later confirmed in another study by Bobyn *et al.* (1980). Inserting plates with pore sizes varying between 5 and 200 μm in a soft tissue bed. Bobyn *et al.* (1982) were able to demonstrate an increasing tissue attachment with increasing pore size and with increasing time of implantation up to the termination of the experiment at 16 weeks.

The early clinically used porous implants had pores all along the implant stem (Engh, 1983; Engh *et al.*, 1984) whereas more modern designs seem to

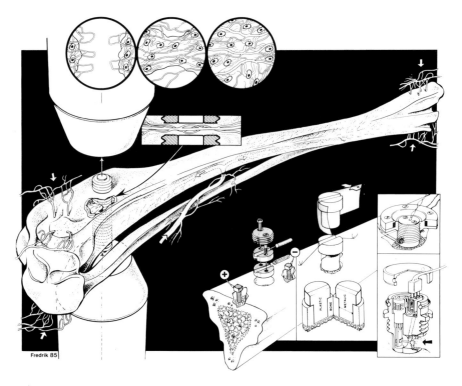

Fig. 4 Various types of experimental implants used by the author to study bone ingrowth under different circumstances.

prefer to have only the proximal portion of the stem porous (Engh and Bobyn, 1985). In an experimental study, Turner *et al.* (1986; 1987) were able to demonstrate that a stem with a circumferential coating seemed to stimulate bone resorption much more than designs with less abundant coatings.

Retrieval Studies of Porous Coated Implants. In the last few years several retrieval studies of porous coated implants have been published. Engh *et al.* (1987) examined 11 retrieved specimens of porous-coated cobalt-chrome femoral implants. The follow-up time varied from 4 weeks to 7 years, the extent of porous coating extended between $^2/_3$ to the entire length of the implants and the pore size was 250 μm with the exception of the two longest followed-up cases that had a pore size of 100 μm. The cases were mainly autopsies, i.e., the retrieval study was not based on failed femoral components. In 9 out of 11 cases there was evidence of bone ingrowth in the pores. The authors indicated that the bone ingrowth primarily occurred at places where the implant was adjacent to cortical structures. There were no exact attempts to quantify the ingrown bone, but it was observed that large portions of the porous surface contained no bone and, thereby, did not contribute to implant fixation. Cook *et al.* (1988) examined 16 femoral porous-coated components from 12 patients that were retrieved in spite of no apparent clinical loosening. The follow-up time in this study spanned over 3 weeks to 24 months (average 10.1 months). The findings were that approximately one third of the hip components had no bone ingrowth or apposition, one third had bone ingrowth in less than 2% of the porous surface area, and the remaining one third had between 2 and 10% of the available porous area ingrown with bone or in apposition with bone. The great proportion of all porous specimens contained soft tissue. The greatest amount of bone was observed in the distal portions of the porous coatings where occasionally there was bone ingrowth to the solid core of the device. The authors concluded that extensive bone ingrowth is not a predictable event in porous-coated femoral stems. In a separate paper, partly based on the same material as that described by Cook *et al.* (1988), Thomas *et al.* (1987) stated that there may be no obvious differences in ingrowth charac- teristics among the different types of porous coatings that were investigated in the study. Bobyn *et al.* (1987) described the retrieval of a porous femoral prosthesis that likewise had very little bone in contact with the metal at a follow-up period of 7 years. Dichiara *et al.* (1987) reported the retrieval of one femoral component after 2 months of implantation when the patient died of unrelated causes. There was a dense fibrous tissue membrane of a thickness of 50 to 100 μm seen along the prosthetic core and surrounding many of the beads. In other locations there was evidence of some woven bone apposing the porous surface. Collier *et al.* (1988), in their examination of 104 femoral porous hip stems that were retrieved for various reasons including loosening, found that at least 28 of their specimens showed regions of bone ingrowth.

Experimental and Retrieval Studies of Mesh Implants.   *Titanium mesh implants* that may be looked upon as a special variety of porous implants were first described by Galante *et al.* (1971) (Fig. 5). Whereas the core of the mesh prostheses generally is manufactured from Ti-6A1-4V, the meshwork itself is made from c.p. titanium. Heck *et al.* (1984), in a canine study, found that different types of soft tissue invaded the meshwork depending on the loading of the prostheses. If there were initial relatively stable conditions a more organized fibrous tissue was found compared to the case where immediate loading was allowed. In another canine study Turner *et al.* (1986) compared various types of porous coatings, among those fiber mesh, with respect to bone ingrowth. There was a substantial bone ingrowth in these components. There was no definite difference in bone response to ordinary porous-coated and mesh implants at 1 month after surgery. However, at 6 months there were indications of an increase of bone invasion in the mesh resulting in a significantly higher proportion of bone in this type of ingrowth prosthesis. Bragdon *et al.* (1989) investigated the bone ingrowth in canine femoral implants where the mesh was confined to the medial, anterior, and posterior surfaces of the proximal half of the implant. At 6 months of follow-up it

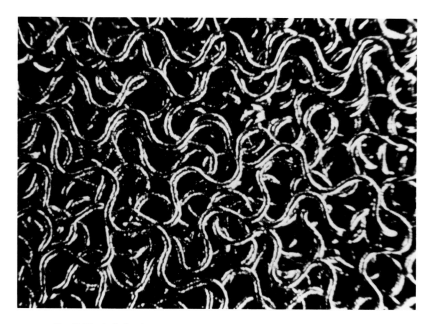

Fig. 5 Typical titanium mesh work used as porous coating on prostheses.

was observed that the percentage of the void space within the porous layer that was occupied by bone varied between 10 and 25%. However, at the same time there was evidence of an average decrease in cortical thickness of some 50%.

In the above summarized retrieval paper by Cook *et al.* (1988), there were three femoral mesh components analyzed. Again, these contained mainly fibrous tissue. Sumner *et al.* (1988), however, analyzed 16 femoral components, with meshwork in the proximal half only, that had been removed from patients for reasons other than loosening between 1 and 33 months after insertion. All these components contained bone in the meshwork, in one case the volume fraction of bone ingrowth was as much as 70%.

Clinical Results of Porous Coated and Mesh Hip Prostheses. Some examples of the clinical outcome of press-fit porous and mesh prostheses will be summarized. It must be observed that the clinical follow-up time is limited to about 2 to 5 years. Engh *et al.* (1987) reported on a study of 307 patients with a 2-year follow-up and 89 patients with a 5-year follow-up of the porous-coated AML-prosthesis. Some 14% of the patients had mid-thigh pain and there was evidence of resorptive remodeling of the proximal part of the femur in many cases. Callaghan *et al.* (1988) reported the clinical outcome of 50 porous-coated anatomic total hip prostheses. Of these, 18 and 16% of the patients complained about pain at 1 and 2 years of follow-up, respectively, and 28% of the patients had a moderate or severe limp. A radiodense femoral line was observed in 41% of the cases and loosened beads in 24%. Galante (1987) reported about 104 mesh hips where 26% of the patients had slight to moderate pain and one patient had severe pain at a follow-up that ranged between 12 and 24 months. Of these patients, 47% had a moderate to slight limp, whereas one patient had a severe limp. Decreased density of the medial femoral cortex was observed in a large number of the patients and radiolucencies were commonly seen around the convex portion of the prosthesis, proximally in the trochanteric region and at the tip of the device.

Granulated Prostheses

Experimental Studies on Macrorough and Microrough Surfaces. Experimental studies with granulated tantalum and niobium femoral stems have been performed by Plenk and co-workers (1983). The stems had conical surface grooves with a diameter of 0.9 mm. After follow-up times of up to 18 months it was found that the majority of the implanted stems were clinically stable and showed evidence of direct bone contact with the metal, either along the entire length of the stem or only in the middle and distal sections of it. There was no exact quantification of the proportion of the bone to metal and soft tissue to metal contact. However, at a longer follow-up of 13 such grooved niobium femoral stems, it was concluded that there was a radiographically observable decrease of apparent bone to implant contact after a follow-up of 12 months. Nevertheless, the majority of the implanted stems remained functional up to the termination of the experiment at 33 months after implantation (Gottsauner-Wolf *et al.*, 1987).

Itami *et al.* (1982) compared various types of granulated surfaces histologically as well as biomechanically. They inserted wedge-shaped implants in canine femora and tested those at 8 to 10 weeks. A non-cemented pagoda-shaped implant was found to have double resistance compared to a cemented similar implant in the tensile test. However, a smooth wedge without fenestrations was found to be much easier to remove than were the cemented implants. A granulated hip prosthesis was inserted by the same authors in dogs for a follow-up of up to 3 years. Mainly soft tissue was found in the stem interface, but there was some evidence of new bone formation as well (Itami *et al.*, 1982).

Schatzker *et al.* (1989) used a Müller type (CoNiCrMo) femoral component very similar to the clinically used version that has longitudinal grooves. They inserted these implants in dogs that were followed up for 4, 8, and 12 months. Prostheses with collar were all stable and direct bone contact was observed in the proximal and distal $^1/_3$ of the implant stem. The proportion of soft and hard tissue in the interface was not determined. However, it was observed that there were no histiocytes or giant cells or any sign of inflammation in the soft tissue.

Clinical Studies of Granulated Prostheses. Refior *et al.* (1988) have summarized their experience with the 1400 PM-type of granulated titanium alloy prostheses. These devices have been used in various surface modifications, one of those provided with a plasmapore c.p. titanium plasma coating in the proximal region of the stem. Clinical results have been positive although the follow-up was limited to 7 years.

The Madreporique hip prosthesis (Lord et al., 1979) is a granulated, macroporous device that has been followed for a long time. The original Madreporique prosthesis had a surface enlargement of small balls all over the stem that was manufactured from a chrome-cobalt alloy. In a dog study it was concluded that prosthesis stability was achieved in most cases although the bone was always separated from the implant by a thin membrane of fibrous tissue. The clinical results of 300 implanted hips were rated as positive over a follow-up period of 1 to 4 years (Lord et al., 1979). In a 7-year follow-up (Lord and Bancel, 1983) 1509 Madreporic implants were reviewed again with a good clinical result. Three Madreporic prostheses were retrieved at 40 days, 11 months, and 2 $1/2$ years after insertion, respectively, in no case because of loosening problems. There was better bone-metal contact in the lower part of the implant. There were patches of a probable direct bone to implant contact, but generally there was a thin soft tissue membrane interposed (Portigliatti Barbos et al., 1987; Portigliatti Barbos, 1988) (Fig. 6a, b).

Wykman (1989) compared two groups, each of 75 matched patients who received either a Charnley cemented or a HP-Garche granulated uncemented prosthesis made of chrome-cobalt alloy. Apart from a more rapid recovery with the cemented patients there were, according to the author, no significant differences between the two groups at a follow-up of 5 years. However, it must be observed that 14 patients had to be re-operated due to loosening after 2 to 5 years of follow-up. Most of these patients had mid-thigh pains.

Another extensively followed granulated (although microrough) cement-free implant system is the Ring hip prosthesis (Ring, 1968). The early Ring design was a metal-on-metal prosthesis which was regarded as the reason for somewhat higher revision percentage than found with cemented implants at 5 years of follow-up (Ring, 1983). Indeed, with a changed plastic on metal (cobalt-chrome) design, the results improved as reported in a 2- to 7-year follow-up of a total of 1488 patients (Nunn, 1988). A similar good success rate of 238 Ring prostheses followed for more than 10 years was reported by Albrecht-Olsen et al. (1989).

Other investigators have preferred ceramic materials such as Al_2O_3 with a microrough surface (Griss and Heimke, 1981) or titanium (to provide stability) coated with aluminum oxide (Trentani et al., 1987). The Zweymüller prosthesis, originally manufactured from Titanium-6Aluminum-4Vanadium alloy, was in 1985 changed to Ti-6Al-7NB material. This latter prosthesis has a microrough granulated surface with material irregularities of the order of 3 to 5 μm (Zweymüller et al., 1988). At insertion of this implant only rasps are required, no rotary drills that are more prone to

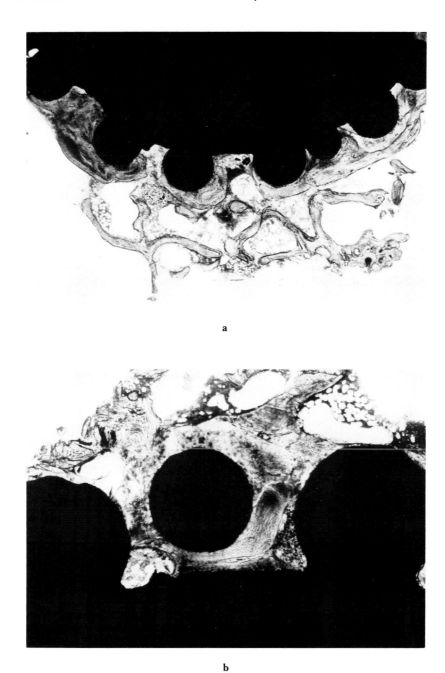

a

b

Fig. 6 (a) Retrieved granulated prostheses generally demonstrate a soft tissue interface between bone and metal. **(b)** Bone may, however, occassionally, invade the granulated coating so that the interface consists of a mixture of soft and hard tissue.

cause thermal damage. Retrieval analyses of two patients who died from pulmonary embolism 3 weeks after implant surgery showed, not surprisingly, old, pre-existing bone trabeculae in contact with the metal stem. However, retrieved specimens from patients analyzed between 3months and 2 years after implantation also showed many zones of the implant in good contact with bone without any interposed soft tissue. However, the exact proportion of bone to implant contact was not quantified. The Zweymüller design does not limit the microroughness to any special part of the stem. The reported clinical results with this prosthesis that in various forms have been inserted in more than 40,000 patients have been very good (Zweymüller, 1986; Zweymüller et al., 1988).

Metal Coating With Bioglass, TCP, or HA Ceramics. Various coating techniques, as a rule producing microrough granulated surfaces, have been advocated too; hydroxyapatite-coating has particularly received some clinical interest (Cook et al., 1988; Geesink, 1988). In principle, of course, coatings may be applied to any type of implant, but the technique has most frequently been used in conjunction with granulated prostheses which is why I will discuss them under this heading. In most studies, coatings of various ceramics have been used as these materials have been regarded as more acceptable to the tissues than are metallic materials. Whether or not this is a correct hypothesis cannot be debated. The reason for not using bulk ceramics is that these materials, as a rule, are too brittle to function mechanically. The first such coating aimed at what has been referred to as "bioactive fixation" was bioglass developed by Hench and co-workers (1971). Although bioglass is interesting from a theoretical standpoint its use as a coating of orthopedic and other similar load-bearing implants has not been realized. According to Hench (1987), the major limitation of bioglass coating is the limited stability of the metal-glass interface. This interface is very susceptible to attack by water and other body fluids. Lemons et al. (1988) have criticized hydroxyapatite-coatings with the same reasoning and coatings with TCP (an HA-related ceramic) have been demonstrated to become loose in clinical retrieval studies (Edge, 1988). Nevertheless, Eschenroder et al. (1987) found a significantly increased resistance of TCP-coated implants at a tensile test 6 months after implantation in dog femurs in comparison to data from uncoated chrome-cobalt rods. Geesink (1988) demonstrated that HA-coated canine hip stems showed direct contact with bone at a follow-up of 2 years. Geesink (1988) furthermore presented clinical results of the first 50 patients followed for up to 2 years. The short-term clinical outcome was good. Other materials that have been used as metal coatings in experimental and clinical studies include proplast (Homsy, 1973) and other polymers (Spector et al., 1988; Magee et al., 1988). Again, direct bone contact has been described in animal experiments and preliminary clinical data have been positive. Various coating materials are indeed interesting, but they are not without risks. The present author agrees with Lemons

(1988) that broad-based human applications for orthopedic devices are still contraindicated. The present clinical use of coated implants should be limited to carefully controlled studies at various university centers (Fig. 7a,b).

Super Press Fit Prostheses

Although ordinary press-fit prostheses may be well adapted to the anchoring site, they are not individualized to the patient and there are definite gaps along the implant stem (Salzer *et al.*, 1983). Noble and co-workers (1988) investigated the anatomy of the femur and came to the conclusion that the shape of the femoral canal is much more variable than most contemporary designs of femoral components would indicate. Poss *et al.* (1988) described the topography of the "average" femur by serial sectioning of 26 cadaver bones, subsequent photography of those, and then digitizing the data. After having checked their findings in biomechanical tests, the authors constructed a "super press fit" femoral stem implant. At the time of reporting their data, however, the clinical follow-up of this design was limited to only six implants that had been followed for more than 6 months (Poss *et al.*, 1988). The further work of this research group has resulted in an optimally (with respect to insertability) shaped press-fit femoral implant (Robertson *et al.*, 1988; Walker and Robertson, 1988).

Another way of individualizing the implant to achieve a super-press fit would be to use a molding technique. Sennerby and co-workers (1987) have demonstrated that alginate can be used without tissue side effects to take *in vivo* "imprints" of bone and joint structures. De Waal Malefijt (1988) has used a mixture of elastomer and xanthopren to achieve a precise print of the femoral canal in animal experiments on pygmé goats. Again, this is an interesting approach that may have clinical possibilities as there are no known side effects of the molding material and this can be easily removed from the marrow cavity.

Threaded Prostheses

Longitudinally directed screws have been used in two hip joint designs to the knowledge of the present author, the Olmed prosthesis and the Engelhardt joint (Engelhardt, 1983). None of these prostheses seem to have been used much internationally. The Engelhardt device consists of an Al_2O_3 threaded femoral component that is aimed for anchorage along the walls of the marrow cavity. A similar approach was suggested for the anchorage of metacarpophalangeal implants by Hagert *et al.* (1986). One potential risk of such endosteally anchored screws is the physiological cortical shift that widens the marrow space, although proponents of longitudinally directed anchorage elements have suggested that the cortical structures will remain intact around a load-bearing implant.

Transversally directed screws are used frequently as fixation for plates, but

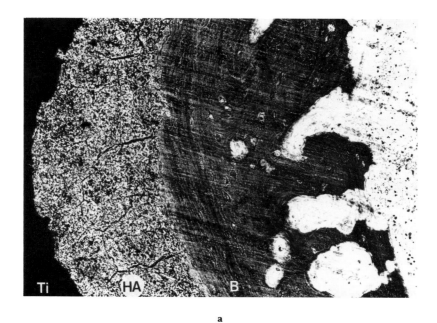

a

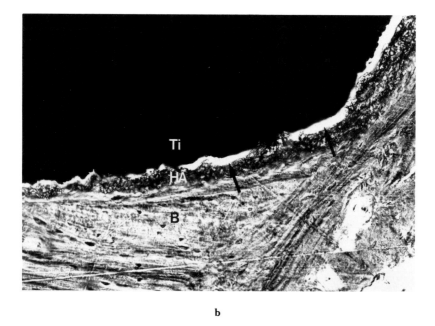

b

Fig. 7 (a) There is no doubt that HA-coated implants show good bone to implant contact. **(b)** However, there is a risk for loosening of the HA-coat (arrows) that may lead to secondary clinical problems.

not to the knowledge of the author for fixation of clinical knee or hip arthroplasties. There is experimental data that verify the possibility of using transversally oriented screws as load-bearing devices (Albrektsson, 1985) and in fixation of dynamically loaded canine knee joints (Albrektsson et al., 1989). An observation of potentially great clinical interest is the tendency to abundant bone conduction around transversally inserted screws (Strid, 1985; Johansson and Albrektsson, 1987; Röstlund et al., 1989). Titanium screws inserted in the mandible of man or the femur or tibia of experimental animals do as a rule elicit a clear condensation of bone around the devices, bone that extend from the cortex down into the medullary space. This means that the screws will be more fixed in the bone with increasing time of implantation. Such bone conduction has been described with other designs than screws and in response to other materials than titanium, but in much less quantities. Strid (1985) used a computerized densitometry technique and could clearly demonstrate that the bone conduction was evident in as good as every clinical case a year or more after implantation insertion. The non-cemented hip, knee, and metacarpophalangeal joint replacements developed at our clinic are all, in part, based on such transversally directed screws (Albrektsson and Albrektsson, 1987; Carlsson, 1989; Röstlund, 1990). The function in experimental animals has been most promising (Röstlund et al., 1989), but all these devices are as yet clinically untested.

Tissue Response to Knee Prostheses

Generally speaking, knee prostheses in the past have shown a less good clinical outcome than have hip prostheses. Particularly problematic has been the fixation of the tibial component. Nevertheless, much of the observations on tissue response to various types of hip implant designs are valid for the knee too. Therefore, I will condense this overview on knee prostheses to three subheadings: experimental observations, retrieval studies, and clinical results.

Experimental observations on knee arthroplasties — Ducheyne and co-workers (1977) found only soft tissue anchoring experimental stainless steel knee joints inserted in the dog. Bobyn et al. (1982) inserted canine porous cobalt-based femoral metal implants articulating against a tibial component of ultra-high molecular weight polyethylene. At animal sacrifice up to 1 year after implantation it was observed that bone had invaded the femoral implant anteriorly as well as posteriorly. However, there was evidence of a gradual femoral bone resorption with time. The plastic tibial component always showed a soft tissue membrane interposed between bone and implant. A similar soft tissue membrane was observed between polyethylene tibial plateau implants and bone in a canine study of ICLH-implants. Also, retrieved clinical specimens showed a similar soft tissue reaction (Freeman et al., 1981) (Fig. 8a through c).

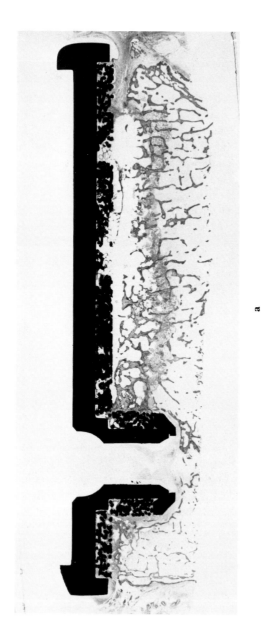

a

Fig. 8 (a) Most commonly, there is poor bone ingrowth in tibial components of knee arthroplasties. **(b)** However, there are locations, particularly at the site of cortical penetrating studs, where bone may be seen invading the porous structures. **(c)** Individual photographs may, therefore, show abundant bone ingrowth. The actual load-bearing capacity of this bone is, however, uncertain. (With permission of Lars Carlsson, M.D., Ph.D.)

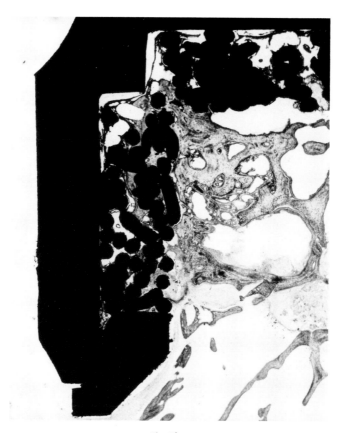

Fig. 8b

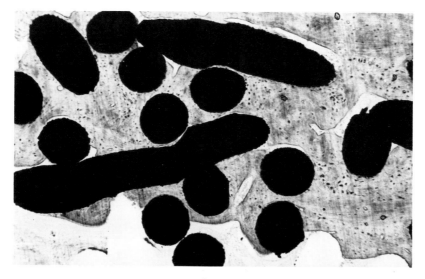

Fig. 8c

The initial mechanical stability of the tibial component is one parameter that will determine its clinical fate. Volz *et al.* (1988) compared four different clinical designs inserted in human cadaver tibias that were loaded in a mechanical apparatus. A design with four central screws only allowed for movements within 100 μm, a titanium mesh prosthesis and one with a central polythylene peg showed a movement of some 200 μm whereas a commonly used porous-coated design with two tilted metallic components for stability showed no less than 500 μm of movement.

Retrieval studies of knee arthroplasties — Cook *et al.* (1986) reported a case with revision of a porous-coated, cobalt-chrome knee arthroplasty after 11 months of clinical function. There was no ingrowth of calcified tissue, but numerous multinucleated giant cells adjacent to the porous metal.

Mayor and Collier (1986) summarized their observations of 60 retrieved knee replacement devices. The authors found no bone ingrowth in the tibial specimens, occasional slight bone ingrowth in the patellar sections and more regular bone ingrowth in the femoral components. Dichiara *et al.* (1987), on the other hand, observed what was referred to as "excellent bone ingrowth" in the posterior portion of the tibial porous coating of two PCA chrome-cobalt implants; however, there was a soft tissue coat all around the prosthetic core and around some of the beads. The femoral components showed some bone ingrowth mainly in the anterior parts at the follow-up of 7 and 13 months, respectively. There was bone ingrowth in the patellar portion too, but again the femoral, as well as the patellar, parts of the prostheses showed a soft tissue membrane lining the core of the devices. The same research group reported about a retrieval analysis of 5 PCA-prostheses from autopsy or amputation cases after 8 to 44 months of clinical function without any signs of loosening. They described the tissue reactions in four different zones: the immediate tissue implant interface where there was a dense fibrous layer (50 to 100 μm thick); the bead tissue interface which predominantly was a loose fibrous connective tissue; the immediate "beadless" marrow space that contained trabecular bone running parallel to the cut section of the prosthesis; the marrow space at a distance greater than 2 mm away from the implant that consisted of essentially normal trabecular marrow. The first two zones being closest to the implant had the lowest percentage of bone, between 6 and 10% average for tibia and femur, respectively. There was more bone ingrowth in the patellar components (Dichiara and Higram, 1987; Vigorita *et al.*, 1989).

Thomas *et al.* (1987) and Cook *et al.* (1988) have presented a retrieval analysis of 62 total knee components from 34 patients. None of the components was removed because of clinical or radiological signs of loosening. The time of implantation varied between 2 weeks and 31 months with an average of 12 months. No component showed more than 10% of the available porous material invaded by bone. In summary, the results very much resembled the findings from bone ingrowth into clinically retrieved porous-coated hip implants published in the same paper: one third of the components contained no bone, one third had an ingrowth in less than 2% of the porous surface, whereas the remaining one third showed bone ingrowth varying between 2 and 10% of the available intra-porous area. In all cases it was observed that the majority of the implant surface was separated from the bone by a dense fibrous tissue layer that could be up to 2 mm in thickness. In some components with a greater bone ingrowth a fibrous tissue orientation in a radial mode away from the implant surface was observed. This seems to be similar to the previous description of fibrous tissue anchorage by Pilliar *et al.* (1981).

In contrast, Sumner *et al.* (1989) examined ten retrieved clinical specimens from titanium mesh tibial plateaus that had been fixed with four screws, i.e., similar to the design shown to have the least movement in the test by Volz *et al.* (1988). None of the components was removed because of loosening. They were analyzed between 6 weeks and 38 months after insertion. Only one implant showed bone ingrowth of less than 5% whereas the remaining nine implants had more than 10% bony ingrowth.

Clinical results of cement-free knee replacements — The present overview is aimed at tissue reactions to non-cemented implants, not at clinical results. Results are difficult to compare because of differing patient materials, various ways of establishing success rates, and varying numbers of drop-out patients in different studies. However, evaluation of clinical results is after all one way to analyze long-term tissue reactions to biomaterials that is not possible in animal experiments that seldom are run more than 1 year. An up-to-date summary of some publications of long-term results with various non-cemented knee replacement devices indicates that most modern techniques of knee arthroplasty have resulted in a clinical success of 75% or more for a follow-up of 5 to 10 years (Barck, 1988; Callea *et al.*, 1986; Donaldson *et al.*, 1988; Kershaw and Themen, 1988; Knutson *et al.*, 1986; Marmor, 1988; Ranawat and Boachie-Adjel, 1988; Rand and Coventry, 1988; Ring, 1988).

On Radiography, Radiolucent Lines, and Implant Micromotion

A very high incidence of radiographical loosening has been reported in cemented arthroplasties. Cotterill *et al.* (1982) described this phenomenon in 73% of all examined hips. Johnston and Crowningshield (1983) did also report on a continuous increase of radiolucency around inserted hip joints but saw no correlation between their radiographical results and the actual incidence of clinical loosening. Hodgkinson *et al.* (1988), on the other hand, saw a strong correlation between radiographically "demarcated" sockets, socket migration, and clinical loosening. Gottsauner-Wolf *et al.* (1987) in their canine experiments with cement-free femoral stems, observed the development of radiographical radiolucency around 5 of 13 operated stems and found those same 5 stems to be clinically loose at sacrifice.

Obviously, it seems difficult to establish any clear correlation between radiographical and clinical loosening. To be at all possible to evaluate it seems that very controlled radiographical techniques will have to be applied (Amstutz, 1985; Bobyn *et al.*, 1988). It has been observed in many cases that the occurrence of a radiolucent line is equivalent to a histologically observed soft tissue interface (Amstutz, 1985; Engh *et al.*, 1987), but not even this statement is necessarily true in all cases. After all, even an optimal radiographical technique has a maximal resolution capacity of 0.1 mm whereas the size of a soft tissue cell is 0.01 mm. Any histological statement based on radiography alone, therefore, remains uncertain. As demonstrated by Hagert *et al.* (1986), there is, furthermore, a tendency of the human eye to overestimate the degree of radiolucency based on the fact that the implant is very radiopaque and that everything else in its vicinity will seem "black" and without bone. Hagert *et al.* (1986) performed a density analysis of implant radiograms with a computerized IBAS system and were able to demonstrate that what was perceived as soft tissue in many cases had the actual density of hard tissue.

Ordinary radiography is not a suitable method for demonstrating implant migration in most cases. Freeman *et al.* (1978) in a study of knee arthroplasty, reported a 12.5% incidence of tibial implant sinkage, a problem that seemed to disappear with the use of larger tibial components. However, with refined techniques involving stereoradiography and tantalum markers, every cemented and non-cemented tibial implant that was investigated in another study did, in fact, migrate (Ryd, 1986). In addition, all prostheses showed inducible micromotion in the study by Ryd (1986) (Fig. 9). It will be of great interest to correlate the degree of observed migration/inducible micromotion with long-term clinical success which will be possible in studies where controlled radiographical techniques are used (Ryd, 1986; Mjöberg, 1986; Zalenski *et al.*, 1989).

On Corrosion, Metal Leakage, Allergy, and Carcinogenesis of Implant Materials

There are several potential metallurgically derived problems with cement-free implants, one of those being the loss of beads from porous coatings. This phenomenon has been reported by several authors and its relation to implant failure has been indicated (Fig. 10) (Buchert *et al.*, 1986; Cheng and Gross, 1988; Davey and Harris, 1988; Morrey and Chao, 1988; Rosenqvist *et al.*, 1986). The purpose of this review is not to give a detailed summary of corrosion, local and systemic metal accumulation, and all possible consequences thereof. The interested reader is referred to the excellent reviews by Williams (1982a, b), Michel (1987), and Finnegan (1989). From these papers it may be concluded that metal ions will always leak out, more or less abundantly, from orthopedic implants and may accumulate locally as well in distant organs such as lung or neural tissue. One risk with such leakage is the development of metal allergy. A metal allergy, irrespective of

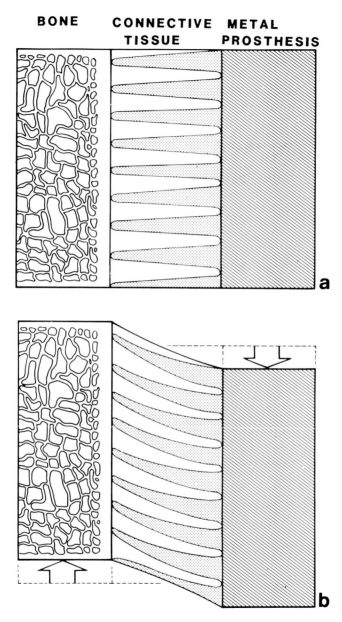

Fig. 9 A soft tissue anchored prosthesis will always show an inducible micromotion when analyzed with controlled two-dimensional radiography.

whether it has been elicited through ion leakage from an implant or through other kinds of metallic exposure may, of course, endanger the fate of hip and knee arthroplasties. In fact, Merrit (1987) estimated that 15% of the normal human population is allergic to metal as manifested by skin testing. Elves *et al.* (1975) and Peltonen (1987) referred to several cases of allergy

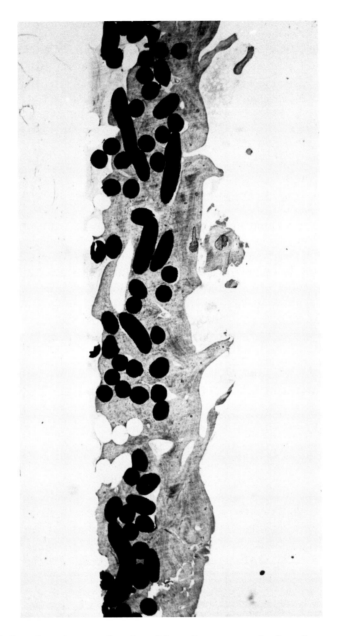

Fig. 10 Sometimes there may be a loss of the entire porous coating from the metallic stem.

to cobalt. For instance, in the study by Elves *et al.* (1975) 28% of the patients having metal-to-metal prostheses had a positive skin test for cobalt in comparison to 1.5% of the control group. To the knowledge of the present author there is only one report of allergy to titanium (Peters *et al.*, 1988).

Also, when tumors in relation to implants are concerned, the great majority have been reported in relation to chrome-cobalt implants (Bago-Granell *et al.*, 1984; Bauer *et al.*, 1987; Dodion *et al.*, 1982; Hughes *et al.*, 1987; vanderList *et al.*, 1988; McDonald, 1981; Penman and Ring, 1984; Swann, 1984) even if there are single reports of sarcoma in association with aluminum oxide implants too (Ryu *et al.*, 1985). Even if the exact proportion of tumors has to be related to the exact amount of implanted devices, it seems as if chrome-cobalt alloy shows more such side reactions than do other commonly used materials.

The problem with tumors and allergy to implant materials is a complicated one. Theoretically, the risk would seem to be greatest, everything else being equal, with cement-free implants that have considerable surface enlargements leading to an extensive contact zone with the tissues, a contact zone that may amount to square meters. On the one hand there are very few reports of allergy and tumors in relation to the annual amount of millions of inserted orthopedic implants, on the other hand most of those have a relatively short-term follow-up and the risk is probably increased with an increased time of exposure. At the present time it seems reasonable only to remind orthopedic surgeons and other clinicians that we are in the first generation of inserting foreign devices in the body and that anyone who does this has a responsibility to carefully monitor all patients and to report possible side effects of the treatment.

On Bone Ingrowth

In summary, many studies have convincingly demonstrated an abundant bone invasion in the pores of canine experimental implants. In the case of human porous-coated implants, retrieved without signs of loosening, there is sparse ingrowth of bone if any at all. One reason for this may, of course, be species related (Hofmann *et al.*, 1988). Another possible explanation is offered by the findings of Magee *et al.* (1989) that young but adult dogs (average age 28.2 months) showed a significantly greater bone invasion in the pores of a femoral implant than did older dogs (average age 79.5 months). The average age of the patients in the study by Engh *et al.* (1987) was 76 years and in the study by Cook *et al.* (1988) 54 years. A third possible explanation is indicated by the findings by Volz *et al.* (1988) that screw fixation of the tibial plateau components showed a greater stability than did other designs (Fig. 11a through c) and the report by Sumner *et al.* (1989) that such screw-fixed tibial plateaus did result in quite a good bone ingrowth in retrieved human specimens. The average insertion time of the clinically retrieved specimens in that study was 16 months.

In summary, it seems that in most, if not all, cases of porous and granular hip and knee implants in current clinical use there is mainly a soft tissue anchorage. In fact, in the great majority of clinically retrieved cases the bone ingrowth is so minor that it seems likely that it has an insignificant

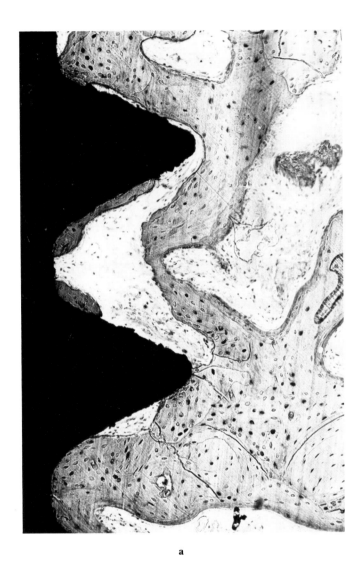

a

Fig. 11 **(a)** When examined after a short follow-up (3 months), there is a lot of soft tissue in
the typical screw interface. Figures 11a—c demonstrate the typical bone response to femoral,
unloaded c.p. titanium transverse screws. **(b)** At 6 months after insertion most of the interface
consists of bone. **(c)** At 12 months after implant insertion there is, generally, more than 90%
bony contact at the cortical passage.

load-bearing function. The load is taken fully by the fibrous tissue. The
occasional observation of some bone to implant contact in the case of
cement-free implants does not seem to be greater than similar observations
with cemented devices (Linder and Hansson, 1983). In neither case is the
use of a terminology such as osseointegration verified (Fig. 12a, b). The

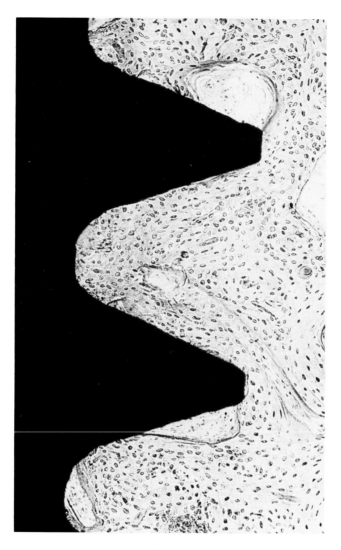

Fig. 11b

present author is of the opinion that such soft-tissue anchored devices are always in the risk zone of overloading and if overloading occurs the soft tissue anchorage will gradually fail. I will conclude this paper by presenting six conditions that will have to be more or less simultaneously controlled to allow for a bone anchorage of an implant and try to give a review of these six factors in relation to the actual situation in today's clinical practice with cement-free implants.

Material Biocompatibility

Of currently used orthopedic implants roughly $1/3$ are made of stainless

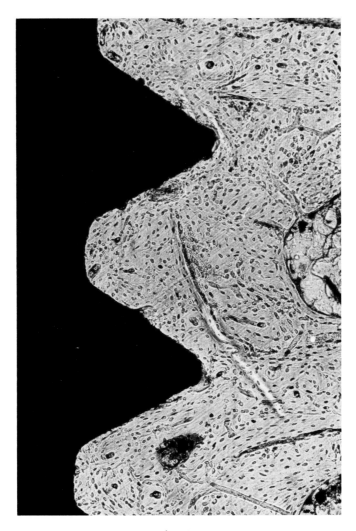

Fig. 11c

steel, $^1/_3$ of chrome-cobalt alloy, and $^1/_3$ of titanium alloy. Stainless steel does corrode in the body and stainless steel, therefore, has not been recommended in newer types of porous-coated implants (Fig. 13). However, chrome-cobalt alloys are neither ideal from a tissue point of view, reflected by the many reports of tumors associated with this material. In a comparison between bone ingrowth into canine and human porous implants of either chrome-cobalt or titanium, it was observed that the latter showed more ingrowth than did chrome-cobalt (Hofmann *et al.*, 1988). The findings by Linder and Lundskog (1975) and Linder (1989) that stainless steel, chrome-cobalt alloy as well as Titanium-6Aluminum-4Vanadium all showed a direct bone-to-implant interface in experimental studies may seem to

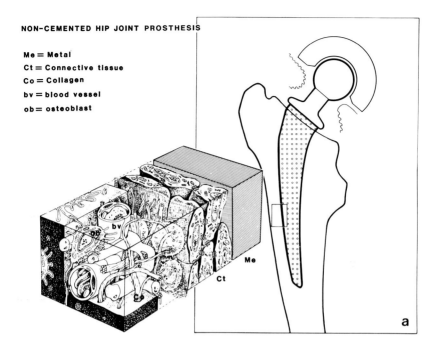

NON-CEMENTED HIP JOINT PROSTHESIS

Me = Metal
Ct = Connective tissue
Co = Collagen
bv = blood vessel
ob = osteoblast

a

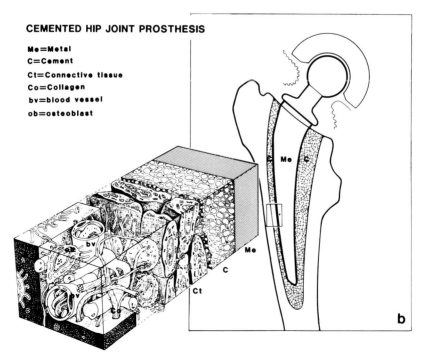

CEMENTED HIP JOINT PROSTHESIS

Me=Metal
C=Cement
Ct=Connective tissue
Co=Collagen
bv=blood vessel
ob=osteoblast

b

Fig. 12 Cemented **(a)** as well as non-cemented **(b)** hip joint implants of conventional designs will, as a rule, demonstrate a soft tissue interface, even if there may be points of direct bony contact.

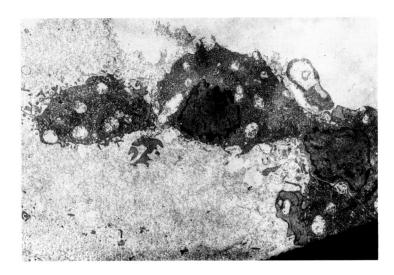

Fig. 13 The interface between bone and stainless steel will often consist of soft tissue with some inflammatory cells.

contradict the notion that currently used metallic biomaterials in hip and knee arthroplasty are not very ideal ones. However, the observations of Linder refer to qualitative studies, not to quantified ones. When the tissue response to Titanium-6Aluminum-4Vanadium was compared to c.p. titanium in a quantified study, the results differed from those of Linder (1989). Johansson et al. (1989; 1990) observed significantly more bone in the interface of their experimental c.p. titanium implants (Fig. 14a, b). Similar findings in favor of c.p. titanium have been reported in comparative studies with gold, stainless steel, and zirconium (Albrektsson et al., 1982; Albrektsson et al., 1983; Albrektsson and Hansson, 1986; Albrektsson et al., 1985), whereas there were no significant differences when c.p. titanium was compared to tantalum or niobium (Johansson et al., 1990). The observed differences in tissue reactions in favor of c.p. titanium compared to currently used implant materials may, thus, seem to be evident, but it must be kept in mind that we don't know if these differences are of a magnitude that is of clinical significance. Nevertheless, the reports of leaking aluminum from titanium-6Al-4V implants may seem to be slightly alarming and no biocompatibility studies of the commercially pure titanium may be regarded as valid for the alloy (Albrektsson and Albrektsson, 1987).

Implant Design

Currently used cement-free implant designs are dominated by porous or granulated stems that do not show an ideal adaptation to the host bed. Carlsson et al. (1986) compared plates, irregular cylinders, and screws of c.p. titanium and found the latter design to show the highest degree of bony contact. The reason for the advantage of the screw may be the better initial fit to the bone bed wit the screw design compared to, for instance, a granulated implant design (Carlsson *et al.*, 1988). However, there is contradictory evidence also exemplified by the experimental study by Maniatoupolous *et al.* (1986) who found that canine porous implants showed a greater resistance to removal than did threaded implants in a directly loading situation.

A screw design may be exactly adapted to the bone bed and receive an immediate mechanical interlock. Fixation pegs or stem devices oriented along the axis of a tubular bone are more prone to interfacial shear stresses than are transversally oriented devices. Due to a mismatch in elastic modulus between a metallic implant and bone, high bending stresses encountered for instance in conventional hip prostheses may result in undue movements between the implant and its bed. An implant model that relies on a series of transversally oriented screws may, on the other hand, have biomechanical advantages that will favor an osseous fixation. There are a great number of clinical reports on the excellent outcome of screw-shaped oral implants that have become directly bone-anchored (Brånemark *et al.*, 1977; Albrektsson *et al.*, 1988a, b; Albrektsson and Lekholm, 1989) (Fig. 15a through c).

Even if previously used hip and knee implants in many cases may be criticized for a relatively poor bone-implant fit, the super-press fit types described above may change this picture. However, we do not know if an initial super-press fit of the implant will be maintained or if bone remodeling with time will lead to less of a good match between bone and foreign material. Cemented implants do, generally, show an initial excellent fit between cement and bone, but due to shrinkage effects of the cement as well as to bone remodeling, this initial good press-fit does not remain.

Implant Surface

Little attention seems to have been given to the implant surface conditions in clinical hip and knee reconstructive surgery. Carlsson *et al.* (1988; 1989) investigated the importance of surface roughness and surface energy. Smooth c.p. titanium screws were found to have less of a good attachment to bone than did rough ones. Artificial increase of the surface energy did not, however, result in an improved implant take in experimental rabbit studies. A clinical study of the effects of surface energy is ongoing. The importance of a careful control of the surface conditions may be indicated by the findings of Albrektsson (1979) and Sennerby *et al.* (1988). The former author reported poor implant take when certain implants were reinserted in animals in spite of careful cleaning and sterilization; whereas the latter authors were able to quantitatively demonstrate an altered and more negative tissue response to reinserted implants in spite of the fact that those were thoroughly cleaned and sterilized.

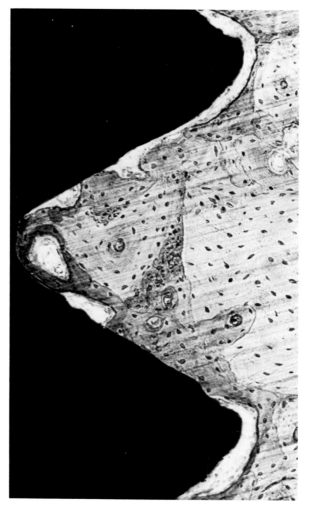

Fig. 14a

The Status of the Host Bed

Hip and knee implants are often introduced to bone beds that are of a potentially poor healing capacity. However, Linder *et al.* (1988) have demonstrated that a bone anchorage of titanium implants is possible in rheumatoid patients. Jacobsson (1985) and Jacobsson *et al.* (1985) have presented experimental evidence of the possibility of having implants bone-anchored in spite of previous irradiation in therapeutic doses, a finding later clinically verified by Jacobsson *et al.* (1988). The administration of various antiinflammatory drugs may also hamper the bone response to an implant (Longo *et al.*, 1989; Trancik *et al.*, 1989).

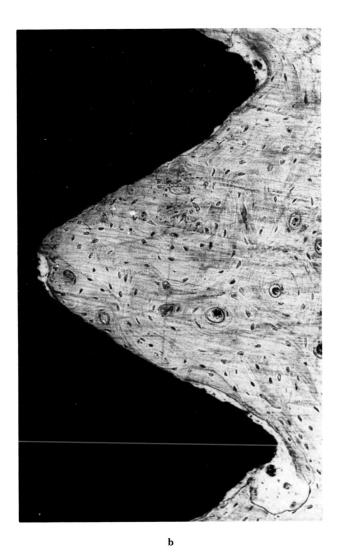

b

Fig. 14 (a) Typical interface between bone and Titanium-6Aluminum-4Vanadium experimental, tibial implant at some months after insertion. Observe the sparse patches of direct bony contact as well as the immature looking bone. **(b)** Typical interface between bone and c.p. titanium experimental, tibial implant at the same time of follow-up. There is a lot of direct bone to implant contact and the bone is much more mature compared to the alloy sample.

Needless to say, the best bone bed for an implant is healthy and without the influence of any disease or drugs. Another question is if it is possible to in one way or the other reinforce the bone healing response. Buch (1985), Buch *et al.* (1986), and Nannmark *et al.* (1985) used direct currents in attempts to stimulate the tissue response around bone implants. There was

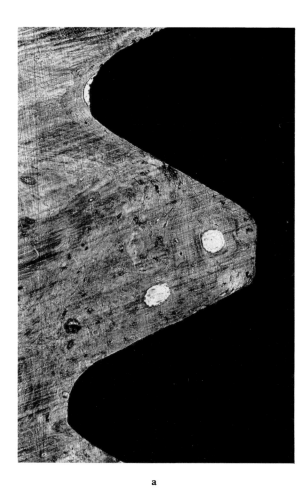

a

Fig. 15 Varying magnifications of a clinically retrieved craniofacial implant after more than 1 year of functional loading.

some evidence of an increased rate of bone healing (Buch *et al.*, 1986) presented after stimulation with 5 or 20 microA over 3 weeks, but it is uncertain if these findings are reproducible in the clinic. Nilsson *et al.* (1988) experimented with increasing the partial pressure of oxygen and found that this resulted in a significantly improved bone healing response as measured in experimental implants (Albrektsson *et al.* 1989). Other ways of accelerating the bone response around implants would be the addition of various types of bone-inducing agents or growth factors. In the clinical situation, however, we still have insufficient data to demonstrate if it is at all possible to accelerate a bone healing response. It could be that our various ways of reinforcements only work in the pathological situation, for instance, when too many vessels have been damaged so that there is a local need for more oxygen that otherwise is best transported through the bloodstream.

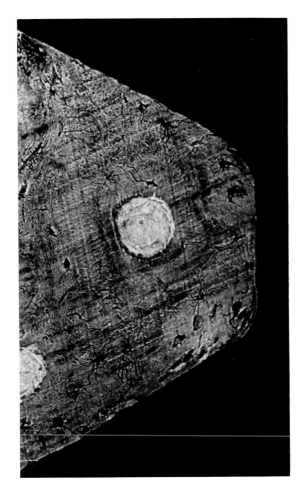

Fig. 15b

Surgical Technique

At the insertion of most conventional cement-free hip and knee implants there is considerable trauma to the tissues. Previous investigators have underestimated the drilling temperature (depending on the fact that most experiments were performed in animals with thin cortices) and overestimated the maximal heat bone tissue will tolerate. For example, at routine clinical insertion of screws to anchor a fracture plate, Eriksson *et al.* (1984) found that the average temperature elevation was around 91°C (Fig. 16), in spite of the fact that profuse cooling was administered. The critical temperature for bone necrosis is not 56°C as suggested by other investigators (Rhinelander *et al.*, 1979) but rather of the order of 47°C at 1 min of exposition (Eriksson and Albrektsson, 1983). Bone preparation as performed

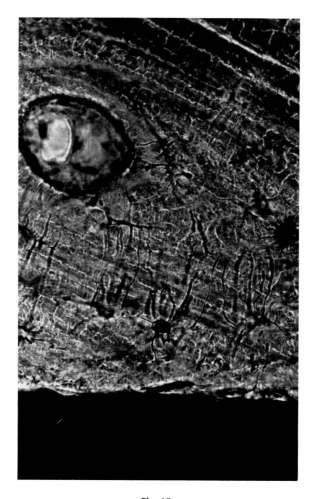

Fig. 15c

at many orthopedic clinics will result in permanent bone damage where bone will not heal as such but as low differentiated scar tissue (Eriksson, 1985).

Lindström *et al.* (1981) summarized several factors of importance to control the trauma in bone surgery. These factors involve the use of sharp instruments, avoid drill speeds above 1500 rpm, ensure profuse saline cooling and the use of a graded series of drill sizes instead of a one-stage large drill. Actually, Eriksson and Adell (1986), following these recommendations, demonstrated that it is quite possible to drill through solid cortical bone in the human mandible without even raising the body temperature. Jönsson *et al.* (1990) investigated another parameter with relevance to the surgical trauma, namely, the power used at insertion of screws. They found that screws inserted with a strong hand (average insertion torque around 35

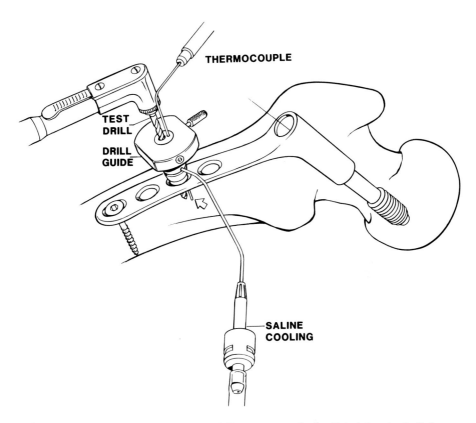

Fig. 16 Experimental design of measuring drill temperatures in the clinical situation by Eriksson et al. (1984). The average temperature at a distance of 0.5 mm away from the drill was 91°C, in spite of profuse saline cooling.

Ncm) became poorly stabilized whereas screws inserted with a gentle hand (around 10 Ncm) showed a rapid increase in torque needed for removal at 4 and 12 weeks after insertion.

Loading Conditions

Most authorities agree that early movements in the implant interface may cause problems for proper bone healing (Uhthoff, 1973; Cameron *et al.*, 1973; Schatzker *et al.*, 1975). At the same time, the obvious ambition for most orthopedic surgeons is to mobilize the hip and knee implant patient as rapidly as possible to avoid various medical complications. Brånemark *et al.* (1977) recommended that implants should remain unloaded for a time of minimally 3 months to allow for bone repair and primary anchorage. Johansson and Albrektsson (1987) have demonstrated that experimental titanium tibial screws that were not subjected to any dynamical load will gradually gain in holding power for at least a year after insertion. At the same time there was morphological evidence of more and more bone formed in the interface. At 3 weeks after insertion, for instance, there was absolutely no bone in the interface and the implant at this stage was in a particularly critical situation with respect to loading.

The way to overcome this seemingly unsolvable dilemma of the clinician's wish to early patient mobilization and the biologist's desire to avoid early loading is to realize that the patient need not be unloaded — only the implant. This may be possible through a specific type of two-stage surgical procedure where the first one does not involve the damaged joint, only the anchorage bone. Furthermore, Röstlund et al. (1989) have demonstrated that, at least in certain joints, a one-stage procedure is possible without preventing the subsequent bone anchorage of the implant. In the knee joint, for instance, it seems possible to use one-stage surgery for femoral components whereas two-stage surgery seems recommendable for tibial anchorage elements (Carlsson, 1989; Röstlund, 1990).

Concluding Remarks

Some authors would strongly suggest that a soft tissue interface is a desired goal in orthopedic implant surgery (Oh, 1987; Walker et al., 1984), whereas others (Albrektsson et al., 1981) see a soft membrane as an indication of imminent failure (Fig. 17). Nevertheless, present day cemented and cement-free implants will almost inevitably be largely anchored to bone through an interposed soft tissue layer (Hori and Lewis, 1982; Lennox et al., 1987). The great advantage of a bony interface is its remodeling capacity: if a full development of a direct bone anchorage will ensue, the long-term loads may be carried out in a far better way than a soft membrane is capable of (Skalak, 1983; Ling, 1986). However, direct bone anchorage necessitates the control of many parameters ranging from material factors to surgical and loading conditions (Figs. 18 through 20). In fact, poor control of only one of those factors will result in soft tissue embedment of a foreign material, no matter how well controlled all other factors are. The outcome of current clinical trials during the 1990s will indicate whether direct bone anchorage of orthopedic implants actually will function as well as the directly bone-anchored oral implants that have revolutionized dental implantology in the 1980s.

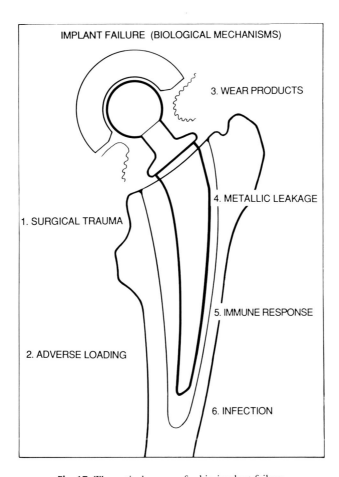

Fig. 17 Theoretical reasons for hip implant failure.

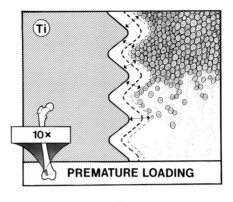

a

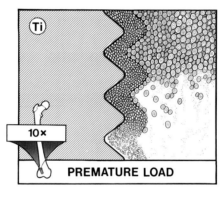

b

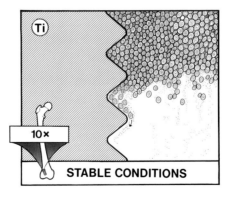

c

Fig. 18 (a) Premature loading leading to interfacial movements will prevent bone formation. (b) The end result of premature load is a soft tissue interface. (c) Stable conditions are necessary for a reliable bone response with subsequent bone conduction (arrow) along the implant.

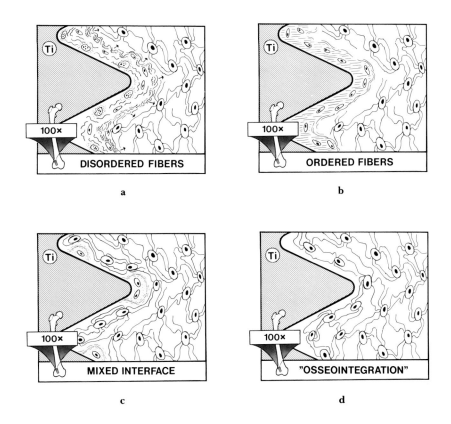

Fig. 19 (a) Implant surrounded by disordered fibers and inflammatory cells are prone to failure because of progressive bone resorption (arrows). (b) It has been discussed whether implants surrounded by ordered fibers with a thread direction perpendicular or oblique to the implant surface represents a clinically positive situation or whether this interfacial arrangement will be transferred to a disordered situation when subjected to overload. (c) The "mixed interface" situation with respect to bone and soft tissue is the one generally observed around bone-anchored screws if the entire interfacial arrangements of the implants are considered. (d) However, if the analysis is confined to certain regions, such as the cortical passage in the case of a transversally oriented screw, between 90 and 100% of the interface may be seen in direct bone contact. This may constitute a structural definition of osseointegration.

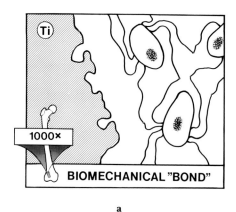

a

b

Fig. 20 **(a)** Provided bone, or perhaps tissue or collagen structures typical of bone, will invade a microrough surface and a biomechanical "bond" may result. There is experimental evidence that such a "bond" may occur with surfaces having irregularities of the size of 1–70 μm, i.e., too small irregularities to permit regular bone ingrowth. **(b)** At higher magnifications osteocyte canaliculae and collagen filaments have been observed approaching the titanium oxide interface with exceptance of a zone of 20–40 nm closest to the implant surface that only consists of cellular ground substance. The oxide surface of the metallic side of the interface seems to grow inwards during clinical conditions (arrows). However, we need more experimental data to verify if such interfacial reactions are generally found with clinically used c.p. titanium implants or whether they are only relevant for special, experimental implants. **(c)** There is a theoretical possibility of a chemical type of bonding between bone and implants. However, more studies will have to be devoted to this interesting area before we can state with any certainty whether such bonds actually occur or not.

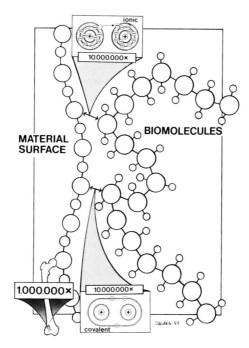

Fig. 20c

References

Albrecht-Olsen, P., Owen-Falkenberg, T., Burgaard, P., and Bögeskov Andersen, P. (1989). Nine-year follow up of the cementless Ring hip. *Acta Orthop.Scand.*, **60**: 77–80.

Albrektsson, B., Albrektsson, T., Carlsson, L., and Röstlund, T. (1989). The bone-anchored knee replacement. In: *The Brånemark Osseointegrated Implant*. Albrektsson, T. and Zarb, G., Eds., Quintessence, Berlin, 251–255.

Albrektsson, T. (1979). Healing of Bone Grafts. In Vivo Studies of Tissue Reactions at Autografting of Bone in the Rabbit Tibia. Ph.D. thesis, University of Gothenburg, Sweden.

Albrektsson, T. (1984). Osseous penetration rate into implants pretreated with bone cement. *Arch. Orthop. Traumatol. Surg.*, **102**: 141–147.

Albrektsson, T. (1985). The response of bone to titanium implants. *CRC Crit. Rev. Biocompat.*, **1**: 53–84.

Albrektsson, T. (1986). Implantable devices for long-term vital microscopy of bone tissue. *CRC Crit. Rev. Biocompat.*, **3**: 25–51.

Albrektsson, T. and Albrektsson, B. (1987). Osseointegration of bone implants. A review of an alternative method of fixation. *Acta Orthop. Scand.*, **58**: 567–577.

Albrektsson, T., Bergman, B., Folmer, T., Henry, P., Higuchi, K., Klineberg, I., Laney, W. R., Lekholm, U., Oikarinen, V., van Steenberghe, D., Triplett, R. G., Worthington, P., and Zarb, G. (1988). A multicenter study of osseointegrated oral implants. *J. Prosthet. Dent.*, **60**: 75–84.

Albrektsson, T., Brånemark, P.-I., Hansson, H.-A., Ivarsson, B., and Jönsson, U. (1982). Ultrastructural analysis of the interface zone of titanium and gold implants. *Adv. Biomat.*, **4**: 167–177.

Albrektsson, T., Brånemark, P.-I., Hansson, H.-A., Kasemo, B., Larsson, K., Lundström, I., McQueen, D., and Skalak, R. (1983). The interface zone of inorganic implants in vivo: titanium implants in bone. *Ann. Biomed. Eng.*, **11**: 1–27.

Albrektsson, T., Dahl, E., Enbom, L., Engevall, S., Engquist, B., Eriksson, R. A., Feldmann, G., Freberg, N., Glantz, P. O., Kjellman, P., Kristersson, L., Kvint, S., Köndell, P.-Å., Plamquist, J., Werndahl, L., and Åstrand, P. (1988). Osseointegrated oral implants. A Swedish multicenter study of 8139 consecutively inserted Nobelpharma implants. *J. Periodontol.* **59**: 287–296.

Albrektsson, T., Eriksson, R. A., Jacobsson, M., Kälebo, P., Strid, K.-G., and Tjellström, A. (1989). Bone repair in implant models. A review with emphasis on the Harvest Chamber for bone remodeling studies. *Int. J. Oral Maxillofac. Impl.*, **4**: 45–54.

Albrektsson, T. and Hansson, H.-A. (1986). An ultrastructural description of the interface between bone and sputtered titanium or stainless steel surfaces. *Biomaterials*, **7**: 201–205.

Albrektsson, T., Hansson, H.-A., and Ivarsson, B. (1985). Interface analysis of titanium and zirconium bone implants. *Biomaterials*, **6**: 97–101.

Albrektsson, T. and Lekholm, U. (1989). Osseointegration: current state of the art. *Dent. Clin. North Am.*, **33** (in press).

Albrektsson, T. and Linder, L. (1984). Bone injury caused by curing bone cement. A vital microscopic study in the rabbit tibia. *Clin. Orthop.*, **183**: 280–287.

Amstutz, H. C. (1985). Arthroplasty of the hip. The search for durable component fixation. *Clin. Orthop.*, **200**: 343–361.

Amstutz, H. C., Kabo, M., Hermens, K., Carroll, P.F., Dorey, F., and Kilgus, D. (1987). Porous surface replacement of the hip with chamber cylinder design. *Clin. Orthop.*, **222**: 140–160.

Amstutz, H. C., Kabo, J. M., Kim, W. C., and Yao, J. (1988). Risk factors for femoral head resurfacing. In: *Non-Cemented Total Hip Arthroplasty.* Fitzgerald, R., Ed., Raven Press, New York, 191–209.

Bobyn, J. D. (1977). The Strength of Fixation of Porous Metal Implants by the Ingrowth of Bone. MSc thesis, McGill University, Montreal.

Bobyn, J. D., Cameron, H. U., Abdulla, D., Pilliar, R. M., and Weatherly, G. C. (1982). Biologic fixation and bone modeling with an unconstrained total knee prosthesis. *Clin. Orthop.*, **166**: 301–312.

Bobyn, J. D., Engh, C. A., and Glassman, A. H. (1987). Histologic analysis of a retrieved microporous-coated femoral prostheses. A seven year case report. *Clin. Orthop.*, **224**: 303–310.

Bobyn, J. D., Pilliar, R. M., Binnington, A. G., and Szivek, J. A. (1987). The effect of proximally and fully porous-coated canine hip stem design on bone modeling. *J. Orthop. Res.*, **5**: 393–408.

Bobyn, J. D., Pilliar, R. M., Cameron, H. U., and Weatherly, G. C. (1980). The optimum pore size for the fixation of porous-surfaced metal implants by the ingrowth of bone. *Clin. Orthop.*, **150**: 263–270.

Bobyn, J. D., Pilliar, R. M., Cameron, H. U., Weatherly, G. C., and Kent, G. M. (1980). The effect of porous surface configuration on the tensile strength of fixation of implants by bone ingrowth. *Clin. Orthop.*, **149**: 291–298.

Bobyn, J. D., Wilson, G. J., MacGregor, D. C., Pilliar, R. M., and Weatherly, G. C. (1982). Effect of pore size on the peel strength of attachment of fibrous tissue to porous-surfaced implants. *J. Biomed. Mater. Res.*, **16**: 571–584.

Boutin, P. (1972). Arthroplastie totale de la hanche par prothese en alumine frittée. *Rev. Chir. Orthop.*, **58**: 229–239.

Bragdon, C. R., Jasty, M., Russotti, G., Cargill, E., Harrigan, T. P., and Harris, W. H. (1989). Patterns of bone ingrowth, cortical porosity, and bone mass in a proximally porous coated canine femoral implant after 6 month implantation. *35th Annu. Meet. Orthop. Res. Soc.*, 378.

Brånemark, P.-I. and afEkenstam, B. (1979). Patent No. 7902035-0, Sweden.

Bago-Granell, J., Aguirre-Canyadell, M., Nardi, J., and Tallada, N. (1984). Malignant fibrous histiocytoma of bone at the site of a total hip arthroplasty. *J. Bone Jt. Surg.*, **66B**: 38–40.

Barck, A. (1988). Uni- and Bicompartmental Knee Replacement. Longitudinal and Predictive Analyses. Ph.D. thesis, Karolinska Hospital. Stockholm.

Bauer, T. W., Manley, M. T., Stern, L. S., Martin, A., and Marks, K. E. (1987). Osteosarcoma at the site of total hip replacement. *13th Annu. Meet. Soc. Biomat.*, 36.

Bell, R. S., Schatzker, J., Fornasier, V. L., and Goodman, S. B. (1985). A study of implant failure in the Wagner resurfacing arthroplasty. *J. Bone Jt. Surg.*, **67A**: 1165–1174.

Brånemark, P.-I., Hansson, B.-O., Adell, R., Breine, U., Lindström, J., Hallén, O., and Öhman, A. (1977). Osseointegrated fixtures in the treatment of the edentulous jaw: experience from a 10-year period. *Scand. J. Plast. Reconstr. Surg. Suppl.*, **16**: 1–132.

Buch, F. (1985). On Electrical Stimulation of Bone Tissue. A Vital Microscopic and Microradiographic Study. Ph.D. thesis, University of Gothenburg, Sweden.

Buch, F., Albrektsson, T., and Herbst, E. (1986). The bone growth chamber for quantification of electrically induced osteogenesis. *J. Orthop. Res.*, **4**: 194–203.

Buch, F., Nannmark, U., and Albrektsson, T. (1986). A vital microscopic description of the effects of electrical stimulation of bone tissue. *J. Bioelectr.*, **5**: 105–128.

Buchert, P. K., Vaughn, B. K., Mallory, T. H., Engh, C. A., and Bobyn, J. D. (1986). Excessive metal release due to loosening and fretting of sintered particles on porous-coated hip prostheses: report of two cases. *J. Bone Jt. Surg.*, **68A**: 606–609.

Callaghan, J. J., Dysart, S. H., and Savory, C. G. (1988). The uncemented porous-coated anatomic total hip prosthesis. *J. Bone Jt. Surg.*, **70A**: 337–346.

Callea, P., Muni, P., Zanelli, F., Lualdi, G., and Minen, D. (1986). *Knee Arthroprosthesis*. Sperri Spa, Udine, Italy.

Cameron, H. U., Pilliar, R. M., and Macnab, I. (1973). The effect of movement on the bonding of porous metal to bone. *J. Biomed. Mater. Res.*, **7**: 301–309.

Campbell, P. A., Namba, R. S., Kilgus, D. J., Kossovsky, N., Nasser, S., and Amstutz, H. A. (1989). Bone ingrowth in human porous surface replacements. *35th Annu. Meet. Orthop. Res. Soc.*, 401.

Campbell, P., Nasser, S., Kossovsky, N., and Amstutz, H. C. (1989). Retrieval analysis of femoral porous coated surface replacements. *Trans. 15th Annu. Meet. Soc. Biomat.*, 33.

Campbell, W. C. (1940). Interposition of vitallium plates in arthroplasties of the knee: preliminary reports. *Am. J. Surg.*, **47**: 639–648.

Carlsson, L. (1989). On the Development of a New Concept for Orthopaedic Implant Fixation. Ph.D. thesis, University of Gothenburg, Sweden.

Carlsson, L., Albrektsson, T., and Berman, C (1989). Bone response to plasma cleaned titanium implants. *Int. J. Oral Maxillofac. Impl.*, **4**: 199–204.

Carlsson, L., Röstlund, T., Albrektsson, B., and Albrektsson, T. (1988). Implant fixation improved by close fit: cylindrical bone implant interface studied in rabbits. *Acta Orthop. Scand.*, **59**: 272–275.

Carlsson, L., Röstlund, T., Albrektsson, B., and Albrektsson, T. (1988). Removal torques for polished and rough titanium implants. *Int. J. Oral Maxillofac. Impl.*, **3**: 21–24.

Carlsson, L., Röstlund, T., Albrektsson, B., Albrektsson, T., and Brånemark, P.-I. (1986). Osseointegration of titanium implants. *Acta Orthop. Scand.*, **57**: 285–289.

Charnley, J. (1979). *Low Friction Arthroplasty of the Hip*. Springer, New York.

Cheng, C. L. and Gross, A. E. (1988). Loosening of the porous coating in total knee replacement. *J. Bone Jt. Surg.*, **70B**: 377–381.

Clemow, A. J. T., Weinstein, A. M., Klawitter, J. J., Koeneman, J., and Anderson, J. (1981). Interface mechanics of porous titanium implants. *J. Biomed. Mater. Res.*, **15**: 73–82.

Collier, J. P., Mayor, M. B., Chae, J. C., Surprenant, V. A., Surprenant, H. P., and Dauphinais, L. A. (1988). Macroscopic and microscopic evidence of prosthetic fixation with porous coated materials. *Clin. Orthop.*, **235**: 173–180.

Cook, S. D., Scheller, A. D., Anderson, R. C., and Haddad, R. J. (1986). Histologic and microradiographic analysis of a revised porous-coated anatomic (PCA) patellar component. A case report. *Clin. Orthop.*, **202**: 147–151.

Cook, S. D., Thomas, K. A., Kay, J. F., and Jarcho, M. (1988). Hydroxyapatite-coated titanium for orthopaedic implant applications. *Clin. Orthop.*, **232**: 225–243.

Cook, S. D., Thomas, K. A., and Haddad, R. J. (1988). Histologic analysis of retrieved human porous-coated total joint components. *Clin. Orthop.*, **234**: 90–101.

Cotterill, P., Hunter, G., and Tile, M. (1982). A radiographic analysis of 166 Charnley-Müller total hip arthroplasties. *Clin. Orthop.*, **163**: 120–133.

D'Ambrosia, R. D., McClain, E. J., Wisiger, H. A., and Riggins, R. S. (1972). Resorption of the femoral head beneath the vitallium mold. *Surg. Forum*, **23**: 465–474.

Davey, J. R. and Harris, W. H. (1988). Loosening of cobalt chrome beads form a porous-coated acetabular component. A report of ten cases. *Clin. Orthop.*, **231**: 97–102.

De Waal Malifijt, J. (1988). Early Features of the Bone Implant Interface in Hip Arthroplasty. *Thesis, University of Nijmegen, Holland.*

Dichiara, J. F. and Higram, P. A. (1987). Histological examination of the bone/metal interface in removed porous coated human prostheses using a new processing method. In: *Biomaterials and Clinical Applications.* Pizzoferrato, A., Marchetti, P. G., Ravaglioli, A., and Lee, A. J. C., Eds., Elsevier, Amsterdam, 63–74.

Dichiara, J. F., Vitolo, J., Higham, P. A., and Vigorita, V. L. (1987). Detailed histologic evaluation of tissue ingrowth into retrieved non-cemented porous coated implants. *13th Annu. Meet. Soc. Biomat.*, 15.

Dodion, P., Putz, P., Amiri-Lamraski, M. H., Efira, A., deMartelaere, E., and Heimann, R. (1982). Immunoblastic lymphoma at the site of an infected vitallium bone plate. *Histopathology*, **6**: 807–813.

Donaldson, W. F., Sculco, T. P., Insall, J. N., and Ranawat, C. S. (1988). Total condylar III knee prosthesis. Long-term follow-up study. *Clin. Orthop.*, **226**: 21–28.

Ducheyne, P., Demeester, P., Aernoudt, E., Martens, M., and Mulier, J. C. (1977). Influence of a functional dynamic loading on bone ingrowth into surface pores of orthopaedic implants. *J. Biomed. Mater. Res.*, **11**: 811–820.

Edge, M. J. (1988). In vivo fracture of the tricalciumphosphate coating from the titanium body of an osseointegrating-type dental implant: a case report. *Int. J. Oral Maxillofac. Impl.*, **3**: 57–58.

Elves, M. W., Wilson, J. N., Scales, J. T., and Kemp, H. B. S. (1975). Incidence of metal sensitivity in patients with total joint replacements. *Br. Med. J.*, **4**: 376–378.

Endler, M. and Endler, F. (1982). Erste Erfahrungen mit einer zementfreien Polyethylenschraubpfanne. *Orthop. Praxis*, **18**: 319–328.

Engelhardt, A. (1982). Uncemented, ceramic-coated, electrically non-conductive implants having a physiologic pattern of stress distribution. In: *Cementless Fixation of Hip Endoprostheses*, Morscher, E., Ed. Springer, New York.

Engh, C. A. (1983). Arthroplasty with a Moore prosthesis with porous coating: a five year study. *Clin. Orthop.*, **176**: 52–61.

Engh, C. A. and Bobyn, J. D. (1985). *Biological Fixation in Total Hip Arthroplasty.* Slack, Thorofare, NJ.

Engh, C. A., Bobyn, J. D., and Gorski, J. (1984). Biological fixation of a modified Moore prosthesis. *Orthopaedics*, **7**: 285–294.

Engh, C. A., Bobyn, J. D., and Glassman, A. H. (1987). Porous coated hip replacement. The factors governing bone ingrowth stress shielding and clinical results. *J. Bone Jt. Surg.*, **69B**: 45–55.

Eriksson, A. R. (1984). Heat-Induced Bone Tissue Injury. An In Vivo Investigation of Heat Tolerance of Bone Tissue and Temperature Rise in the Drilling of Cortical Bone. Ph.D. thesis, University of Gothenburg, Sweden.

Eriksson, A. R. and Adell, R. (1986). Temperatures during drilling for the placement of implants using the osseointegration technique. *J. Oral Maxillofac. Surg.*, **44**: 4–7.

Eriksson, A. R. and Albrektsson, T. (1983). Temperature threshold levels for heat-induced bone tissue injury: a vital microscopic study in the rabbit. *J. Prosthet. Dent.*, **50**: 101–107.

Eriksson, A. R., Albrektsson, T., and Albrektsson, B. (1984). Heat caused by drilling cortical bone. Temperatures measured in vivo in patients and animals. *Acta Orthop. Scand.*, **55**: 629–631.

Eschenroder, H. C., Jr., McLaughlin, R. E., and Reger, S. I. (1987). Enhanced stabilization of porous-coated metal implants with tricalcium phosphate granules. *Clin. Orthop.*, **216**: 234–246.

Finnegan, M. (1989). The tissue response to internal fixation devices. *CRC Crit. Rev. Biocompat.*, **5**: 1–11.

Freeman, M. A. R., Blaha, J. D., Brown, G., Day, W., Insler, H. P., and Revell, P. A. (1981). Cementless fixation of a tibial compåonent for the knee. *27th Annu. Meet. Orthop. Res. Soc.*, 157.

Freeman, M. A. R. and Bradley, G. W. (1982). ICLH double cup arthroplasty. *Orthop. Clin. North Am.*, **13**: 799–811.

Galante, J. O. (1977). Cementless prosthesis: clinical experience. In: *Biomaterials and Clinical Applications*. Pizzoferrato, A., Marchetti, P. G., Ravaglioli, A., and Lee, A. J. C., Eds., Elsevier, Amsterdam, 131–139.

Galante, J. O., Rostoker, W., Lueck, R., and Ray, R. D. (1971). Sintered fiber metal composites as a basis for the attachment of implants to bone. *J. Bone Jt. Surg.*, **53A**: 101–110.

Geesink, R. G. (1988). Hydroxyl-apatite Coated Hip Implants. Ph.D. thesis, University of Maastricht, Holland.

Gerard, Y. (1978). Hip arthroplasty by matching cups. *Clin. Orthop.*, **134**: 25–34.

Gerard, Y., Chelius, Ph., and Legrand, A. (1985). Arthroplastie de hanche par cupeles coupleés non scellées, 14 ans d'experience. *Rev. Chir. Orthop. Suppl.*, **11**: 82.

Gootsauner-Wolf, G., Dallant, P., Pflüger, G., Plenk, H., Jr., Grundschober, F., and Schider, S. (1987). Histomorphometrical and roentgenological evaluations of bone reactions to cementless niobium femoral stems in dogs. In: *Biomaterials and Clinical Applications*, Pizzoferrato, A., Marchetti, P. G., Ravaglioli, A., and Lee, A. J. C., Eds., Elsevier, Amsterdam, 753–758.

Griss, P. and Heimke, G. (1981). Five-years experience with ceramic metal composite hip endoprostheses. *Arch. Orthop. Traumatol. Surg.*, **98**: 157–164.

Griss, P., Jentschura, G., and Heimke, G. (1978). Technik der Pfannenimplantation bei dysplastischem Acetabulum. *Arch. Orthop. Traumatol. Surg.*, **93**: 57–66.

Haddad, R. J., Cook, S. D., and Thomas, K. A. (1987). Biologic fixation of porous-coated implants. *J. Bone Jt. Surg.*, **69A**: 1459–1466.

Hagert, C.-G., Brånemark, P.-I., Albrektsson, T., Strid, K.-G., and Irstam, L. (1986). Metacarpophalangeal joint replacement with osseointegrated endoprostheses. *Scand. J. Plast. Reconstr. Surg.*, **20**: 207–218.

Head, W. C. (1981). Wagner surface replacement of the hip. Analysis of fourteen failures in forty-one hips. *J. Bone Jt. Surg.*, **63A**: 420–429.

Heck, D. A., Nakajima, I., Chao, E. Y., and Kelly, P. J. (1984). The effect of immobilization on biologic ingrowth into porous titanium fibermetal prostheses. *30th Annu. Meet. Orthop. Soc.*, 178.

Hench, L. L. (1987). Cementless fixation. In: *Biomaterials and Clinical Applications*. Pizzoferrato, A., Marchetti, P. G., Ravaglioli, A., and Lee, A. J. C., Eds., Elsevier, Amsterdam, 22–34.

Hench, L. L., Splinter, R. J. M., Allen, W. C., and Greenlee, T. K. (1971). Bonding mechanisms at the interface of ceramic prosthetic materials. *J. Biomed. Mater. Res. Symp.*, **2**: 117–141.

Herberts, P., Lansinger, O., and Romanus, B. (1983). Surface replacement arthroplasty of the hip. Experience with the ICLH method. *Acta Orthop. Scand.*, **54**: 884–890.

Hodgkinson, J. P., Shelley, P., and Wroblewski, B. M. (1988). The correlation between the roentgenographic appearance and operative findings at the bone-cement junction of the socket in Charnley low friction arthroplasties. *Clin. Orthop.*, **228**: 105–109.

Hofmann, A. A., Bachus, K. N., and Dauterman, L. A. (1988). Canine and human cancellous bony ingrowth into titanium and cobalt chrome porous coated test plugs implanted into the proximal tibia. *Soc. Biomat. Symp. Retrieval and Analysis of Surgical Implant and Biomat.*, 31.

Homsey, C. A. (1973). Implant stabilization. Chemical and biological considerations. *Orthop. Clin. North Am.*, **4**: 295–304.

Hori, R. Y. and Lewis, J. L. (1982). Mechanical properties of the fibrous tissue found at the bone-cement interface following total joint replacement. *J. Biomed. Mater. Res.*, **16**: 911–920.

Hughes, A. W., Sherlock, D. A., Hamblen, D. L., and Reid, R. (1987). Sarcoma at the site of a single hip screw. *J. Bone Jt. Surg.*, **69B**: 470–472.

Huiskes, R. (1987). Finite element analysis of acetabular reconstruction. Noncemented threaded cups. *Acta Orthop. Scand.*, **58**: 620–625.

Hulbert, S. F., Klawitter, J. J., Talbert, C. D., and Fitts, C. T. (1969). Materials of construction for artificial bone segments. In: *Research in Dental and Medical Materials*, Korostoff, E., Ed., Plenum Press, New York, 19–67.

Itami, Y., Akamatsu, N., Tomita, Y., and Nagai, M. (1982). A cementless system of total hip prosthesis. *Arch. Orthop. Traumatol. Surg.*, **100**: 183–189.

Itami, Y., Akamatsu, N., Tomita, Y., and Nagai, M. (1982). The direct fixation system of total hip prosthesis. *Arch. Orthop. Traumatol. Surg.*, **100**: 11–17.

Jacobsson, M. (1985). On Bone Behaviour after Irradiation. Ph.D. thesis, University of Gothenburg, Sweden.

Jacobsson, M., Jönsson, A., Albrektsson, T., and Turesson, I. (1985). Short- and longterm effects of irradiation on bone regeneration. *Plast. Reconstr. Surg.*, **76**: 841–848.

Jacobsson, M., Tjellström, A., Thomsen, P., Albrektsson, T., and Turesson, I. (1988). Integration of titanium implants in irradiated bone. A histologic and clinical study. *Ann. Otol. Rhinol. Laryngol.*, **97**: 337–340.

Jasty, M. and Harris, W. H. (1988). Observations of factors controlling bony ingrowth into weight-bearing, porous, canine total hip replacements. In: *Non-Cemented Total Hip Arthroplasty*, Fitzgerald, R., Jr., Ed., Raven Press, New York, 175–189.

Johansson, C. and Albrektsson, T. (1987). Integration of screw implants in the rabbit. A 1-year follow up of removal torque of titanium implants. *Int. J. Oral. Maxillofac. Impl.*, **2**: 69–75.

Johansson, C., Hansson, H.-A., and Albrektsson, T. (1990). A qualitative, interfacial study between bone and tantalum, niobium or commercially pure titanium. *Biomaterials*, **11**: 277–280.

Johansson, C., Lausmaa, J., Ask, M., Hansson, H.-A., and Albrektsson, T. (1989). Ultrastructural differences of the interface zone between bone and Ti-6Al-4V or commercially pure titanium. *J. Biomed. Eng.*, **11**: 3–8.

Johansson, C., Thomsen, P., and Albrektsson, T. (1990). Removal torques of c.p. titanium and titanium alloy screw-shaped implants. *Advances in Biomaterials*, **9**: 87–92.

Johnston, R. C. and Crowninshield, R. D. (1983). Roentgenologic results of total hip arthroplasty. *Clin. Orthop.*, **181**: 92–98.

Jönsson, A., Gottlander, M., and Albrektsson, T. (1990). Insertion versus removal torque of experimental implants. Submitted.

Judet, J. and Judet, R. (1950). The use of an artificial femoral head for arthroplasty of the hip joint *J. Bone Jt. Surg.*, **32B**: 166–175.

Judet, J., Judet, R., Lagrange, J., and Dunoyer, J. (1954). *Resection-Reconstruction of the Hip. Arthroplasty with an Acrylic Prosthesis.* Churchill Livingstone, Edinburgh.

Kershaw, C. J. and Theemen, A. E. G. (1988). The Attenborough knee, A four to ten-year review. *J. Bone Jt. Surg.*, **70B**: 89–93.

Kim, W. C., Rechl, H., Amstutz, H. C., Hermens, K., O'Carroll, P. F., and Kabo, M. (1986). Results of a stemmed bone ingrowth hip resurfacing arthroplasty in the canine. *Mater. Res. Soc. Symp.*, **55**: 197–202.

Knutson, K., Lindstrand, A., and Lidgren, L. (1986). Survival of knee arthroplasties. A nationwide, multicentre investigation of 8000 cases. *J. Bone Jt. Surg.*, **68B**: 795–803.

Lemons, J. E. (1988). Hydroxyapatite coatings. *Clin. Orthop.*, **235**: 220–223.

Lemons, J. E., Ramsay, N. Z., and Chamoun, E. K. (1988). Dental implant device retrievals. *Trans. Soc. Biomat. Symp. Retrieval and Analysis of Surg. Implants and Biomat.*, 4.

Lennox, D. W., Schofield, B. H., McDonald, D. F., and Riley, L. H. (1987). A histologic comparison of aseptic loosening of cemented, press-fit and biologic ingrowth prostheses. *Clin. Orthop.*, **225**: 171–191.

Lewis, J. L. and Galante, J. O., Eds. (1985). A Workshop on the bone-implant interface. Proc. Conf. held in Chicago, September 13–16, 1983. American Academy of Orthopaedic Surgeons.

Linder, L. (1982). The tissue response to bone cement. In: *Biocompatibility of Orthopaedic Implants*, Vol. II, Williams, D. F., Ed., CRC Press, Boca Raton, FL, 1–23.

Linder, L. (1989). Osseointegration of metallic implants. I. Light microscopy in the rabbit. *Acta Orthop. Scand.*, **60**: 129–134.

Linder, L., Carlsson, Å., Marsal, L., Bjursten, L.-M., and Brånemark, P.-I. (1988). Clinical aspects of osseointegration in joint replacement. A histological study of titanium implants. *J. Bone Jt. Surg.*, **70B**: 550–555.

Linder, L. and Hansson, H.-A. (1983). Ultrastructural aspects of the interface between bone and cement in man. Report of three cases. *J. Bone Jt. Surg.*, **65B**: 646–649.

Linder, L. and Lundskog, J. (1975). Incorporation of stainless steel, titanium and vitallium in bone. *Injury*, **6**: 277–285.

Lindström, J., Brånemark, P.-I., and Albrektsson, T. (1981). Mandibular reconstruction using the preformed autologous bone graft. *Scand. J. Plast. Reconstr. Surg.*, **15**: 29–38.

Ling, R. S. M. (1986). Observations on the fixation of implants to the bony skeleton. *Clin. Orthop.*, **210**: 80–96.

Lintner, F. (1983). Die Ossifikationsstörung an der Knochen-Zement-Knochengrenze. Histologische und Chemische Untersuchung-Experiment und Klinik. *Acta Chir. Austr. (Suppl.)*, **48**: 3–17.

Longo, J. A., Magee, F. P., Hedley, A. K., and Weinstein, A. M. (1989). The effect of chronic indomethacin on fixation of porous implants. *15th Annu. Meet. Soc. Biomat.*, 88.

Lord, G. and Bancel, P. (1983). The madreporique cementless total hip arthroplasty. *Clin. Orthop.*, **176**: 67–76.

Lord, G. A., Hardy, J. R., and Kummer, F. J. (1979). An uncemented total hip replacement. Experimental study and review of 300 Madreporique arthroplasties. *Clin. Orthop.*, **141**: 2–16.

Magee, F. P., Longo, J. A., and Hedley, A. K. (1989). The effect of age on the interface strength between porous coated implants and bone. *35th Annu. Meet. Orthop. Res. Soc.*, 575.

Magee, F. P., Weinstein, A. M., Longo, J. A., Koeneman, J. B., and Yapp, R. A. (1988). A canine composite femoral stem. *Clin. Orthop.*, **235**: 237–252.

Maniatopoulos, C., Pilliar, R. M., and Smith, D. C. (1986). Threaded versus porous-surfaced designs for implant stabilization in bone endodontic implant model. *J. Biomed. Mater. Res.*, **20**: 1309–1318.

Marmor, L. (1988). Unicompartmental knee arthroplasty. Ten- to 13-year follow up study. *Clin. Orthop.*, **226**: 14–20.

Mayor, M. B. and Collier, J. P. (1986). The histology of porous coated knee prostheses. *Orthop. Trans.*, **10**: 441–442.

McDonald, I. (1981). Malignant lymphoma associated with internal fixation of a fractured tibia. *Cancer*, **48**: 1009–1011.

Merritt, K. (1987). Allergic reactions to materials used in prosthetic surgery. In: *Biomaterials and Clinical Applications*. Pizzoferrato, A., Marchetti, P. G., Ravaglioli, A., and Lee, A. J. C., Eds., Elsevier, Amsterdam, 711–716.

Michel, R. (1987). Trace metal analysis in biocompatibility testing. *CRC Crit. Rev. Biocompat.*, **3**: 235–317.

Mittelmeier, H. (1983). Ceramic total hip replacement with self-locking anchorage. In: *Cementless Fixation of Hip Endoprostheses*. Morscher, E., Ed., Springer, New York.

Mittelmeier, H. and Singer, L. (1956). Anatomische und histologische Untersuchung-en von Arthroplastikgelenken mit Plexiglas-Endoprothesen. Möglichkeiten und Grenzen der Gelenkneubildung. *Arch. Orthop. Unfall Chir.*, **48**: 519–528.

Mittelmeier, T. and Walter, A. (1987). The influence of prosthesis design on wear and loosening phenomena. *CRC Crit. Rev. Biocompat.*, **3**: 319–419.

Mjöberg, B. (1986). Loosening of the cemented hip prosthesis. The importance of heat injury. *Acta. Orthop. Scand. Suppl.*, **221(57)**: 1–40.

Morrey, B. F. and Chao, E. Y. (1988). Fracture of the porous-coated metal tray of a biologically fixed knee prosthesis. *Clin. Orthop.*, **228**: 182–189.

Morscher, E. W. (1983). Cementless total hip arthroplasty. *Clin. Orthop. Rel. Res.*, **181**: 76–91.

Nannmark, U., Buch, F., and Albrektsson, T. (1985). Vascular reactions during electrical stimulation. Vital microscopy of the hamster cheek pouch and the rabbit tibia. *Acta Orthop. Scand.*, **56**: 52–56.

Nilsson, P. Granström, G., and Albrektsson, T. (1987). The effect of hyperbaric oxygen treatment of bone regeneration. An experimental study in the rabbit using the bone harvest chamber (BHC). *Int. J. Oral Maxillofac. Impl.*, **3**: 43–48.

Noble, P. C., Alexander, J. W., Lindahl, L. J., Yew, D. T., Granberry, W. M., and Tullos, H. S. (1988). The anatomic basis of femoral component design. *Clin. Orthop.*, **235**: 148–165.

Nunn, D. (1988). The Ring uncemented plastic-on-metal total hip replacement. Five year result. *J. Bone. Jt. Surg.*, **70B**: 40–44.

Oh, I. (1987). Design rationale of interference-fit total hip prostheses. In: *Biomaterials and Clinical Applications.* Pizzoferrato, A., Marchetti, P. G., Ravagliolo, A., and Lee, A. J. C., Eds., Elsevier, Amsterdam, 141–153.

Peltonen, L. (1987). Can endoprostheses cause allergic skin reactions?, *Nord. Med.*, **102**: 89–91.

Penman, H. G. and Ring, P. A. (1984). Osteosarcoma in association with total hip replacement. *J. Bone Jt. Surg.*, **66B**: 632–634.

Peters, M. S., Schroeter, A. L., vanHale, H. M., and Broadbent, J. C. (1988). Pacemaker contact sensitivity. *Contact Dermatitis,* **11**: 214–218.

Pilliar, R. M. (1987). Porous surfaced metallic implants for orthopaedic applications. *J. Biomed. Mater. Res.*, **21**: 1–33.

Pilliar, R. M., Cameron, H. U., and Macnab, I. (1975). Porous surface layered prosthetic devices. *Biomed. Eng.*, **10**: 126–135.

Pilliar, R. M., Cameron, H. U., Welsh, R. P., and Binnington, A. G. (1981). Radiographic and morphologic studies of load-bearing porous surfaced structured implants. *Clin. Orthop.*, **156**: 249–257.

Plenk, H., Jr., Pflüger, G., Böhler, N., Gottsauner-Wolf, F., Grundschober, F., and Schider, S. (1984). Long-term anchorage of cementless tantalum and niobium femoral stems in canine hip-joint replacements. In: *Biomaterials and Biomechanics.* Ducheyne, P., vanderPerre, G., and Aubert, A. E., Eds., Elsevier, Amsterdam, 61–66.

Portagliatti Barbos, M. (1988). Bone ingrowth into Madreporique prostheses. *J. Bone Jt. Surg.*, **70**: 85–88.

Portagliatti Barbos, M., Baudrocco, F., Iulita, P., and Rossi, P. (1987). Adaptive bone remodelling in Madreporic hip prostheses. In: *Biomaterials and Clinical Application.* Pizzoferrato, A., Marchetti, P. G., Ravagliolo, A., and Lee, A. J. C., Eds., Elsevier, Amsterdam, 171–176.

Poss, R., Robertson, D. D., Walker, P. S., Reilly, D. T., Ewald, F. C., Thomas, W. H., and Sledge, C. B. (1988). Anatomic stem design for press-fit and cemented application. In: *Non-Cemented Total Hip Arthroplasty,* Fitzgerald, R. H., Jr., Ed., Raven Press, New York, 343–363.

Ranawat, C. S. and Boachie-Adjei, O. (1988). Survivorship analysis and results of total condylar knee arthroplasty. *Clin. Orthop.*, **226**: 6–13.

Rand, J. A. and Coventry, M. B. (1988). Ten-year evaluation of geometric total knee arthroplasty. *Clin. Orthop.*, **232**: 168–173.

Refior, J. H., Parhofer, R., Ungethüm, M., and Blömer, W. (1988). Special problems of cementless fixation of total hip-joint endoprostheses with reference to the PM type. *Arch. Orthop. Traumatol. Surg.*, **107**: 158–171.

Reissis, N., Dendrinos, G., Reissis, E., and Ring, P. A. (1988). The Ring total knee replacement. *Arch Orthop. Traumatol. Surg.*, **107**: 309–315.

Rhinelander, F. W., Nelson, C. L., Stewart, R. D., and Stewart, C. L. (1979). Experimental reaming of the proximal femur and acrylic cement implantation. Vascular and histologic effects. *Clin. Orthop.*, **141**: 74–83.

Ring, P. A. (1968). Complete replacement arthroplasty of the hip by the Ring prosthesis. *J. Bone Jt. Surg.*, **50B**: 720–731.

Ring, P. A. (1983). Ring UPM total hip arthroplasty. *Clin. Orthop.*, **176**: 115–123.

Robertson, D. D., Walker, P. S., Hirano, S. K., Zhou, X. M., Granholm, J. W., and Poss, R. (1988). Improving the fit of press-fit hip stems. *Clin. Orthop.*, **228**: 134–140.

Rosenqvist, R., Bylander, B., Knutson, K., Rydholm, U., Rosser, B., Egund, N., and Lidgren, L. (1986). Loosening of the porous coating of biocompartmental prostheses in patients with reumatoid arthritis. *J. Bone J.t Surg.*, **68A**: 538–542.

Ryd, L. (1986). Micromotion in knee arthroplasty. A roentgen stereophotogrammetric analysis of tibial component fixation. *Acta Orthop. Scand. Suppl.*, **220(57)**: 1–80.

Ryu, R. K., Bovill, E. G., Jr., Skinner, H. B., and Murray, W. R. (1987). Soft tissue sarcoma associated with aluminum oxide ceramic total hip arthroplasty. A case report. *Clin. Orthop.*, **216**: 207–212.

Röstlund, T. (1990). On the Development of a New Arthroplasty. With Special Emphasis on the Gliding Elements in the Knee. Ph.D. thesis, University of Gotherburg, Sweden.

Röstlund, T., Carlsson, L., Albrektsson, B., and Albrektsson, T. (1989). Osseointegrated knee prostheses. An experimental study in rabbits. *Scand. J. Plast. Reconstr. Surg.*, **23**: 43–46.

Salzer, M., Knahr, K., and Frank, P. (1983). Radiologic and clinical follow up of un-cemented femoral endoprostheses with and without collars. In: *The Cementless Fixation of Hip Endo-prostheses*, Morsher, E., Ed., Springer, New York, 161–170.

Schatzker, J., Anderson, G., Sumner-Smith, G., Hearn, T., and Fornasier, V. (1989). An experimental investigation in the dog into the mode of osseous integration of total joint implants. *Arch. Orthop. Traumatol. Surg.*, **108**: 132–140.

Schatzker, J., Horne, J. G., and Sumner Smith, G. (1985). The effect of movement on the holding power of screws in bone. *Clin. Orthop.*, **111**: 257–262.

Sennerby, L., Lekholm, U., and Eriksson, L. E. (1988). Soft tissue response to clinically retrieved titanium implants reimplanted in the rat's abdominal wall. *Soc. Biomater. Symp. Retrieval and Analysis Surg. Implants and Biomater.*, 27.

Sennerby, L., Röstlund, T., Albrektsson, B., and Albrektsson, T. (1987). Acute tissue reactions to potassium alginate with and without colour/flavour additives. *Biomaterials*, **8**: 49–52.

Skalak, R. (1983). Biomechanical considerations in osseointegrated prostheses. *J. Prosthet. Dent.*, **49**: 843–848.

Smith-Petersen, M. N. (1939). Arthroplasty of the hip. A new method. *J. Bone Jt. Surg.*, **21**: 269–278.

Spector, M., Heyligers, I., and Roberson, J. A. (1988). Porous polymers for biological fixation. *Clin. Orthop.*, **235**: 207–219.

Strid, K. G. (1984). Radiographic results. In: *Tissue Integrated Prostheses*. Brånemark, P.-I., Zarb, G., and Albrektsson, T., Eds., Quintessence, Berlin, 187–198.

Sumner, D. R., Jacobs, J. J., Turner, T. M., Urban, R. M., and Galante, J. O. (1989). The amount and distribution of bone ingrowth in tibial components retrieved from human patients. *35th Annu. Meet. Orthop. Res. Soc.*, 375.

Sumner, D. R., Jacobs, J. J., Turner, T. M., Urban, R. M., and Galante, J. O. (1989). Quantitative study of bone ingrowth in tibial components retrieved from human patients. *15th Annu. Meet. Soc. Biomater.*, 89.

Sumner, D. R., Jasty, M., Turner, T. M., Urban, R. M., Galante, J. O., Bragdon, C., and Harris, W. H. (1987). Bone ingrowth in porous-coated cementless acetabular components retrieved from human patients. *Trans. Orthop. Res. Soc.*, **12**: 509.

Swann, M. (1984). Malignant soft-tissue tumour at the site of a total hip replacement. *J. Bone Jt. Surg.*, **66-B**: 629–631.

Thomas, K. A., Cook, S. D., and Haddad, R. J. (1987). Histologic analysis of retrieved human total joint components. *13th Annu. Meet. Soc. Biomater.*, 14.

Tooke, S. M., Nugent, P. J., Chotivichit, A., Goodman, W., and Kabo, J. M. (1988). Comparison of in vivo cementless acetabular fixation. *Clin. Orthop.*, **235**: 253–260.

Trancik, T., Mills, W., Vinson, N., and Borg, T. (1989). The effect of several therapeutic agents on bone ingrowth into a porous coated implant. *15th Annu. Meet. Soc. Biomater.*, 87.

Trentani, C., Montagnani, A., and Vicenzi, G. (1987). Ten year follow up of uncemented total hip prosthesis with alumina acetabulum and titanium femoral stem by plasma jet technique. In: *Biomaterials and Clinical Applications*. Pizzoferrato, A., Marchetti, P. G., Ravaglioli, A., and Lee, A. J. C., Eds., Elsevier, Amsterdam, 177–182.

Turner, T. M., Sumner, D. R., Urban, R. M., and Galante, J. O. (1987). A comparison of uncoated and porous coated press fit femoral components in a canine total hip arthroplasty (THA) model. *13th Annu. Meet. Soc. Biomater.*, 2.

Turner, T. M., Sumner, D. R., Urban, R. M., Rivero, D. P., and Galante, J. O. (1986). A comparative study of porous coating in a weight-bearing total hip arthroplasty model. *J. Bone Jt. Surg.*, **68A**: 1396–1409.

Uhthoff, H. K. (1973). Mechanical factors influencing the holding power of screws in compact bone. *J. Bone Jt. Surg.*, **55-B**: 633–639.

vanderList, J. J., vanHorn, J. R., Sloof, T. J., and tenCate, L. N. (1988). Malignant epithelioid hemangioendothelipoma at the site of a hip prosthesis. *Acta Orthop. Scand.*, **59**: 328–330.

Vigorita, V. J., Dichiara, J. F., Minkowitz, B., and Higham, P. A. (1989). Histomorphometric analysis of bone ingrowth in five retrieved, unfailed, unloosened non-cemented porous-coated implants. *35th Annu. Meet. Orthop. Res. Soc.*, 403.

Volz, R. G., Nisbet, J. K., Lee, R. W., and McMurtry, M. G. (1988). The mechanical stability of various noncemented tibial components. *Clin. Orthop.*, **226**: 38–42.

Wagner, H. (1978). Surface replacement arthroplasty of the hip. *Clin. Orthop.*, **134**: 102–130.

Walker, P. S. and Robertson, D. D. (1988). Design and fabrication of cementless hip stems. *Clin. Orthop.*, **235**: 25–34.

Walldius, B. (1957). Arthroplasty of the knee using an endoprosthesis. *Acta Orthop. Scand. Suppl.*, **24**: 1–112.

Welsh, R. P., Pilliar, R. M., and Macnab, I. (1971). Surgical implants — the role of surface porosity in fixation to bone and acrylic. *J. Bone Jt. Surg.*, **53A**: 963–972.

Willems, W. J., Eulderbrink, F., Rozing, P. M., and Obermann, W. R. (1988). Histopathologic evaluation in failed Gerard double cup arthroplasty. *Clin. Orthop.*, **228**: 123–133.

Williams, D. F. (1982). Corrosion of orthopaedic implants. In: *Biocompatibility of Orthopaedic Implants*, Vol. I. Williams, D. F., Ed., CRC Press, Boca Raton, FL, 197–229.

Williams, D. F. (1982). Tissue reaction to metallic corrosion products and wear particles in clinical orthopaedics. In: *Biocompatibility of Orthopaedic Implants*, Vol. I. Williams, D. F., Ed., CRC Press, Boca Raton, FL, 231–248.

Wykman, A. (1989), Cemented and non-cemented total hip arthroplasty. Ph.D. thesis, Karolinska Hospital, Stockholm, Sweden.

Zalenski, E., Jasty, M., O'Connor, D. O., Page, A., Krushell, R., Bragdon, C., Russotti, G., and Harris, W. H. (1989). Micromotion of porous-surfaced, cementless prostheses following 6 months of in vivo bone ingrowth in a canine model. *35th Annual Meet. Orthop. Res. Soc.*, 377.

Zweymüller, K. A. (1983). First clinical experience with a cementless modular femoral prosthesis system with a wrought Ti-67Al-4V stem and an Al_2O_3 ceramic ball head. In: *Cementless Fixation of Hip Endoprostheses*. Morscher, E., Ed., Springer, New York.

Zweymüller, K. A. (1986). Das Zementfreie Hüftendoprothesen System Zweymüller-Endler. Facultas Universitätsverlag, Wien.

Zweymüller, K. A., Lintner, F. K., and Semlitsch, M. F. (1988). Biologic fixation of a press-fit titanium hip joint endoprosthesis. *Clin. Orthop.*, **235**: 195–206.

6

Bone Inductive Molecules and Enhancement of Repair and Regeneration

L. KALEVI KORHONEN and KALERVO VÄÄNÄNEN
Department of Anatomy
University of Oulu
Oulu, Finland

> "The goal for many years when a bone graft is studied is to see if we can do better than just wait for the natural "fate" to proceed. As clinicians we like to have better control of the system to improve the final outcome". (Muzal B. Habal, Bone Grafts and Bone Substitutes. From Basic Science to Clinical Application. An International Symposium, Tampa, Florida, January 26–29, 1989.)

Introduction

Substantial knowledge has accumulated in recent years concerning the regulation of bone cells and their functions. This subject occupies a key position for the understanding not only of the development, maintenance, and repair of the skeleton but also for its treatment and the prevention of skeletal disorders. Bone growth, repair, and remodeling are known to be influenced by a variety of genetic, endocrinological, and other systemic and local factors, and also by nutrition and mechanical stress. The present review discusses research carried out into bone inductive factors and the possibilities for using these in the treatment of skeletal disorders. The main emphasis is placed on the effects of decalcified bone matrix as a bone-inductive material and on the isolation and characterization of the inductive factor(s) in it. Investigations in a number of laboratories, especially by Marshall Urist and research team, have shed light on many aspects of cartilage and bone induction by factors present in bone matrix. Elizabeth Wang and group have succeeded in isolating highly purified bone inductive factors from bovine bone and preparing its complementary DNAs (cDNAs) and corresponding human recombinant polypeptides (Wozney *et al.*, 1988).

Bone inductive factors can be understood to represent a subgroup of growth factors (see Volume 1, Chapter 4). Generally speaking, growth factors are mitogenic agents which either stimulate mitoses or decelerate differentiation, enabling the mitoses of non-differentiated cells to continue. Several growth factors have been identified in recent times, but since they are often bound to non-specific carrier proteins, their estimated size and other characteristics are largely dependent on the methods used for isolating them.

Growth factors are operationally defined as agents that increase cell replication, although they may also affect differentiated functions (James and Bradshaw, 1984). Most known growth factors are polypeptides that are synthesized by a variety of cell systems and tissues, including the skeleton. In some instances they act as systemic agents, but often they are primarily local regulators. Recent investigations have shown that the skeletal tissue is a rich source of growth factors which may also mediate the effects of systemic factors such as hormones. In addition, they may have important effects in the coupling of bone formation and resorption. Bone is a heterogeneous tissue containing a mixed cell population that includes fibroblasts, osteoprogenitor cells, osteoblasts, bone surface lining cells, osteoclasts, and the cells of the marrow tissue. Bone-derived growth factors may originate or affect any of these cells, while bone matrix may selectively trap systemic factors which could then act as putative local regulators of bone growth and remodeling.

Bone-Related Growth Factors

A variety of growth factors have been isolated from bone. Hauschka *et al.* (1986) estimate that bovine bone free of blood and cartilage contaminants has a volume concentration of mitogens up to 20 times greater than serum, while Hauschka *et al.* (1988) refer in general to bone-derived growth factor (BDGF), the group present in bone (Tables 1 and 2 and also see Volume 1, Chapter 4). These can be divided into two topics of study: exogenous, outside the skeleton produced factors which act on specific target cells in

Table 1.
Factors Affecting Bone and Cartilage Growth

	Mr
Fibroblast growth factors (FGF)	
acidic FGF (aFGF)	16 to 20 kD
basic FGF (bFGF)	16 to 20 kD
Endothelial cell growth factor (ECGF)	17 kD
Growth Factors from Skeletal and Cartilage Cells	
Transforming growth factors (TGF)	
TGF-β-1 (= cartilage inducing factor A)	5.6 kD
TGF-β-2 (= cartilage inducing factor B or BDGF I)	25 kD
Insulin-like growth factors (IGF)	
IGF I (= somatomedin C)	7.6 kD
IGF II (= MSA, multiplication stimulating activity)	
Beta-2-microglobulin (β-2-m)	11.8 kD
(= bone derived growth factor II, BDGF II)	
Platelet-derived growth factor (PDGF)	27 to 30 kD
Cartilage derived factor (CDF), probably closely related with IGF II	11 kD
Cartilage-derived growth factor (CDGF), related to bFGF	18 to 22 kD or 16.4 kD
Human skeletal growth factor (hSGF, SGF)	83 kD
Bone morphogenetic protein (BMP)	30 kD, 18 kD, and 16 kD
Blood-cell Derived Factors	
Interleukin 1 (IL-1)	17 kD
Macrophage-derived growth factor (MDGF)	10, 40 kD
Tumor necrosis factor alpha (TNF-α)	17 kD
Tumor necrosis factor beta (TNF-β)	

Derived from Canalis (1985), Marks and Popoff (1988), and Simmons (1985).

bone, and endogenously produced local factors with possible autocrine or paracrine action. Of the generally known growth factors, only IGF-I, TGF-β, and β-2-microglobulin have been found to be expressed in bone, since no mRNAs for aFGF or bFGF, for instance, have been found there (for the abbreviations, see Table 1). A specific group among the growth factors are those with an osteoinductive capacity, and it is these that are discussed in more detail in this paper.

As a general effect in bone, BDGFs cause a wave of proliferation of cells and extracellular matrix with decreased osteocalcin secretion and a reduction in $1,25\text{-}(OH)_2$ vitamin D_3-stimulated osteocalcin synthesis, reduced specific activity of alkaline phosphatase, decreased cyclic AMP responsive-

Table 2.
Effects of Some Growth Factors on Bone

	On Bone Collagen (Matrix) Synthesis		DNA Synthesis and Cell Replication	Bone Resorption	Alkaline Phosphatase Activity	Mitogenic On			
	Direct Effect	Secondary to Mitogenesis				Fibroblasts	Chondroblasts	Osteoblasts	Endothelial Cells
EGF									
aFGF	—	nd	+	+	—	+	+	nd	nd
bFGF	—	+	+	nd	—	+	+	+	+
ECGF	—	+	+	nd	—	+	+	+	+
TGF-β	—	+	+	nd	nd	nd	nd	+	+
TGF I	—	+	+	+	—	—	+	±	nd
β-2-m	+	nd	+	nd	nd	+	+	+	nd
PDGF	+	nd	+	nd	nd	+	nd	nd	nd
hSGF	+	nd	+	+	nd	+	nd	+	—
(BDGF)	+	nd	+	nd	nd	—	+	+	nd
CDF	+	nd	+	nd	nd	+	+	+	+
CDGF	nd	nd	nd	nd	nd	+	+	nd	nd
BMP	—	nd	+	nd	—	+	nd	nd	—
Interleukin 1	±	nd	+	+	nd	+	nd	+?	nd
MDGF	nd	nd	nd	nd	nd	—	+	+	nd
Prostaglandins	±	nd	±	nd	nd	nd	nd	nd	nd
TNF-α	—	nd	+	+	nd	nd	nd	+	nd

nd = not determined

ness to parathyroid hormone, and increased type I collagen synthesis (Hauschka *et al.*, 1988). A few other BDGFs which act as osteoinductive factors are discussed briefly in the following. The terminology in this area, as in many other cases, is confusing, and the identity of certain factors is questionable. The following summary is largely based on reviews by Canalis *et al.* (1989) and Hauschka *et al.* (1988).

FGF appears in two major forms, acidic and basic. They are products of different genes but have 50% amino acid sequence homology. They bind to the same receptors and have similar biological effects, being angiogenic and mitogenic for a variety of cell types, including osteoblasts. Slight inhibition of collagen type I synthesis and lowering of alkaline phosphatase activity has been reported. Both aFGF and bFGF have been isolated from bone matrix, but no information exists on their synthesis by bone cells. Several molecular subforms with a M_r from 16 to 20 kDa are known.

TGFs are polypeptides that stimulate anchorage-dependent cells to lose contact inhibition and undergo anchorage-independent growth in soft agar cultures. They were first found in the media of transformed cell cultures but are also produced by normal cells.

TGF-α shares extensive amino acid sequence homology with EGF and acts through EGF receptors, causing similar effects. A like EGF, TGF-α, has not been isolated from bone tissue but is mitogenic in bone cell cultures. It has a M_r of 5.6 kDa.

TGF-β, with a M_r of 25 kDa, consists of two subunits, each with a M_r of 12.5 kDa. It is a highly conserved polypeptide, and displays only minimal differences in amino acid sequences among various species. Three forms have been identified: TGF-β-1, TGF-β-2, and TGF-β-1,1, and also two homodimers and one heterodimer. Beta-1 and beta-2 forms have been isolated from bone matrix and were first characterized by their cartilage-inducing properties *in vitro,* consequently being named cartilage-inducing factor A and B, respectively. TGF-β is highly concentrated in bone and is estimated to exceed 200 µg/kg tissue. It is mitogenic for bone cells, stimulates collagen type I synthesis and increases the number of cells capable of expressing the osteoblastic phenotype in cell cultures. TGFs are characterized by their property of increasing the production of cartilage-specific macromolecules by fibroblasts *in vitro,* but they do not lead to any new cartilage or bone formation when tested *in vivo.*

Both IGF-I and IGF-II are growth hormone-dependent polypeptides which are structurally closely related to insulin. They are mitogenic for chondrocytes, bone cells, myoblasts, and fibroblasts, and stimulate cartilage growth, proteoglycan synthesis in cartilage, and collagen type I synthesis in bone in particular. Bennett *et al.* (1984) demonstrated a specific receptor for IGF-I in cultured fetal rat osteoblast-like bone cells with binding characteristics similar to those in human fibroblasts, while Isgaard *et al.* (1986) demonstrated the local growth-promoting effects of both IGF-I and growth hormone. IGF-I receptor concentrations are increased by exposure to glucocorticoids, which may affect the rate of mitosis. IGFs are synthesized by many different tissues, including bone and cartilage, and locally produced IGF-I may play a more significant role in skeletal and cartilage growth than its systemic counterpart. The two forms of IGF have a M_r of 7.6 kDa and exhibit similar biochemical and physiological properties. Serum contains IGF-binding proteins with M_r from 35 to 150 kDa.

A factor originally termed BDGF II is identical to β-2-m. It stimulates bone collagen and DNA synthesis simultaneously, and is found on the surface of almost all mammalian cells, non-covalently associated with membrane proteins, particularly with the major histocompatibility antigens and a series of differentiation antigens. β-2-m complexes probably act by modulating the binding of other growth factors to their receptors. β-2-m displays a M_r of 11.8 kDa.

PDGF is mitogenic for fibroblasts and bone cells, requires the presence of a progression factor, e.g., insulin or IGF, stimulates the synthesis of proteins, is chemotactic for various cells and stimulates the synthesis of prostaglandins. Several normal and neoplastic tissues, including bone cells, synthesize PDGF, which has M_r values ranging from 27 to 30 kDa.

CDF and the recently demonstrated low M_r form, skeletal growth factor, all have a M_r of 11 kDa and are similar in their biological effects. This suggests that they may be closely related if not identical; they are probably identical to IGF-II (Canalis et al., 1989).

Azizkhan and Klagsburn (1980) isolated CDGF, which is a non-histone protein found in intracellular and extracellular loci and has a molecular weight of 16.4 kDa. CDGF stimulates mitogenic activity in 3T3 fibroblasts, chondrocytes, and capillary epithelial cell lines but inhibits the incorporation of 35-sulfate into GAG. Kato et al. (1981) found a similar fetal cartilage-derived factor that is mitogenic for cultured chondrocytes and osteoblast precursors but enhances GAG synthesis.

Chondrogenic stimulating activity (CSA) is a highly soluble acidic protein isolated from bone, and displays a M_r of 31 kDa. It initiates the conversion of mesenchymal cells into chondrocytes and stimulates proteoglycan synthesis (Syftestad et al., 1985). It may be identical to BMP.

Bab et al. (1988) partially purified a preparation with a potent growth-promoting activity with respect to osteogenic cells from healing bone marrow conditioned culture media. This preparation displays M_r values from 10 to 35 kDa, and the authors claim that it differs in its characteristics from all other known growth factors in bone.

Factors originally named BDGFs (bone-derived growth factors) have been isolated from rat calvaria cultures. BDGF I later proved to be identical to TGF-β, and BDGF II to be beta-2-microglobulin (Canalis et al., 1989).

hSGF is a high M_r polypeptide (83 kDa in size) which stimulates DNA and type I collagen synthesis in bone (Farley and Baylink, 1982). It has also been postulated to link bone formation and bone resorption, and for this reason it is called a coupling factor. A level of 0.3 μg/ml of hSGF increases DNA synthesis more than twofold, the growth rate of chicken embryonic bone almost twofold and that of human bone more than tenfold.

BMP is mitogenic for fibroblasts and embryonic myoblasts but not for endothelial cells, and causes differentiation of cultured embryonic myoblasts into cartilage. Bone does not develop in cell culture, but cartilage induced *in vitro* will cause the formation of heterotopic bone when implanted in experimental animals. BMP coprecipitates with matrix Gla-protein and promotes DNA synthesis and cell proliferation in bone organ cultures. A crude preparation in the form of decalcified bone matrix gelatin, or partially purified preparations, will cause the formation of heterotopic bone when implanted in muscle pouches. Reddi and colleagues (Sampath *et al.*, 1987) called their preparation osteogenin. Human recombinant BMP polypeptides to bovine BMP display M_r of 30, 18, and 16 kDa, and all of them induce cartilage when implanted in the muscles of rats (Wozney *et al.*, 1988).

hSGF (Farley and Baylink, 1982) stimulates osteoprogenitor cells to proliferate in serum-free tissue culture media, while BMP initiates the covert stage by inducing the differentiation of mesenchymal-type perivascular cells into cartilage. The hydrophilic hSGF which is secreted into the media of bone cells in culture advances the covert stage of bone development by stimulating DNA synthesis, proline transformation into hydroxyproline, sulfate uptake, and other metabolic processes. BMP-induced development is irreversible, while SGF growth stimulation is reversible and comparable overall to the effects of somatomedin. According to Urist " . . . the two growth factors, BMP and hSGF, may be complementary for bone repair and other applications, with the former initiating the differentiation of new bone cells and the latter regulating the total number of bone cells produced" (Maugh, 1982).

BMP initiates cell differentiation, while other growth factors stimulate a somatomedin-like proliferation of a differentiated cell population. Growth hormone, or somatomedin, is a requirement for the action of BMP, which has to be met in tissue culture by the addition of 10% fetal calf serum to produce the chondrogenic response of mesenchymal cells to BMP.

Some other agents involved in the process of bone formation are worth remembering in addition to growth factors. Mikulski and Urist (1975) isolated a hydrophobic glycopeptide from bone which has an antimorphogenetic effect and displays a M_r of 5 kDa, while Somerman *et al.* (1983) isolated a chemotactic factor from decalcified bone matrix which may play a role in the recruitment of osteoprogenitor cells. Minkin *et al.* (1985) extracted several chemotactic factors of macrophages from bone.

Formation of Heterotopic Cartilage and Bone

The formation of new bone after implantation of autogenous living bone fragments was first reported during the last century by Barth (1893) and Bonome (1886). A number of other tissues and cells have been shown to cause the formation of heterotopic bone and/or cartilage since then. Neuhof discovered at the beginning of this century (Neuhof, 1917) that the urinary tract epithelium caused heterotopic bone formation, and Huggins studied the induction of bone by urinary bladder and gallbladder epithelia in his classical investigations in the 1930s (Huggins, 1930; 1931; 1969; Huggins and Sammet, 1933). These phenomena were later confirmed by Friedenstein and colleagues (Abdin and Friedenstein, 1972). Implanted malignant epithelial cells (Anderson, 1976) and virus transformed cell lines (Wlodarski *et al.*, 1971) will also induce heterotopic bone formation *in vivo*. Contrary to these established effects of certain epithelial cell types, chicken limb ectoderm conditioned collagen gel is inhibitory to chondrogenesis (Zanetti and Solursh, 1986).

Subcutaneously implanted dentin will induce bone formation (Bang and Urist, 1967), and the transplantation of whole epiphyseal cartilage or its cells subcutaneously into tolerant hosts has been employed in a number of studies on the induction of endochondral bone formation. This is a specific property of epiphyseal plate cells, as articular chondrocytes from the same animal do not undergo this sequence. Heat-killed chondrocytes also failed to yield any cartilage or bone formation (for references, see Wright *et al.*, 1985).

The formation of cartilage and bone may also be seemingly a non-specific reaction to trauma or necrotizing agents, but this may be a species-dependent quality (Anderson, 1976) and the amorphous calcification of necrotic tissue should be distinguished from ossification. Heterotopic bone formation has been described in nearly every tissue in the body, that in the muscle tissue of comatose patients and that occurring as a complication of total hip arthroplasty operations being common examples. These incompletely understood problems have been recently discussed in a review by Urist (1989).

Decalcified Bone Matrix as an Osteoinductive Material

Demineralized bone or dentin matrix implanted into muscle pouches causes the formation of heterotopic cartilage which eventually calcifies, vascularizes, and is replaced by bone with hemopoetic marrow (see references in Harakas, 1984; Urist *et al.*, 1983; Urist, 1989). In fact, demineralized bone matrix is an even more effective agent for the induction of bone in rats than is whole living or preserved bank bone (Oikarinen and Korhonen, 1979). (The terms demineralized and decalcified are used interchangeably in the following. The treated bone matrix also still retains protein-bound calcium, only the bone mineral has been removed.) Similarly, chondrogenesis is observed when muscle explants are cultured on bone matrix *in vitro* (Nogami and Urist, 1974; Terashima and Urist, 1977) but endochondral cascade does not occur (Nogami and Urist, 1970).

It was originally believed that bone collagen itself was the active inducing agent, but it is evident that collagens from non-calcified tissues do not substitute for bone collagen and dentin (Reddi, 1976; Reddi and Anderson, 1976), and collagenase-treated bone matrix is still active in inducing chondrogenesis as osteogenesis (Nogami and Urist, 1974). Since 1952 Urist and team have proposed that the inductive capacity of decalcified bone matrix is caused by a specific chemical substance or substances which they named bone morphogenetic protein or BMP (Urist and Strates, 1971). In contrast, Reddi and co-workers have proposed that geometry and electrical surface charges are the key ingredients for the osteoinductive capacity of decalcified bone and dentin (Reddi and Huggins, 1972; 1973), and suggest that the collagenous matrix may provide a suitable substratum for anchorage-dependent proliferation and differentiation of cells.

In an extensive series of investigations, Urist and group have discovered that consistent osteoinduction can be achieved by means of decalcified bone implants when controlled conditions are used in preparing them. The methods used vary somewhat among investigators, but the essential steps are defatting with organic solvents and decalcification (usually in 0.6 N HCl). Subsequently, the material may be converted to an insoluble matrix gelatin by extraction with concentrated $CaCl_2$ to remove protein and polysaccharide moieties and LiCl as a denaturant (Harakas, 1984; Urist, 1989). Endogenous proteolysis should be inhibited during preparation.

The particle size is critical when demineralized bone matrix or gelatin is used as an inductive factor. Urist *et al.* (1968) suggested that small particles of less than 400 μm^3 are phagocytosed or dispersed too rapidly, while Reddi and Huggins (1973) proposed that pulverization destroys the geometric configuration and electric surface structure which they thought essential for induction. Syftestad and Urist (1979) demonstrated that the yield of new bone from implants of pulverized demineralized whole bone matrix and bone matrix gelatin declines as the particles decreased in diameter below 125 μm. When a narrow range of particle sizes is used, e.g., from 100 to 250 μm, the process of induction is very regular.

Phases in Bone Induction

The process of bone induction proceeds through two major steps. Hyaline cartilage is formed on the surfaces of implanted pieces of matrix at the first stage, and bone forms thereafter. Thus it is possible that the specific inductive property actually concerns only the induction of cartilage, and that the formation of bone is a secondary phenomenon caused by other factors.

The sequential histological differentiation which takes place in the induc-

Table 3.
Phases in the Induction of Cartilage and Bone by Decalcified Bone Matrix
in Muscle Pouches

Days After Implantation	Phases
1	Polymorphonuclear leucocytes + +
3	Polymorphonuclear leucocytes +, fibroblasts + + + +
5	Fibroblasts + + +, chondroblasts + (immature cartilage progenitor cells and cartilage in small amounts), no giant cells
7	Chondrocytes + + + (cartilage abundant), cartilage begin to calcify
9	Hypertrophy and calcification of chondrocytes. Incursion of capillaries into the plaques, chondrolysis begins, early hemocytoblasts
10	Osteoblasts + + +, chondrolysis
12	Bone + + +, few cartilage cells
14	Most of the cartilage disappeared, bone + + + +, osteoclasts, bone marrow
18	All cartilage vanished
40	Red hematopoietic bone marrow regularly present

Modified from Inoue *et al.*, 1986; Reddi and Anderson, 1976; Reddi and Huggins, 1972; Steinman and Reddi, 1980.

tion of cartilage and bone goes through the following stages: (1) chemotaxis and migration of leukocytes, followed by mesenchymal cells within the first 2 days; (2) mesenchymal cells differentiate into chondrocytes between the 2nd and 18th day; (3) hypertrophy of the chondrocytes and calcification of the matrix followed by vascular invasion and woven bone development between the 10th and 20th days; (4) hemopoietic bone marrow develops beginning from the 14th up to the 30th day (Inoue *et al.*, 1986; Reddi and Anderson, 1976; Sampath and DeSimone, 1982; Urist, 1965). The progress of osteoinduction *in vivo* and chondrogenesis *in vitro* can be monitored by radiographs and by collecting samples for histological and chemical investigation. Tests such as the incorporation of ^{45}Ca, ^{35}S, alkaline phosphatase activity, analysis of hydroxyproline, and collagen types have been employed. The main steps in the histomorphological changes, which are carefully described in a number of investigations, are presented in Table 3 and a selection of biochemical events is recorded in Table 4.

The series of collagen types synthesized during cartilage and bone induction recapitulates the embryonic development of long bones (Steinmann and Reddi, 1980). The changes in proteoglycan types during matrix-induced cartilage and bone development also correspond roughly to the changes in growth cartilage. Proteoglycan synthesis at the beginning of induction corresponds to the types found in chicken limb chondrogenesis or mesenchymal limb bud cell cultures (von der Mark and Conrad, 1979; Reddi *et al.*, 1978).

Table 4.
Events During the Chondro-Osteogenesis Induced by Demineralized Bone Matrix

Day	Alkaline Phosphatase	^{45}Ca Incorporation	^{32}P Incorporation
1	∓	nd	—
3	∓	±	—
5	∓	±	—
7	+	+	+
9	+	+ +	+ +
10	+ +	+ + +	+ + + +
11	+ +	+ + + +	+ + +
12	+ +		+ + +
14	+	+ + + +	+ + +
18	+	+ + + +	+ + +
21	+	+ + + +	+ + +

From Reddi and Anderson, 1976.

Histological, ultrastructural, and biochemical observations on BMP-induced cartilage formation have demonstrated the induction of typical hyaline cartilage, containing proteoglycans and type II collagen (Anderson and Griner, 1977; Reddi *et al.*, 1977; 1978). The change in the phenotypes of the fibroblasts to osteoblasts is a stable transformation, as living bone with hemopoietic bone marrow is found even on day 700, long after the transforming agent has disappeared.

Isolation and Characteristics of Bone Morphogenetic Protein (BMP)

It has been shown in organ culture experiments and when using implanted diffusion chambers that the factor inducing cartilage differentiation is a diffusible substance (Buring and Urist, 1967; Goldhaber, 1961; Heiple *et al.*, 1968; Nagakawa and Urist, 1977; Urist *et al.*, 1977). This factor or factors, BMP, is transferred from the bone matrix to a responsive mesenchymal-like cell population within 24 h of implantation (Nakagawa and Urist, 1977). Diffusion chamber experiments demonstrate that the inductive agent may diffuse a distance of at least 2 mm (Nogami and Terashima, 1976), although diffusion chamber experiments can easily produce erroneous results if not properly controlled (Lehtonen *et al.*, 1975).

Considerable difficulty was encountered when attempting to solubilize the osteoinductive factor, and consequently elucidation of its biochemical properties virtually came to a standstill by the late 1970s. The first steps in the isolation and purification of BMP were taken when Urist and team solubilized it with purified bacterial collagenase (Urist *et al.*, 1979), or with the use of a non-polar solvent, ethylene glycol (Urist and Mikulski, 1979). Several methods were later developed for isolating active BMP, which

Table 5.
Relative Molecular Weights Reported from Preparations of BMP

Source	Molecular Weight	Reference
Bovine bone	17.5 kD (24 kD, 34 kD)	Mizutani and Uris, 1982
	18 kD	Urist et al., 1983
	17.5 kD	Urist et al., 1984
Rat bone	<14 kD, and ca. 22 kD	Sampath et al., 1982
Human bone	17 to 18 kD	
	BMP-1 30 kD	Wozney et al., 1989
	BMP-2A 18 kD	
	BMP-2B	
	BMP-3 16 kD	
Rabbit bone	21 kD, 14.3 kD	Urist et al., 1979
	24 kD	Takahashi et al., 1987
Rabbit dentin	12–30 kD	Wu and Hu, 1988
		Conover and Urist, 1981
Osteosarcoma	12.5 kD, 16 kD	Hanamura et al., 1980
	22 kD	Takaoka et al., 1982
Porcine	19.7 kD	Wu and Hu, 1988

can be done from whole acid-demineralized bone matrix or by first converting this into gelatin by means of lithium chloride to facilitate the extraction. Use of chaotropic reagents such as 4 M guanidine HCl (GuHCl) or 6 M urea enables the hydrophobic inductive agent to be extracted from the decalcified matrix (Harakas, 1984; Urist, 1989). The BMP should be protected from endogenous proteolysis, alkaline hydrolysis, etc. during the isolation. The chemicals and procedures used for preparation ensure satisfactory sterility of the inductive material for experimental purposes, but if further sterilization is necessary, the precautions mentioned in a review by Harakas (1984), for example, should be noted.

Different sources (cortical bone, dentin, and osteosarcoma tissues) and different preparative methods result in BMP preparations with somewhat varying molecular weights and other characteristics (Table 5). Urist (1989) defines the general characteristics of these preparations as follows: a non-collagenous *in vitro* protein component of bone matrix is designated BMP if it induces chondrogenesis, while an *in vivo* preparation is BMP if it induces differentiation of both cartilage and later bone with functional bone marrow.

Elizabeth Wang and research group have obtained a highly purified (approximately 300,000-fold) preparation of BMP from GuHCl extracts of demineralized bovine bone (Wang et al., 1988). The activity resided in a single band after SDS-polyacrylamide gel electrophoresis under non-re-

duced conditions, corresponding to a molecular size of 30 kDa. This protein
is basic and glycosylated, composed of disulfide-linked subunits and yields
proteins of 30, 18, and 16 kDa on reduction. The authors derived the amino
acid sequence from it and produced full-length complementary DNAs
(cDNAs) encoding the human equivalents of three polypeptides originally
purified from bovine bone. In addition, human recombinant BMP polypeptides were produced by means of Chinese hamster ovary cells or *E. coli* and
tested for the biological activity in rats (Wozney *et al.*, 1988). Amino acid
analysis of BMP preparations obtained from rat bone (Sampath and Reddi,
1984), bovine bone (Urist *et al.*, 1984), and human bone (Urist *et al.*, 1983),
and also the terminal amino acid sequence of bovine BMP (Urist *et al.*,
1984), differ considerably from the properties of BMP reported by Wang *et
al.* (1988) and Wozney *et al.* (1988). These last mentioned preparations
display the best criteria of purity, potency, and specificity so far reported
for BMP, and their specific activity is at least an order of magnitude greater
than the figures previously reported. Some interesting features of the BMP
isolated and produced by Wang and colleagues are commented on briefly
in the following.

The human recombinant BMP polypeptides corresponding to the three
fractions mentioned above were designated BMP-1, BMP-2A, and BMP-3.
The researchers identified a further closely related protein designated BMP-
2B by cross-hybridization with a BMP-2A probe. Structurally, BMP-1 appears to be unrelated to other known growth factors, but both BMP-2A and
BMP-3 are closely related to proteins involved in embryonic morphogenesis
and the authors regard them as new members of the growth factor family,
which includes TGF-β and inhibin. The fourth preparation, BMP-2B, seems
to be yet another member of this family.

The first amino acid residues in BMP-1 are hydrophobic and characteristic of the leader sequence of a secreted protein. This polypeptide consists
of 730 amino acid residues grouped into five domains. Domain A probably
contains protease activity, three other domains (B1, B2, B3) are regions of
internal sequence similarity, and domain E resembles sequences found in
EGF, probably functioning in calcium binding and in protein-protein
interactions.

BMP-2A and BMP-2B are 396 and 408 amino acid residues long, respectively, and BMP-3 has a length of 472 amino acid residues. All three are
new members of the TGF-β family of growth factors. BMP-2A and BMP-
2B display about 75% sequence identity with the *Drosophila* dpp protein,
which is involved in dorso-ventral specification and the development of the
imaginal disc during embryogenesis. One or both of these polypeptides may
represent the human homolog of the dpp polypeptide, considering the evo-
lutionary distance between the species concerned. Both polypeptides also
show about 57% sequence similarity to Vgl protein, which is thought to
function as a signal from the endodermal cell to initiate ectodermal cell
differentiation into mesoderm during early amphibian embryogenesis.

Osteoinduction may depend on more than one factor, since bone matrix is a rich source of growth factors and osteoinduction may depend on many cellular functions. In any event, BMP very probably occurs as a protein-protein aggregate in tissues in the native state. Wozney *et al.* (1988) consider it quite likely that BMP activity may represent the combined action of multiple factors. BMP-1 may also activate or bind other BMP components. The pure preparation of BMP will allow better opportunities for practical applications in the treatment of skeletal defects, and can also be expected to facilitate research into the significance of bone inductive growth factors, e.g., for osteoporosis.

Target Cells and the Mechanism of Action

Bone is one of the exceptional tissues in the bodies of higher vertebrates which are able to differentiate continuously, remodel internally, and regenerate completely after injury. How much of this capacity can be attributed to proliferation of predifferentiated osteoprogenitor cells and how much to induced differentiation of mesenchymal-type cells is one of the basic problems in studying induction.

Although cartilage and bone cells are both derived from a common pool of mesenchymal progenitor cells, these two cell lineages are not interconvertible. A chondrocyte is never differentiated into an osteoblast or osteocyte. Cartilage sets up the broad shape of bone during embryonic development, but cartilage is not the progenitor of new bone in a cellular sense. It has been demonstrated that the potential for generating cells which differentiate into chondrocytes exists in many non-chondrogenic cell types throughout the lifetime of an animal (Beresford, 1989; von der Mark and Conrad, 1979).

The induction of bone by decalcified bone matrix has often been compared with the development of bone in embryos, but it must be recognized that this bone formation is influenced by factors which reside in the bone itself, some of which may not be present when embryonic mesenchymal cells first differentiate into cartilage at the site where the cartilage will first differentiate into the anlage for future bone. The bone matrix-directed chondrogenesis of muscle *in vitro* as compared with chondrogenesis in early embryos has been reviewed extensively by Nathanson (1985).

The osteoinductive competence of mesenchymal cells with respect to decalcified bone inductive material varies from organ to organ. Expressed in terms of positive results (%) and bone yields, we obtain the following series: bone and bone marrow > skeletal muscle > subcutaneous tissue > dermis > brain > lung > anterior chamber of eye > testes > pancreas > ovary (Urist *et al.*, 1969). These authors also observed that endodermally derived organs could not support chondrogenesis when bone matrix was implanted directly into them, whereas a reactive cell type separated from its normal microenvironment retains its developmental potential (Nathanson, 1985).

Skeletal muscle is most often used in experiments on osteoinductive capacity *in vivo*, which demonstrate that connective tissue cells of both this muscle and cloned mononucleated myoblasts or their precursors can be the target cells for the inducing molecules (Nathanson *et al.*, 1978). Under cell culture conditions, BMP is able to reactivate the muscle cells and push them towards differentiation into chondroblasts, thus demonstrating their phenotypic instability.

In monolayer cultures, however, chondrogenic development is inhibited by binding of the cells to the plastic culture dish. Indeed, the interaction of the cells with a plastic surface appears to promote the dedifferentiation of chondrogenic cells into cells with a fibroblastic morphology that no longer synthesize cartilage proteoglycan or type II collagen. When stage 24 chicken embryo limb mesenchymal cells are plated into culture, a density-dependent phenotypic expression is observed. Cells plated at low density develop into myotubes, those plated at higher density differentiate into bone cells, and those plated at very high density exhibit chondrogenic phenotypes (Caplan *et al.*, 1983). Differentiation and differentiated functions are also dependent on the cell shape. The investigation by Takigawa *et al.* (1984) and others suggest that the intactness of the microtubules and the disruption of the microfilaments are factors involved in regulating the expression of the differentiated phenotype of chondrocytes in culture.

One factor of importance in the microenvironment of differentiating mesenchymal cells is fibronectin. This is a major cell surface glycoprotein which works as a cell attachment factor for cell-substratum, usually cell-collagen, interaction. Weiss and Reddi (1981) observed that one early event after the implantation of decalcified bone matrix was the binding of circulating plasma fibronectin to the collagenous matrix. When this was inhibited by treating the implant with anti-fibronectin, osteoinductive capacity was markedly reduced (Weiss and Reddi, 1981).

Allogeneic implantation of rat demineralized bone matrix results in a local differentiation of endochondral bone, xenogeneic implants of human, monkey, or bovine bone matrices are reported to display only weak or noninducing capacity. This species-specificity of xenogeneic matrices is due to immunogenic or inhibitory components in extracellular bone matrices, as purified, reconstituted bone-inducing proteins are equally efficient regardless of their source (Sampath and Reddi, 1983).

It should also be noted that the usual cascade in bone induction by decalcified bone matrix or BMP prepared from it passes through a previous stage of chondrogenesis *in vivo*, and that only chondrogenesis is observed *in vitro*, without osteogenesis, as described previously in this paper. These facts and the presence of alkaline phosphatase at early stages in chondrogenesis suggest that there may be another process of differentiation apart from chondrocyte differentiation. Once the chondroblasts are stimulated by the demineralized matrix, they may produce some agent in the matrix, or secrete some factor, that acts on a different progenitor cell and pushes it towards the osteoblast phenotype. Another possibility is that angiogenic factors such as FGF may be produced, stimulating the vascular invasion by which the osteoprogenitor cells arrive and the differentiation of bone tissue starts. Progenitor cells of this type are absent in muscle cell cultures. It should also be noted that the presence of bone marrow greatly enhances osteoinduction by decalcified bone matrix.

The observations that cartilage and bone induction by BMP is based on a chemically diffusible factor are reminiscent of the proposal made over 50 years ago by Spemann and others (Spemann, 1938) working on embryonic induction, while the proposal that BMP may be a polypeptide is in agreement with the hypothesis of Slack (1980) that cell repair and regeneration is coded by cell membrane glycoproteins. The cell membrane dissociates during damage, fixed glycoproteins are freed from it and redistributed to start the healing and regeneration processes. The great diversity of glycoproteins in a given cell membrane makes them primary candidates for the large number of entities that are required for promoting differentiation of a given cell type into a number of different functional cells, a probable requirement for wound healing and organ regeneration. In the case of bone tissue, some of these specific glycoproteins may be secreted and trapped in the bone matrix.

Experimental and Clinical Applications of Osteoinductive Factors

Of all the materials available for osseous repair and reconstruction, fresh autogenous bone should be preferred because of its compatibility and efficacy. The limitations on its use nevertheless include the time required for the harvesting procedure, its associated morbidity, and the inadequate amount of transplantable, osteogenic bone, particularly in infants, children, and frail adults. Especially in facial bone surgery, the autogenous bone may also be difficult to shape and fix for restoration of a symmetrical facial contour. Even a small piece of autogenous bone graft in dental surgery requires the use of an operating theater rather than the dentist's chair (Glowacki et al., 1981; Oikarinen, 1981). The risk of sequestration should also be taken into account when large transplants are used. The ideal material for bone grafting should be easy to sterilize, easy to shape, available in sufficient amounts and optimally it should be possible to store it at room temperature.

Results obtained with the use of experimental animals and our limited clinical experience suggest that decalcified bone matrix and/or active agents prepared from it may represent an alternative material worth consideration for bone grafting. Experimental results suggest that inflammatory and immunological reactions are minimal or absent, even in the case of xenografts, if purified inductive material is used (Muthukumaran et al., 1985, Sampath and Reddi, 1983). Although decalcified bone matrix is in itself a non-living material, it does not hinder the cellular invasion, is quickly resorbed, is not sequestrated, and causes *de novo* bone formation at the transplant site (Oikarinen, 1981).

As Urist (1989) puts it, waves of enthusiasm have risen and fallen with regard to the use of implants of demineralized bone matrix for reconstructive bone surgery. The first wave to be recorded occurred at the turn of the century, the second was between 1950 and 1960, and the most recent one has been from 1980 onwards. Recent experimental achievements in the identification of active agents have also resulted in their first applications to clinical use. It may be mentioned in passing that Senn was already using acid-demineralized bone matrix for the treatment of osteomyelitic cavities in 1889, and believed that this treatment was successful because the decalcified implanted bone was rendered antiseptic by the acid treatment.

Extensive reviews on bone growth and regulation, fracture healing, bone grafting, and related subjects with emphasis on growth factors and the phenomena of bone induction and their clinical applications, have been published by Urist (1989), Harakas (1984), and Simmons (1985). We will underline just a few points on the subject in this paper.

The results obtained by means of animal experiments require careful consideration prior to any attempt at clinical application. First of all, there are considerable differences between species. The capacity of the rat to regenerate bone in response to allogeneic demineralized bone matrix implants is extraordinary. Einhorn *et al.* (1984) obtained good results when replacing segmental defects representing 20% of the shaft of the femur with demineralized allogeneic bone matrix implants, 6 mm resection defects of the mid-fibula were completely regenerated (Narang *et al.*, 1973) and fibular defects too large to heal even with autogenic bone grafts were repaired by means of allogeneic bone matrix implants (Oikarinen and Korhonen, 1979). In other species such as the guinea pig, dog, monkey, or man, allogeneic bone matrix induces only minor deposits of bone, and only after a lag phase of several weeks, even though the bone marrow stroma cells will enhance new bone formation by demineralized matrix.

Selected examples of clinical applications of the use of bone inductive material in reconstructive surgery are given below. Urist (1968) reported 26 cases with clinical evaluations involving totally decalcified allogeneic bone in 16 cases and surface-decalcified bone in 10 cases and compared them with 9 cases treated with undemineralized bone. Although the outcome was in general successful, Urist was still apprehensive as to whether conclusive clinical results had been achieved (Urist, 1972). Osbon *et al.* (1976) reported six successful clinical cases in which a surface-decalcified bone graft had been used to reconstruct maxillary and mandibular defects. Allogeneic materials or combinations of allogeneic and autologous materials had been used. Glowacki *et al.* (1981) reported 26 successful clinical cases in which they used allogeneic decalcified bone implants to repair craniofacial defects, and the same group also reported 44 cases of maxillocraniofacial defects corrected successfully with allogeneic demineralized bone grafts (Mulliken *et al.*, 1981) and 50 successful jaw defect repairs (Kaban *et al.*, 1982). Libin *et al.* (1975) treated three clinical cases successfully using demineralized pulverized bone allografts to repair periodontal defects, while Pearson *et al.* (1981) published a controlled study with seven patients subjected to periodontal surgery which clearly demonstrated the usefulness of demineralized allogeneic cancellous bone grafts. Sonis *et al.* (1983) treated 22 patients with periodontal defects using allogeneic demineralized bone powder as an adjunct to the treatment. Demineralized dentin material has been used in few clinical cases (Register *et al.*, 1972).

A separate type of bone graft is represented by allogeneic, antigen-extracted, surface-demineralized bone material, which also displays bone-inductive capacity. The results of clinical applications have been reviewed by Urist (1989).

A few clinical trials have been performed using a purified BMP preparation, with promising results (Urist, 1986); e.g., successful treatment of 12 patients with resistant femoral non-unions with implants of a purified BMP preparation combined with bone grafts (Johnson *et al.*, 1988). These trials show that purified preparations can be used in human beings.

An interesting experiment on the regeneration of articular cartilage is also worth mentioning in this connection, namely, that in which bone matrix implanted into the joint space of condylectomized mandibles in rats induced regeneration of the entire condyle complete with a cartilaginous cap (Narang and Wells, 1973). In our own laboratory, Oikarinen (1981) obtained promising results with the use of demineralized bone matrix implants for the restoration of experimental defects in the knee-joint articular cartilage of rabbits. No comparable regenerative capacity has been reported in species with a longer life-span.

Most research has been done with allogeneic decalcified rodent bone, which incites minimal antigenic immunological reactions (Reddi and Huggins, 1972; Urist, 1965). Xenogeneic material may produce an adverse immune response (Urist, 1973; Urist *et al.*, 1968; Urist, 1973), but such implants have also been used (Thieleman *et al.*, 1978; 1982), in spite of the fact that they may give a very much weaker response or no response at all (Sampath and Reddi, 1983). In contrast, purified BMP is not species-specific between rats and rabbits, and a similar nonspecificity has been reported in the case of human and bovine purified BMP (Urist and Mikulski, 1979; Urist *et al.*, 1979; Sampath and Reddi, 1981; 1983).

It has been suggested that the process of bone resorption and replacement may be mediated by a chemical substance released from the bone matrix during resorption. This coupling agent could then stimulate the synthesis of new bone (see Jaworski, 1984). Osteoclastic resorption can solubilize polypeptide growth factors from bone matrix, as demonstrated by Pfeilschifter *et al.* (1986) in the case of TGF-β. One unanswered question concerns which growth factor can be liberated from the bone matrix and what growth factor fraction may survive proteolytic degradation by osteoclasts? The acidic microenvironment created by the activity of osteoclasts may also activate BMP. Do the different growth factors have different physiological roles, e.g., some regulating the maintenance and remodeling functions and others signaling actual growth stimulation? Obviously a hierarchy of control and differential responses may be anticipated with at least six potential osteoblastic mitogens present in the bone matrix, and probably more.

Any break in the coordinated process of resorption and replacement of bone, or the coupling process, will obviously result in an increased loss of bone material, as in osteoporosis. It is interesting to note in this connection that the bones of elderly individuals, both experimental animals and human beings, seem to contain less BMP than those of young individuals while the bones of women after menopause have less BMP (Urist, 1989). Whether these findings reflect one of the reasons for osteoporosis is a question that remains to be resolved.

Growth factors may be important in the linkage or coupling of bone formation and bone resorption, and may mediate the effects of systemic hormones. Hormones may therefore act on skeletal cells either directly, or indirectly, by modulating the synthesis or effect of local factors, which could in turn stimulate or inhibit bone formation or bone resorption. As Hauschka *et al.* (1988) put it: "Systemic responses of the skeleton to endocrine signals alone do not explain the complex patterns of bone growth and remodelling, which are exquisitely sensitive to local and physical stresses. In a dense, labyrinthine mineralized bone tissue, with many barriers to the free diffusion of circulating hormones, it is an exciting prospect that these local responses may be regulated by the reservoir of specific growth factors in the matrix".

References

Abdin, M. and Friedenstein, A. Y. (1972). Electron microscopic study of bone induction by the transitional epithelium of the bladder in guinea pigs. *Clin. Orthop. Rel. Res.*, **82**: 182–194.

Anderson, H. C. (1976). Osteogenetic epithelial-mesenchymal cell interactions. *Clin. Orthop. Rel. Res.*, **119**: 211–223.

Anderson, H. C. and Griner, S. (1977). Cartilage induction *in vitro*. *Dev. Biol.*, **60**: 351–358.

Azizkhan, J. C. and Klagsburn, M. (1980). Chondrocytes contain a growth factor that is localized in the nucleus and is associated with chromatin. *Proc. Natl. Acad. Sci. U.S.A.*, **77**: 2762–2766.

Bab, I., Gazit, D., Muhlrad, A., and Stheyer, A. (1988). Regenerating bone marrow produces a potent growth-promoting activity to osteogenic cells. *Endocrinology*, **123**: 345–352.

Band, G. and Urist, M. R. (1967). Bone induction in excavation chambers in matrix of decalcified dentin. *Arch. Surg.*, **94**: 781–789.

Bennett, A., Chen, T., Feldman, D., Hintz, R. L., and Rosenfeld, R. G. (1984). Characterization of insulin-like growth factor I receptors on cultured rat bone cells: regulation of receptor concentration by glucocorticoids. *Endocrinology*, **115**: 1577–1583.

⁶⁶A

Beresford, J. N. (1989). Osteogenic stemm cells and the stromal system of bone and marrow. *Clin. Orthop. Rel. Res.*, **240**: 270–280.

Buring, K. and Urist, M. R. (1967). Transfilter bone induction. *Clin. Orthop.*, **54**: 235–242.

Canalis, E. (1985). Effect of growth factors on bone cell replication and differentiation. *Clin. Orthop. Rel. Res.*, **193**: 246–263.

Canalis, E., Centrella, M., and Urist, M. R. (1985). Effect of partially purified bone morphogenetic protein on DNA synthesis and cell replication in calvarial and fibroblast cultures. *Clin. Orthop. Rel. Res.*, **193**: 289–296.

Canalis, E., McCarthy, T., and Centrella, M. (1989). The regulation of bone formation by local growth factors. In: *Bone and Mineral Research*, Vol. 6. Peck, W. A., Ed., Elsevier, Amsterdam, 27–56.

Caplan, A. I., Syftestad, G., and Osdoby, B. (1983). The development of embryonic bone and cartilage in tissue culture. *Clin. Orthop. Rel. Res.*, **174**: 243–263.

Einhorn, T. S., Lane, J. M., Burstein, A. H., Kopman, C. R., and Vigorita, V. J. (1984). The healing of segmental bone defects induced by demineralized bone matrix. *J. Bone Jt. Surg.*, **66A**: 274–279.

Farley, J. R. and Baylink, D. J. (1982). Purification of a skeletal growth factor from human bone. *Biochemistry*, **21**: 3502–3507.

Glowacki, J., Kaban, L. B., Murray, J. E., Folkman, J., and Mulliken, J. B. (1981). Application of the biological principle of induced osteogenesis for craniofacial defects. *Lancet*, **8227**: 959–963.

Goldhaber, P. (1961). Osteogenic induction across millipore filter in vitro. *Science*, **133**: 2065–2067.

Hanamura, H., Higuchi, Y., Nakagava, M., Iwata, H., and Urist, M. R. (1980). Solubilization and purification of bone morphogenetic protein (BMP) from Dunn osteosarcoma. *Clin. Orthop. Rel. Res.*, **153**: 232–240.

Harakas, N. K. (1984). Demineralized bone-matrix-induced osteogenesis. *Clin. Orthop.*, **188**: 239–251.

Hauschka, P. V., Chen, T. L., and Mavrakos, A. E. (1988). Polypeptide growth factors in bone matrix. In: *Cell and Molecular Biology of Vertebrate Hard Tissues*. Ciba Foundation Symp. 136, Wiley, Chichester, 207–225.

Hauschka, P. V., Mavrakos, A. E., Iafrati, M. D., Doleman, S. E., and Klagsburn, M. (1986). Growth factors in bone matrix. Isolation of multiple types by affinity chromatography on heparin-sepharose. *J. Biol. Chem.*, **261**: 12665–12674.

Heiple, K. G., Herndon, C. H., Chase, S. W., and Wattleworth, A. (1968). Osteogenic induction by osteosarcoma and normal bone in mice. *J. Bone Jt. Surg.*, **50A**: 311–325.

Huggins, C. B. (1930). Experimental osteogenesis — influence of urinary tract mucosa on the experimental formation of bone. *Proc. Soc. Exp. Biol. Med.*, **27**: 349–353.

Huggins, C. B. (1931). The formation of bone under the influence of epithelium of the urinary tract. *Arch. Surg.*, **22**: 377–408.

Huggins, C. B. (1969). Epithelial osteogenesis — a biological chain reaction. *Proc. Am. Phil. Soc.*, **113**: 458–463.

Huggins, C. B. and Sammet, J. F. (1933). Function of the gall bladder epithelium as an osteogenic stimulus, and the physiological differentiation of connective tissues. *J. Exp. Med.*, **58**: 393–400.

Inoue, T., Deporter, D. A., and Melcher, A. H. (1986). Induction of chondrogenesis in muscle, skin, bone marrow, and periodontal ligament by demineralized dentin and bone matrix in vivo and in vitro. *J. Dent. Res.*, **65**: 12–22.

Isgaard, J., Nilsson, A., Lindahl, A., Jansson, J.-O., and Isaksson, O. G. P. (1986). Effect of local administration of GF and IGF-1 on longitudinal bone growth in rats. *Am. J. Physiol.*, **250**: E367–E372.

James, R. and Bradshaw, R. A. (1984). Polypeptide growth factors. *Annu. Rev. Biochem.*, **53**: 259–292.

Jaworski, Z. F. G. (1983). Coupling of bone formation to bone resorption: a broader view (editorial). *Calcif. Tissue Int.*, **36**: 531–535.

Johnson, E. E., Urist, M. R., and Finerman, A. M. (1988). Bone morphogenetic protein augmentation grafting of femoral nonunions: a preliminary report. *Clin. Orthop. Rel. Res.*, **230**: 257–265.

Kaban, L. B., Mulliken, J. B., and Glowacki, J. (1982). Treatment of jaw defects with demineralized bone implants. *J. Oral Maxillofac. Surg.*, **40**: 623–626.

Kato, Y., Nomura, Y., Tsuji, M., Kinoshita, M., Ohane, H., and Suzuki, F. (1981). Somatomedin-like peptide(s) isolated from fetal bovine cartilage (cartilage-derived-factor): isolation and some properties. *Proc. Natl. Acad. Sci. U.S.A.*, **78**: 6831–6835.

Lehtonen, E., Wartiovaara, J., Nordling, S., and Saxen, L. (1975). Demonstration of cytoplasmic processes in millipore filters permitting kidney tubule induction. *J. Embryol. Exp. Morphol.*, **33**: 187–203.

Libin, B. M., Ward, H. L., and Fishman, L. (1975). Decalcified, lyophilized bone allografts for use in human periodontal defects. *J. Periodontol.*, **46**: 51–56.

von der Mark, K. and Conrad, G. (1979). Cartilage cell differentiation. *Clin. Orthop. Rel. Res.*, **139**: 185–205.

Marks, S. J. R. and Popof, S. N. (1988). Bone cell biology: the regulation of development, structure, and function in the skeleton. *Am. J. Anat.*, **183**: 1–44.

Maugh, T. H. (1982). Human skeletal growth factor isolated. *Science*, **217**: 819.

Mikulski, A. J. and Urist, M. R. (1975). An antigenic antimorphogenetic bone hydrophobic glycopeptide. *Prep. Biochem.*, **5**: 21–39.

Minkin, C., Bannon, D. J., Jr., and Pokers, S. (1985). Bone-derived macrophage chemotactic factors: methods of extraction and further characterization. *Calcif. Tissue Int.*, **37**: 63–72.

Mizutani, H. and Urist, M. R. (1982). The nature of bone morphogenetic protein (BMP) fractions derived from bovine bone matrix gelatin. *Clin. Orthop. Rel. Res.*, **171**: 213–223.

Mulliken, J. B., Glowacki, J., Kaban, L. B., Folkman, J., and Murray, J. E. (1981). Use of demineralized allogeneic bone implants for the correction of maxillocraniofacial deformities. *Ann. Surg.*, **194**: 366–372.

Muthukumaran, N., Sampath, T. K., and Reddi, A. H. (1985). Comparison of bone inductive proteins of rat and porcine bone matrix. *Biochem. Biophys. Res. Commun.*, **131**: 37–41.

Nagakawa, M. and Urist, M. R. (1977). Chondrogenesis in tissue cultures of muscle under the influence of diffusible component of bone matrix. *Proc. Soc. Exp. Biol. Med.*, **154**: 568–572.

Narang, R., Wells, H., and Lloyd, W. S. (1973). Demineralization of bone transplants *in vivo*. *Oral Surg. Oral Med., Oral Pathol.*, **36**: 291–305.

Nathanson, M. A. (1985). Bone matrix-directed chondrogenesis of muscle *in vitro*. *Clin. Orthop. Rel. Res.*, **200**: 142–158.

Nathanson, M. A., Hilfer, S. R., Searls, R. (1978). Formation of cartilage by nonchondrogenic cell types. *Dev. Biol.*, **64**: 99–117.

Neuhof, H. (1917). Fascia transplantation in visceral defects. *Surg. Gynecol. Obstet.*, **24**: 383–427.

Nogami, H. and Terashima, Y. (1976). Diffusion of bone morphogenetic activity from the residue of collagenase digested bone matrix gelatin through interstitial fluid. *Clin. Orthop. Rel. Res.*, **115**: 268–273.

Nogami, H. and Urist, M. R. (1970). A substratum of bone matrix for differentiation of mesenchymal cells into chondro-osseous tissue *in vitro*. *Exp. Cell Res.*, **63**: 404–410.

Nogami, H. and Urist, M. R. (1974a). Substrata prepared from bone matrix for chondrogenesis in tissue culture. *J. Cell Biol.*, **62**: 510–519.

Nogami, H. and Urist, M. R. (1974b). Explants, transplants and implants of cartilage and bone morphogenetic matrix. *Clin. Orthop. Rel. Res.*, **103**: 235–251.

Oikarinen, J. (1981). Decalcified bone matrix as a substitute material for bone grafting. *Acta Univ. Ouluensis Ser. D. Med.*, **76(14)**: 1–44.

Oikarinen, J. (1982). Experimental spinal fusion with decalcified bone matrix and deep-frozen allogeneic bone in rabbits. *Clin. Orthop. Rel. Res.*, **162**: 210–218.

Oikarinen, J. and Korhonen, L. K. (1979). The bone inductive capacity of various transplanting materials used for treatment of experimental bone defects. *Clin. Orthop. Rel. Res.*, **140**: 208–215.

Osbon, D. B., Lilly, G. E., Thompson, C. W., and Jost, T. (1976). Bone grafts with surface decalcified allogeneic and particulate autologous bone: report of ten cases. *J. Oral Surg.*, **35**: 276–284.

Pearson, G. E., Rosen, S., and Deporter, D. A. (1981). Preliminary observations on the usefulness of a decalcified, freeze-dried cancellous bone allograft material in periodontal surgery. *J. Periodontol.*, **52**: 55–59.

Pfeilschifter, J., D'Souza, S., and Mundy, G. R. (1986). Transforming growth factor β is released from resorbing bone and stimulates osteoblast activity. *J. Bone Miner. Res.*, 1 (Suppl. 1):294 (abstr.).

Reddi, A. H. (1976). Collagen and cell differentiation. In: *Biochemistry of Collagen.* Ramachandran, G. R. and Reddi, A. H., Eds., Plenum Press, New York, 449–478.

Reddi, A. H. and Anderson, W. A. (1976). Collagenous bone matrix-induced endochondral ossification and hemopoesis. *J. Cell Biol.*, **69**: 557–571.

Reddi, A. H., Gay, R., Gay, S., and Miller, E. J. (1977). Transitions in collagen types during matrix induced cartilage, bone and bone marrow formation. *Proc. Natl. Acad. Sci. U.S.A.*, **74**: 5589–5592.

Reddi, A. H., Hascall, V. C., and Hascall, G. K. (1978). Changes in proteoglycan types during matrix-induced cartilage and bone development. *J. Biol. Chem.*, **253**: 2429–2436.

Reddi, A. H. and Huggins, C. B. (1972). Biochemical sequences in the transformation of normal fibroblasts in adolescent rats. *Proc. Natl. Acad. Sci. U.S.A.*, **69**: 1601–1605.

Reddi, A. H. and Huggins, C. B. (1973). Influence of geometry of transplanted tooth and bone on transformation of fibroblasts. *Proc. Soc. Exp. Biol. Med.*, **143**: 634–637.

Register, A. A., Scopp, I. W., Kassouny, D. Y., Pfau, F. R., and Peskin, D. (1972). Human bone induction by allogeneic dentin matrix. *J. Periodontol.*, **43**: 459–467.

Sampath, T. K., Muthukumaran, N., and Reddi, A. H. (1987). Isolation of osteogenin, an extracellular matrix-associated, bone inductive protein, by heparin affinity chromatography. *Proc. Natl. Acad. Sci. U.S.A.*, **84**: 7109–7113.

Sampath, T. K. and Reddi, A. H. (1981). Dissociative extraction and reconstruction of extracellular matrix. Components involved in local bone differentiation. *Proc. Natl. Acad. Sci. U.S.A.*, **78**: 7599–7603.

Sampath, T. K. and Reddi, A. H. (1983). Homology of bone-inductive proteins from human, monkey, bovine and rat extracellular matrix. *Proc. Natl. Acad. Sci. U.S.A.*, **80**: 6591–6595.

Sampath, T. K. and Reddi, A. H. (1984). Importance of geometry of the extracellular matrix in endochondral bone differentiation. *J. Cell Biol.*, **98**: 2192–2197.

Sampath, T. K. and De Simone, D. P. (1982). Extracellular bone matrix-derived growth factor. *Exp. Cell Res.*, **142**: 460–464.

Simmons, D. J. (1985). Fracture healing perspectives. *Clin. Orthop. Rel. Res.*, **200**: 100–112.

Slack, J. M. W. (1980). A serial threshold theory of regeneration. *J. Theor. Biol.*, **82**: 105–140.

Somerman, M., Hewitt, A. T., Varner, H. H., Schiffman, E., Termine, J., and Reddi, A. H. (1983). Identification of a bone-matrix-derived chemotactic factor. *Calcif. Tissue Int.*, **35**: 481–485.

Sonis, S. T., Kaban, L. B., and Glowacki, J. (1983). Clinical trial of demineralized bone powder in the treatment of periodontal defects. *J. Oral Med.*, **38**: 117–122.

Spemann, H. (1938). *Embryonic Development and Induction.* Yale University Press, New Haven.

Steinmann, B. U. and Reddi, A. H. (1980). Changes in synthesis of types-I and -III collagen during matrix-induced endochondral bone differentiation in rat. *Biochem. J.*, **186**: 919–924.

Syftestad, G. T., Kujawa, M. J., Carrino, D. A., and Caplan, A. I. (1985). Isolation and characterization of a bioactive factor from adult bone which stimulates chondrogenesis. *J. Cell Biol.*, **101(5P2)**: 29.

Syftestad, G. and Urist, M. R. (1979). Degradation of bone matrix morphogenetic activity by pulverization. *Clin. Orthop. Rel. Res.*, **141**: 281–286.

Takahashi, S., Iwata, H., and Hanamura, H. (1987). Nature of bone morphogenetic protein (BMP) from decalcified rabbit bone matrix. *J. Jpn. Orthop. Assoc.*, **61**: 197–218.

Takigawa, M., Takano, T., Shirai, E., and Suzuki, F. (1984). Cytoskeleton and differentiation: effects of cytochalasin B and colchisine on expression of the differentiated phenotype of rabbit costal chondrocytes in culture. *Cell Differ.*, **14**: 197–204.

Terashima, M. D. and Urist, M. R. (1977). Chondrogenesis in outgrowths of muscle tissue onto modified bone matrix in tissue culture. *Clin. Orthop. Rel. Res.*, **127**: 248–255.

Thieleman, F. W., Schmidt, K., and Koslowski, L. (1982). Osteoinduction. II. Purification of the osteoinductive activities of bone matrix. *Arch. Orthop. Traumatol. Surg.*, **100**: 73–78.

Thieleman, F., Veihelmann, D., and Schmidt, K. (1978). The induction of new bone formation after transplantation. *Arch. Orthop. Traumatol. Surg.*, **91**: 3–9.

Urist, M. R. (1965). Bone formation by autoinduction. *Science*, **150**: 893–899.

Urist, M. R. (1968). Surface-decalcified allogeneic bone (SDAB) implants. *Clin. Orthop. Rel. Res.*, **56**: 37–50.

Urist, M. R. (1972). Osteoinduction in undemineralized bone implants modified by chemical inhibitors of endogenous matrix enzymes. *Clin. Orthop. Rel. Res.*, **87**: 132–137.

Urist, M. R. (1973). A bone morphogenetic system in residues of bone matrix in the mouse. *Clin. Orthop. Rel. Res.*, **91**: 210–220.

Urist, M. R. (1989). Bone morphogenetic protein, bone regeneration, heterotopic ossification and the bone-bone marrow consortium. In: *Bone and Mineral Research*, Vol. 6. Peck, W. A., Ed., Elsevier, Amsterdam, 57–112.

Urist, M. R., Granstein, R., Nogami, H., Svanson, L., and Murphy, R. (1977). Transmembranic bone morphogenesis across multiple-walled diffusion chambers. New evidence for a diffusible bone morphogenetic property. *Arch. Surg.*, **112**: 612–619.

Urist, M. R., DeLange, R. J., and Finerman, G. A. M. (1983). Bone cell differentiation and growth factors. *Science*, **220**: 680–686.

Urist, M. R., Dowell, T. A., Hay, P. H., and Strates, B. S. (1968). Inductive substrates for bone formation. *Clin. Orthop. Rel. Res.*, **59**: 59–96.

Urist, M. R., Hay, P. H., Duruc, F., and Buring, K. (1969). Osteogenetic competence. *Clin. Orthop. Rel. Res.*, **64**: 194–220.

Urist, M. R., Huo, Y. K., Brownell, A. G., Hohl, W. M., Buyske, J., Lietze, A., Tempst, P., Hunkapiller, M., and DeLange, R. J. (1984). Purification of bovine morphogenetic protein by hydroxyapatite chromatography. *Proc. Natl. Acad. Sci. U.S.A.*, **81**: 371–375.

Urist, M. R., Lietze, A., Mizutani, H., Takagi, K., Triffit, J. T., Amstutz, J., DeLange, R., Termine, J., and Finerman, G. A. M. (1982). A bovine low molecular weight bone morphogenetic protein (BMP) fraction. *Clin. Orthop. Rel. Res.*, **162**: 219–232.

Urist, M. R. and Mikulski, A. J. (1979). A soluble bone morphogenetic protein extracted from bone matrix with a mixed aqueous and nonaqueous solvent (40616). *Proc. Soc. Exp. Biol. Med.*, **162**: 48–53.

Urist, M. R., Mikulski, A., and Lietze, A. (1979). Solubilized and insolubilized bone morphogenetic protein. *Proc. Natl. Acad. Sci. U.S.A.*, **76**: 1828–1832.

Urist, M. R., Sato, K., Brownell, A. G., Malinin, T. I., Lietze, A., Huo, Y.-K., Prolo, D. J., Oklund, S., Finerman, G. A. M., and DeLange, R. J. (1983). Human bone morphogenetic protein (hBMP) (41630). *Proc. Soc. Exp. Biol. Med.*, **173**: 194–199.

Urist, M. R. and Strates, B. S. (1971). Bone morphogenetic protein. *J. Dent. Res.*, (Suppl. 6 **50**: 1392–1406.

Wang, E. A., Rosen, V., Cordes, P., Hewick, R. M., Kriz, M. J., Luxenberg, D. P., Sibley, I S., and Wozney, J. M. (1988). Purification and characterization of other distinct bon inducing factors. *Proc. Natl. Acad. Sci. U.S.A.*, **85**: 9484–9488.

Weiss, R. E. and Reddi, A. H. (1980). Synthesis and localization of fibronectin during collagenous matrix-mesenchymal cell interaction and differentiation of cartilage and bone in vivo. *Proc. Natl. Acad. Sci. U.S.A.*, **77**: 2074–2078.

Weiss, R. E. and Reddi, A. H. (1981). Role of fibronectin in collagenous matrix-induced mesenchymal cell proliferation and differentiation *in vivo*. *Exp. Cell Res.*, **133**: 247–254.

Wlodarski, K., Poltorak, A., and Kazirowska, J. (1971). Species specificity of osteogenesis induced by WISH cell line and bone induction by vaccinia virus transformed human fibroblasts. *Calcif. Tissue Res.*, **7**: 345–352.

Wozney, J. M., Rosen, V., Celeste, A. J., Mitsock, L. M., Shitters, M. J., Kritz, R. W., Hewick, R. M., and Wang, E. (1988). Novel regulators of bone formation: molecular clones and activities. *Science*, **242**: 1528–1534.

Wright, G. C., Jr., Miller, F., and Sokoloff, L. (1985). Induction of bone by xenografts of rabbit growth plate chondrocytes in the nude mouse. *Calcif. Tissue Res.*, **37**: 250–256.

Wu, Z. Y. and Hu, X.-B. (1988). Separation and purification of porcine bone morphogenetic protein. *Clin. Orthop. Rel. Res.*, **230**: 229–236.

Zanetti, N. C. and Solursh, M. (1986). Epithelial effects on limb chondrogenesis involve extracellular matrix and cell shape. *Dev. Biol.*, **113**: 110–118.

7

Growth Plate Distraction and Response of Growth Plates to Trauma

A. TURNER
University of Liverpool
New Cross Hospital
Wolverhampton Health Authority
Wolverhampton, United Kingdom

AND

J. ANDERSON
University of Liverpool
Liverpool, United Kingdom

Slow growth plate distraction
Summary
Acknowledgments
References

Introduction

The morphological and clinical effects of fractures in and around the growth plates of long bones in children are well known (Salter and Harris, 1963). More subtly, iatrogenic fracture through the growth plate by the application of a longitudinal distracting force using an external fixator attached to the limb, in order to increase bone length, has been used in the management of leg length inequality (Ring, 1958; Monticelli and Spinelli, 1981b; Ilizarow and Soybelman, 1969).

In this process, termed distraction epiphysiolysis, both the speed of distraction and the magnitude of the distracting force are relatively large. The result is a fracture through the layer of hypertrophic chondrocytes. The fracture gap so produced is reconstituted in the same way as the healing of any long bone fracture, with the formation of primary callus and its eventual conversion to lamellar bone within the metaphysis.

More recently, De Bastiani et al. (1984) have used the term "chondrodiatasis" to describe a slower and less forceful distraction of the growth plate which they claim results in physiological stimulation of growth plate activity rather than growth plate fracture per se. (De Bastiani et al., 1986a).

Theoretically, longitudinal mechanical distraction across the growth plate may cause an increase in bone length by one or more of the following mechanisms:

(1) Direct mechanical stretching of either the cellular or intercellular components
(2) Macro- or micro-fracture of the plate
(3) Physiological stimulation of the growth mechanism of the plate

These mechanisms may also be influenced by, or influence, changes in the intricate blood supply to the various cellular components of the plate. It has been hypothesized by the present authors and others, that the vascular architecture of the growth plate and changes in it caused by mechanical distraction, have a fundamental bearing, both upon the physiological effects and clinical results of growth plate distraction.

It is because of the latter hypothesis that the first part of this chapter will describe in detail the morphology of the growth plate including its vascular supply and the effects on growth plate morphology of changes in the latter brought about by experimental damage.

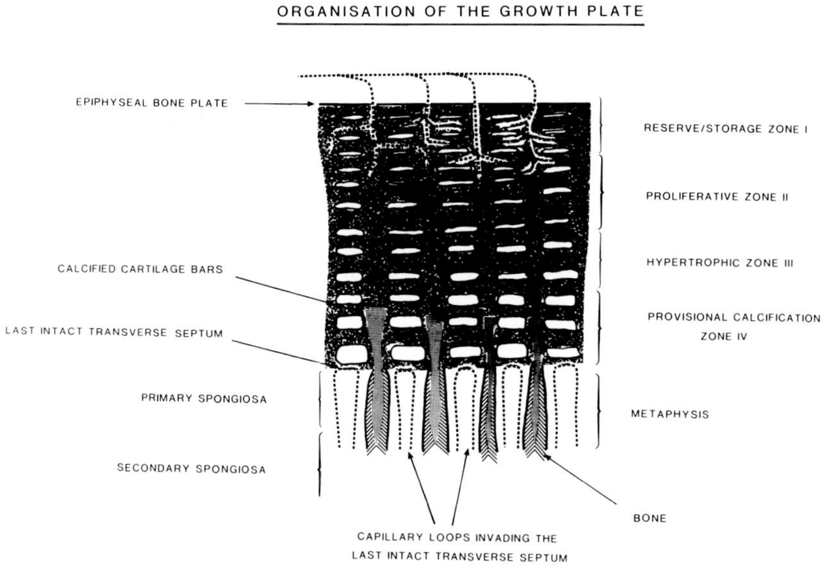

ORGANISATION OF THE GROWTH PLATE

Fig. 1 General morphology of the growth plate including its blood supply.

Growth Plate Morphology

In the mammalian growth plate cellular morphology and vascular supply are essentially similar between species despite minor variations (Brighton, 1984). The morphology of the plate with clearly arranged cellular layers and columns (Fig. 1) is not well recognizable until the ossific nucleus of the epiphysis is well developed and has expanded to define the cellular area which will be the future growth plate sandwiched between the bone of the metaphysis and the developing ossific nucleus of the epiphysis. By this time, blood vessels have grown into the latter and a layer of bone has condensed on its surface facing the growth plate and termed the "epiphyseal bone plate". In addition, blood vessels have grown up from the nutrient artery and metaphyseal arteries towards the growth plate from the metaphyseal aspect.

The basic components of the growth plate are:

(1) Cellular (cartilage cells)
(2) Bony (the epiphyseal bone plate on the epiphyseal side and the metaphyseal bone immediately adjacent to the growth plate on the metaphyseal side)
(3) Fibrous (circumferential fibrous components and intercellular collagenous architecture)
(4) Vascular (the blood vessels of the epiphyseal and metaphyseal circulations)

The Cellular (Cartilaginous) Component

The cartilaginous cells of the growth plate are arranged in three layers (Fig. 1):

(1) The storage (reserve) zone (adjacent to the epiphysis)
(2) The proliferative zone
(3) The hypertrophic zone (adjacent to the metaphysis)

The Storage (Reserve) Zone

This zone has previously been described as the reserve or resting zone. It was formerly believed that cells from this zone were contributing to the next layer (proliferative zone). However, it seems much more likely that these cells store substrates necessary for metabolic processes going on in the adjacent (proliferative) zone since they are high in lipids, have a relatively high metabolic activity, and a rich vascular supply.

The Proliferative Zone

This zone has cells arranged in columns. The area adjacent to the storage zone has a high oxygen content and the cells here form glycogen and adenosine triphosphate rapidly through aerobic respiration. These cells thus require a rich blood supply which comes through the epiphyseal vessels (see below). The main metabolic and cellular activity of the growth plate occurs in this area. Cell division proceeds quickly, resulting in an increase in growth plate thickness and the formation of longitudinal columns.

The Hypertrophic Zone

This layer is often subdivided into three subzones.

(1) Maturation
(2) Degeneration
(3) Provisional calcification

Maturation. Cells in this layer enlarge up to five times their size in the proliferative zone before entering in the next zone of degeneration.

Degeneration. The cartilage cells in this zone show metabolic changes indicative of impending cell death. This is presumably due to the poor blood supply in this area (see below) and is associated with the preparation of the intercellular matrix for calcification in the next subzone.

Provisional Calcification. Here the intercellular matrix is calcified prior to ossification in the metaphysis. Calcification and ossification take place in close relationship to the metaphyseal blood vessels (see below). It is in this zone that the metabolic environment is such that calcification occurs in the cartilaginous trabeculae with the release of calcium from mitochondria.

The Bony (Metaphyseal) Component

The primary spongiosum (Fig. 1) consists of bone deposited upon calcified cartilaginous trabeculae and is included as the most proximal layer of the growth plate next to the true metaphysis.

The Fibrous Component

This consists of:

(1) The perichondrial ring of Lacroix
(2) The groove of Ranvier
(3) The intercellular collagenous architecture

The Perichondrial Ring of Lacroix

This circumferential layer of fibrous tissue is continuous both with the periosteum of the metaphysis and with the perichondrium of the epiphysis. It supports the growth plate circumferentially and provides considerable resistance under conditions of growth plate distraction.

The Groove of Ranvier

This area consists of a number of cell systems contributing towards the cellular component of the plate to allow for circumferential and radial growth. It also contributes collagen fibers to the perichondrial ring.

The Intercellular Collagenous Architecture

A number of collagen fiber systems have been identified within the growth plate arranged in radial, longitudinal, and circumferential fashion (Speer, 1982). These contribute towards plate stability and towards stability of the adjacent metaphysis and epiphysis. Cellular hypertrophy and lack of collagen fibers in the hypertrophic zone of the plate may account for the separation of the plate at this level under conditions of distraction, or shear (slipped upper femoral epiphysis).

The Vascular Component (Fig. 1)

This has been examined in considerable detail, chiefly by the use of microinjection techniques followed by microradiography or Spalteholz processing. Traditionally, the blood supply of the growth plate has been described as follows:

(1) Epiphyseal
(2) Metaphyseal
(3) Perichondrial

The Epiphyseal Blood Vessels

These vessels provide the main nutritional supply to the growth plate, supplying those areas where high metabolic activity is occurring (the storage and proliferative zones); thus a high oxygen tension is required. These vessels are derived from the blood supply to the epiphysis and are theoretically likely to be damaged during placement of an external fixator screw for the purposes of growth plate distraction. They are branches of the vessels to the epiphyseal nucleus which pass through the epiphyseal bone plate and arborize in the storage and proliferative layers. Each branch of an epiphyseal vessel ends above a cell column of the proliferative zone. Vessels are formed which pass back through the bone plate to join the epiphyseal veins.

The Metaphyseal Blood Vessels

The arrangement of the metaphyseal circulation near the growth plate consists of hairpin loops derived from (1) the nutrient artery in the central portion of the plate and (2) the metaphyseal and periosteal arteries at the periphery. Each loop is associated with one cell column in the zone of provisional calcification (Fig. 1). The loop apex ends just below the last intact transverse septum and hence near the last degenerating cartilage cell of that particular column. There has been some debate as to whether the terminal loops are closed throughout their extent or whether they rupture to form an extravascular circulation which corresponds with degeneration of the last chondrocyte in the column. Between the loops are the vertical cartilage septa undergoing calcification prior to ossification in the metaphysis. It is the metaphyseal circulation which is concerned with cartilage calcification rather than with nutrition of the plate, the latter function being the responsibility of the epiphyseal supply under normal conditions.

The Perichondrial Blood Vessels

These vessels are supplied from the perichondrial ring of vessels surrounding the circumference of the plate and pass through the perichondrium into the outer layers of the plate supplying it on both the metaphyseal and epiphyseal sides as well as supplying the perichondrial ring of Lacroix and the groove of Ranvier.

Under normal conditions, no communication exists between the epiphyseal and metaphyseal vessels. However, communicating vessels do cross the plate in the fetal state, following growth plate closure at maturity and following injury in association with the formation of bony bridges across the plate.

The growth plate thus functions as a factory for the production of cartilage cells. These cartilage cells produce an intercellular matrix which in the deeper layers of the plate is prepared for provisional calcification. An increase in the length of the bone therefore occurs by cartilage proliferation, and its conversion to bone is really a secondary phenomenon. It is important to grasp the concept of cartilage cells being produced on one side of the plate and being destroyed on the other. There is of course no actual movement of cells through the zones. This is an illusion based on the fact that new cells are being produced on one side and destroyed on the other and hence the growth plate is always moving away from the anatomical center of the diaphysis. The epiphyseal and metaphyseal circulations thus have separate rolls and are intimately bound with this process. Experimental manipulation of this blood supply has not only enabled us to learn a great deal about growth plate physiology but has also revealed the differing functions of these two vascular territorial areas.

Damage to the Epiphyseal Circulation

Trueta and Amato (1960) showed that growth plate morphology can be altered by surgical interference with specific parts of the growth plate circulation.

Using a number of mammalian species, these workers interfered with the epiphyseal circulation by destroying the blood vessels immediately adjacent to the epiphyseal bone plate, either temporarily or permanently with the insertion of plastic sheets, and studied subsequent plate morphology. This maneuver caused the height of the plate to decrease because further growth and division of cells in the proliferative zone ceased, while cartilage degeneration with provisional calcification continued on the metaphyseal side.

Interruption for a relatively short period of time caused the plate to thin temporarily and then return to normal when the epiphyseal blood supply was restored. If interruption was for a longer period, whole columns of cells died (Fig. 2) and blood vessels grew in from surrounding columns and from the metaphysis to eventually form a bony bridge. Interruption of a few vessels to part of the plate only had much less of an effect than if the whole epiphyseal circulation was destroyed, when growth plate closure occurred prematurely.

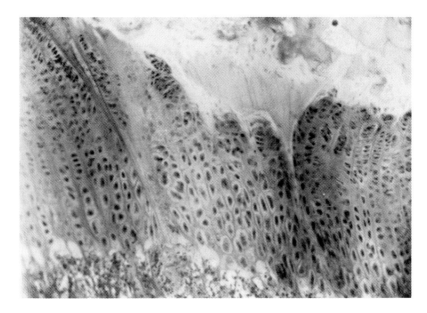

Fig. 2 Changes in growth plate structure following damage to the epiphyseal blood supply showing death of whole cell columns.

Damage to the Metaphyseal Circulation

Interruption to the metaphyseal circulation had the opposite effect in Trueta and Amato's experiments (Fig. 3). The plate thickened because normal cartilage production continued from the epiphyseal side. However, provisional calcification did not occur and the cartilage accumulated. If this was a temporary interruption the plate returned to normal thickness when the blood supply was restored; permanent destruction resulted in a bony bridge following ingrowth of vessels and communication across the plate. An interruption of the blood supply to a substantial part of the plate once more resulted in premature closure of the entire plate.

This account of growth plate morphology and blood supply is important for subsequent understanding of the events occurring in growth plate damage due either to trauma or mechanical distraction. It is believed that growth plate activity following such damage is strongly dependent upon their effect on the blood supply to the growth plate.

The Effects of Physical Forces on the Growth Plate

For well over 100 years the effects of force upon the skeleton have interested scientific workers. Such observations have been mainly upon the growth of bone as a whole without specific reference to the growth plate. Lately,

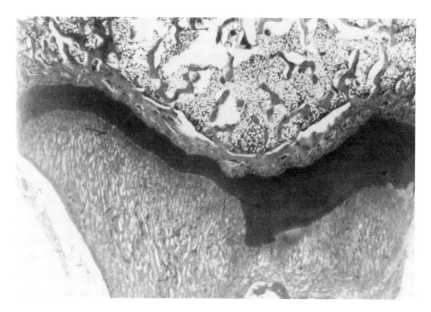

Fig. 3 Changes in growth plate structure following damage to the metaphyseal blood supply showing thickening of the growth plate due to failure of metaphyseal calcification.

the growth plate has become more of a focus of interest, chiefly because of the effect of pressure and compression, rather than tension per se. There is, of course, an extensive literature on the morphological and clinical effects of injury to the growth plate.

Hueter (1862) first noted the relatively greater growth of bone when the compressive force upon it was less and vice versa. This is often referred to as the Hueter-Volkmann Law. Continuous traction may stimulate bone growth at a growth disc as observed on the concave side of a scoliosis during conservative treatment.

Keith (cited in Bassett, 1971) noted many years ago that bone responded to changes in compressive or tensile forces upon it by changing the formation or behavior of long chain polymers within its substance.

Compression may affect cellular behavior by retarding or accelerating cellular responses on the basis of the Theory of Arrhenius. Nucleic acid and protein synthesis may be affected in the osteoblast and chondroblast. Small variations in pressure across the cell membrane do seem to affect sodium transport. It is reasonable to assume that tensile forces will have an effect upon cell function in just the same way as compressive forces of which much more is known, albeit that the mechanism and result may differ.

Mechanical energy may affect cell function in three ways — by piezo-electricity (stress on bone), solid state physical effects (crystalline in nature), and streaming potentials (occurring due to the rapid movement of cells past each other containing charged ions or molecules).

Bourret and Rodan (1975) found that a hydrostatic pressure of 60 g/cm^2 inhibited the accumulation of cyclic adenosine monophosphate in cells of the proliferative zone of the chick growth plate.

A number of other studies have investigated the effects of compression upon the physiological activity of the growth plate, compared with the relatively small amount of work done on the effects of tension or distraction. However, such observations are still valid if one considers that distraction is merely a reduction in pressure as opposed to an increase. On this basis, Ehrlick *et al.* (1972) studied the biochemical and physiological events during closure of the stapled distal femoral epiphyseal growth plate in rats. Compression appeared to be a regulatory mechanism for cellular responses with DNA synthesis and lysosomal enzyme production appearing to be exquisitely sensitive.

Many other experiments have been designed to study the effects of compression and tension on the growth plate both mechanically and biochemically. Gelpke (1951) used a rather crude experiment to obtain both compression and tension. He passed wire around the lower growth plate of growing dogs' femurs. As growth continued the wire got tighter and the growth plate thinner. A force of 1 kg was needed to deform the wire. The femur subjected to compression remained shorter and histology showed disappearance of the growth cartilage and irregularity of the plate. The histological changes could be reversed if the compression was released soon enough. Tension was also applied to a growth plate by passing a wire loop through the patella and through a hole in the nearby femoral shaft. This exerted a force on the tibial apophysis as the femur grew. This was a crude experiment but histology showed no change after 3 months. Wire was also passed through the olecranon and humeral shafts to exert tension on the olecranon apophysis. After 15 weeks, irregularity and narrowing of the growth plate occurred. Tension, like compression, appeared to damage the plate and this was confirmed histologically and there was certainly no increase in longitudinal growth. Smith and Cunningham (1957) used Holstein calves with a turn-buckle device fitted to the upper tibia in an attempt to remove compressive forces. An increase in the height of the growth plate was noted. They did not mention how much distraction was used, nor for how long. Histologically the cartilage cell columns became large, rectangular, and elongated.

Harsha (1962) implanted spring distracting devices across the physis in dogs. This did not appear to influence growth in any way.

Hert and Liskova (1964) stapled the radius and ulna of young rabbits together so producing, by differential growth, increased pressure on the proximal radial growth plate and decreased pressure on the distal radial growth plate. In all cases, unloaded cartilage increased its growth activity and compressed cartilage diminished it. These observations were made purely by measurement and X-rays, and no histological detail was available. Hert (1969) further placed distracting springs across the growth plates of rabbits and found an acceleration of growth as measured on X-ray. However, 3 months later the growth rate had slowed down and the operated side often ended up shorter than the control side, possibly indicating cellular damage. Premature growth plate closure on the unloaded side was seen. Histologically the unloaded growth plates showed a thicker cartilage with a larger number of cell columns. It was postulated that changes in loading influenced mitotic activity in the growth plate, possibly by changes in hydration. It was found that the load needed to be decreased by at least a quarter of the body weight.

Hinrichsen and Storey (1968) placed helical torsion springs across the growth plates of guinea pigs' tibiae, used injected tetracycline as a marker for bone growth, and measured changes on standardized radiographs. A force of 150 g was applied. Longitudinal growth was inhibited slightly and the growth plate was no longer at right angles to the axis of the tibia due to the construction of the springs. The force seemed to have had little effect upon the growth plate.

Growth Plate Distraction

This process has been studied extensively in the literature both experimentally and clinically. The main effect is the formation of a fracture through the plate with the production of a fracture gap. This process has been termed "distraction epiphysiolysis" and is the result of rapid distraction (greater than 1 mm/day) using relatively large forces. More recently, De Bastiani et al. (1984; 1986a,b) suggested that a slower distraction rate may be used with resultant physiological growth stimulation of the plate rather than fracture. These latter workers coined the term "chondrodiatasis" to describe this process although others had previously investigated the concept (Sledge and Noble, 1978).

Distraction Epiphysiolysis

Many reports have been published concerning this process (Ring, 1958; Ilizarow and Soybelman, 1969; 1970; Monticelli et al., 1981b). It is used in the field of leg lengthening and to a lesser extent for the correction of angular deformity. Its reported advantages over diaphyseal lengthening are

(1) Its ease of performance without recourse to open surgical osteotomy
(2) Management mainly on an out-patient basis following application of an external fixator, with a short hospitalization time
(3) Good quality new bone formation without the need for bone grafting
(4) No necessity for internal fixation

(5) Theoretically, the continuing viability of the growth plate following the procedure, thus allowing growth to continue post-operatively and the procedure to be repeated on the same growth plate if necessary

Those features of this process of special interest are

(1) The amount of force necessary to fracture the growth plate
(2) The optimum rate or speed of lengthening
(3) The quality of the new bone formed and the mechanism of reconstruction of the fracture gap
(4) The amount of lengthening obtained
(5) The most desirable growth plates to be used
(6) The age at which the procedure is best performed
(7) The viability of the plate following the procedure

Forces Involved in Distraction Epiphysiolysis

These have varied widely as measured in the experimental animal and in the human. Gelpke (1951) noted that a force of 1 kg was necessary to deform wires passed around the growth plate in dogs. Janovek and Fait (1981) found a force of 214 newtons necessary to distract the epiphysis from the metaphysis in 10-year-old children. Monticelli and Spinelli (1981a) used 18 ± 4 kg to induce epiphyseal separation in sheep and found a force of 80 to 105 kg necessary in children. Noble (1982) looked at the breaking force of the rabbit growth plate and studied the application of this to epiphyseal distraction. It was felt that forces likely to be safe and effective in growth plate distraction work *in vivo* were only 5 to 10% of those occurring *in vitro*. Noble (1978) also noted a force of 6 to 8 kg as necessary to produce a Salter Harris type one fracture in rabbits.

It is obvious that the amount of force required to fracture the growth plate will vary with the experimental animal and also with age. Associated with this is the advisability of detaching the periosteum prior to growth plate distraction as has been studied by Houghton (1982). He found that less final growth was obtained if the periosteum was surgically released at the time of distraction, possibly due to scar formation and further tethering of the periosteum.

Taking all the literature into account it would appear that a considerable force is necessary to obtain detachment of the plate, a conclusion that is certainly borne out by the clinical studies of Monticelli and Spinelli (1981b) who found that during distraction epiphysiolysis in children a sudden increase in pain occurred some days after initiation of the process due to sudden detachment of the plate. In some cases pain was so intense as to lead workers to induce a mechanical distraction with the production of a fracture gap under anesthetic prior to gradual lengthening.

Speed or Rate of Distraction

It appears that epiphysiolysis is produced by distraction at the rate of 1 to 2 mm/day. This also appears to be a safe speed clinically without major neurovascular damage, (Peltonen *et al.*, 1984; Monticelli and Spinelli, 1981b; Li *et al.*, 1985; Grill, 1984; Eydelshteyn *et al.*, 1973; Bensahel *et al.*, 1983).

Even at 0.5 mm/day De Pablos *et al.* (1986) found evidence of a fracture gap, a rate at which De Bastiani *et al.* (1986) suggested physiological stimulation only.

Reconstitution of the Distracted Growth Plate

Separation of the growth plate occurs between the zone of degenerating chondrocytes and calcified cartilage layer (De Pablos *et al.*, 1986; De Bastiani *et al.*, 1986a; Monticelli and Spinelli, 1981a; Ring, 1958). Fishbane and Riley (1978) noted separation through the layer of primary bone trabeculae in the metaphysis distal to the growth plate in growing puppies. Much of this work is therefore in agreement with the classical studies showing separation through the same level in slipped upper femoral epiphysis (Harris and Hobson, 1956). However, there is good evidence to suggest that there may be varying patterns of failure in and around the physis when the direction of stress is varied. Moen and Pelker (1984) studied compression, tension, shear, and torque individually applied in immature bovine femora and tibiae. The results showed that the histological failure pattern did vary with each type of applied load. Compression resulted in failure in the zone of provisional calcification and the metaphysis, rather than in the previously hypophysized germinal zone. Tension loads caused failure in the upper zone of columnation. Failure between the upper zone of columnation and lower zone of hypertrophy was caused by shear load. Torque resulted in varied failure through all zones.

Following separation, the fracture gap fills with blood clot and organizes from the periphery, first by the formation of fibrous tissues and then by conversion to bone. The center of the distracted area is the last to ossify. In sheep, De Pablo *et al.* (1986) noted that ossification started at 20 days following epiphysiolysis and was completed in 4 months. They also noted that a fracture gap was created at all speeds, that is, from 2 to 0.5 mm/day, although by 6 weeks only the gap at the slowest speed had recalcified. Recalcification and ossification were slower at faster speeds. They also found that at the slowest speed of 0.5 mm/day, a higher trabecular density and more cortical bone was formed than at the faster speed of 2 mm/day.

Eydelshteyn *et al.* (1973) noted six radiological phases in the reconstruction of the fracture gap with gradual opacification of the area.

Ilizarow and Soybelman (1970) noted gradual reconstitution of the fracture gap in puppies over 4 to 6 months. Monticelli *et al.* (1981a) noted a similar process in sheep. Three phases were described:

(1) Epiphysiolysis and hematoma formation
(2) Resorption and fibrous tissue formation
(3) Ossification of the fibrous tissue and reconstitution of the periosteal bone

As the fibrous tissue developed, the cartilaginous segment which had been dislocated downwards with the metaphysis gradually disappeared, becoming partly reabsorbed by penetrating blood vessels. Small islands of cartilage were sometimes found in the connective tissue. The time required for reconstitution of the fracture gap depended very much on the rate of distraction and the total amount of lengthening obtained. The greater these were, the longer consolidation took. When bone lengthening was 3 to 4 cm it took 2 months for the cortex to form after completion of lengthening. One year after the start of distraction the neometaphysis had acquired a complete bone structure.

Startseva and Gorbunova (1982) investigated epiphysiolysis in young puppies and found an age dependence concerning the level of separation and the morphological structure following reconstitution.

It appears that in no cases have bone grafts of the epiphyseal area been needed, nor thought necessary. Bensahel (1983) carried out lengthenings of up to 11 cm in children without the need for such bone grafting.

The Amount of Lengthening Obtained

This is variable and depends upon the pathology of the cause of the leg length discrepancy. Letts and Meadows (1978) carried out manual epiphysiolysis and produced an immediate 6% increase in the length of a rabbit tibia. Figures between 4 and 18 cm have been quoted in children. (Bensahel *et al.*, 1983; Berchiche and Wittek, 1983; Franke *et al.*, 1984; Grill and Altenhuber, 1984; Li *et al.*, 1985; Fischenko *et al.*, 1976; Monticelli and Spinelli, 1981b).

Which Growth Plate

In children this process has chiefly been confined to the lower femoral, upper tibial, and lower tibial growth plates. De Bastiani *et al.* (1986b) found that distraction through the upper tibial growth plate tended to produce knee subluxation and so confined their tibial lengthenings to the lower tibial epiphysis.

The Optimum Age for the Performance of Epiphysiolysis

Most workers have performed this process towards the end of growth. This is because there is considerable disquiet concerning damage to the growth plate following the process. Most advise that the procedure be done as late as possible in order that possible premature closure will not adversely affect the final length obtained (Besahel, 1983; Fishbane and Riley, 1978; Monticelli and Spinelli, 1981b).

Growth Plate Viability Following Distraction

De Pablos *et al.* (1986) found that morphological changes within the growth plate were directly related to the speed of distraction. Six months after distraction up to 2 cm and at a rate of 2 mm/day, bony bridges occurred across the physis in sheep accompanied by morphological evidence of damage. Eydelshtyn *et al.* (1973) in a 5-year follow-up found no retardation of growth in younger patients. Fishbane and Riley (1978) found premature fusion in five puppies followed to maturity.

Hert (1969) noted premature fusion of an unloaded plate. Jani (1984) found severe histological damage in rabbits following distraction epiphysiolysis; all lost the length originally obtained. In Letts and Meadows (1978) series all plates were non-viable and although Monticelli and Spinelli (1981a) found that there was a translucent line at the growth plate following distraction and stated that the plate continued to function post-operatively, they still advocated the procedure towards the end of growth. Growth apparently continued in eight out of ten pigs distracted by Peltonen (Peltonen *et al.*, 1984), but all Ring's dogs stopped growing (Ring, 1958). Startseva and Gorbunova (1982) noted complete loss of function.

Complications

Recorded complications are similar to those of diaphyseal leg lengthening and include distal neurovascular compromise, infection, loss of alignment, failure of adequate new bone formation, loss of length obtained, and joint stiffness. However, they appear to be less severe than in diaphyseal lengthening.

Of special concern is fracture of the lengthened segment and loss of length obtained. This is best prevented by plaster fixation post-operatively and the need for non-weight bearing for a considerable period (Franke *et al.*, 1984). In addition, these latter authors also noted a large incidence of superficial pin track infection in their cases, but this almost never progressed to serious bone infection.

Monticelli and Spinelli (1981b) noted that all their elongations consolidated without fracture. Post-operative management in their cases consisted of plaster being applied some 4 months following distraction. Weight-bearing was not allowed for 8 months following elongation. Complications included anomalous separation of the epiphysis when the procedure was done at too late an age. Tomograms of the growth plate were advised to make sure that it was open prior to attempting distraction.

In conclusion, therefore, distraction epiphysiolysis has a definite place in the management of leg length inequality provided it is done at an age when the growth plate is definitely open throughout its area but when premature fusion is not a serious consideration.

Slow Growth Plate Distraction (Chondrodiatasis)

De Pablos et al. (1986) carried out growth plate distraction at 3 speeds; 2, 1, and 0.5 mm/day. They found no signs to indicate physiological stimulation of growth and noted that even at the slowest speed, fracture occurred across the plate through the layer of hypertrophic chondrocytes. At speeds of 1 or 2 mm/day, epiphysiolysis occurred, although they did also recognize that reconstitution of the fracture gap occurred more rapidly at the slowest speed.

Noble et al. (1978) applied distraction springs to Kirschner wires placed on either side of the femoral growth plate of the rabbit. They noted that a force of 6 to 8 kg in the springs produced a Salter-Harris type I fracture in all cases. With forces of 1 to 2 kg some partial fractures occurred but, in two thirds of the rabbits, either microscopic fracture or no fracture at all was seen. The measured growth increase in these rabbits was highly significant, the average being 216%. Striking histological changes with enormous thickening of the growth plate and increased new bone formation as demonstrated by tetracycline labeling were seen. There was also a significant increase in cell division detected by tritiated thymidine and in matrix synthesis using radioactive sulfate. It was concluded that increased linear growth, increased new bone formation and accelerated cellular formation in the growth plate occurred in response to distraction. The springs used by Noble and co-workers were an ingenious device which allowed a more or less constant force of distraction to be applied. It is to be noted that in a simple distraction device using a screw mechanism, at whatever speed is used between 2 and 0.5 mm/day, there will be a sudden dramatic force applied to the growth plate on turning the screw, which of course will rapidly diminish as the tissues accommodate to the increase in tension. Using a spring-loaded mechanism, a more or less constant tension force can be maintained, although admittedly as the tissues lengthen, together with the spring, tension is slightly decreased. Noble was able to maintain a constant tension from day to day by incorporating a separate screw mechanism into his spring distractors which allowed the tension force in the spring to be kept constant. It would seem that the biological effects of such constant vs.

intermittent distraction will be considerable, but very little work has been done on this aspect of distraction to date and there is room for considerable research in this area.

De Bastiani et al. (1984) revived, strengthened, and considerably advanced the idea of slow growth plate distraction, coining the term chondrodiatasis. They developed their methods in conjunction with the production of the orthofix external fixator, a monolateral fixator capable of controlled and symmetrical distraction. They noted fracture between the calcified zone and degenerate zone in experimental animals distracted at 1 mm/day using a prototype orthofix distractor. When a speed of 0.5 mm/day was employed, however, there was neither evidence of fracture 28 days following distraction nor was there any evidence of cellular damage. It was concluded that there was a biological effect of distraction at this speed on bone formation and growth plate function. In addition, it was also concluded that the plate remained viable following distraction at this slower speed. A further conclusion was that the growth plate continues to grow normally, albeit at a slower rate, following the end of distraction in the immature animal.

Although these findings are certainly true to a large extent, a close analysis of the paper by De Bastiani et al. (1986a) does reveal that the histological appearance of the growth plate following distraction, although admittedly remaining viable, is certainly not normal. The growth plate is thickened, there are many more layers of cells and the normal architecture is not maintained. Second, there are as yet no clear studies to show that the growth plate regularly remains open following distraction and continues to grow normally.

De Bastiani et al. (1986b) went on to describe the clinical application of their method in the elongation of children with both leg length discrepancy and short-limbed dwarfism. They obtained an increase in length of 36% in the non-achondroplastics and 65% in the achondroplastics. They confined the technique to the last 2 years of growth, although there was an age range of 6 to 16 years.

Aldegheri et al. (1989) reported 75 children who had undergone chondrodiatasis, 41 with leg length discrepancy and 34 with achondroplasia. There were 170 bony segments altogether. In those children with leg length discrepancy, a mean increase in length of 3.4 cm (10.9% of the total bone length) was obtained and 7.4 cm (34% of the total bone length) was obtained in achondroplastics. In those with leg length discrepancy, there were 6 complications in 48 segments (3 asymmetrical distractions, 1 stiff knee, and 2 early fusions of a fibular osteotomy), and in those with achondroplasia there were 27 complications in 122 segments (4 screw site infections, 2 fractures through the lengthening site, 7 malunions of the distraction site, and 8 premature fusions of the fibular osteotomy).

Kenwright and Spriggins (1986) recognized the little knowledge available concerning the relationship between different mechanical distraction regimes and the biological responses of the growth plate. They demonstrated

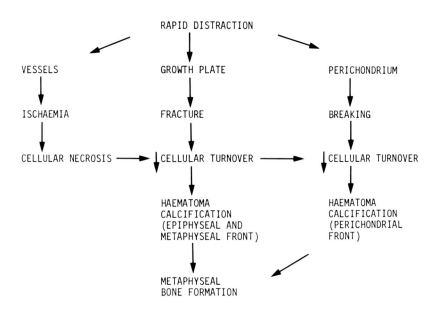

Fig. 4 Theoretical results of rapid distraction of the growth plate.

two patterns of growth plate distraction. In one group of rabbits close to skeletal maturity and measuring the axial force placed upon the growth plate using strain gauges bonded on to an external fixator, they noted that forces increased to 25 to 38 newtons and then suddenly decreased to 16 to 20 newtons during distraction, indicating fracture. The fracture pattern was random through the growth plate. In another group of rabbits using the same technique lower peak forces of 10 to 17 newtons were recorded and hyperplasia of the growth plate was seen histologically without fracture. They concluded that hyperplasia of the growth plate can occur with distraction and that the critical force level below which hyperplasia will occur without fracture can be defined accurately.

It is possible that one of the chief factors related to the speed of distraction may be a change in the blood supply to the growth plate. It may be that under conditions of rapid distraction, a vascular stretching or rupture occurs which produces a reduction in growth plate function, together with direct damage to the growth plate itself and to the surrounding perichondrium (Fig. 4). Conversely, slow distraction may have much less of an effect upon the vasculature, which is able to accommodate distraction easily. At the same time there may be a direct stimulation of cellular turnover, both in the growth plate and in the perichondrium (Fig. 5).

In order to study the effect of distraction upon the growth plate vasculature more closely, the authors of the present chapter carried out experi-

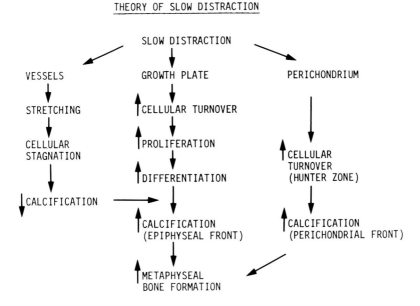

Fig. 5 Theoretical results of slow distraction of the growth plate.

ments on the growth plates of lambs. The histology of the growth plate and
its vascular supply at varying distraction rates were studied (Turner and
Anderson, 1986). The histology of the plate was studied following distraction and the blood supply was also looked at by vascular injection techniques. Nine lambs, normally maturing at 15 to 18 months of age, had a
prototype orthofix external fixator applied across the left lower femoral
growth plate (Fig. 6). Control screws were placed in the opposite femur
without distraction. Three lambs underwent distraction at 2 mm/day, three
at 1 mm/day, and three at 0.5 mm/day, each plate being distracted to 1 cm
in total. One animal was studied immediately at the end of the distraction
period, one 6 weeks later, and one long-term lamb 6 months later. India
ink was injected under pressure into the abdominal aorta just prior to
sacrifice to fill the capillaries of the growth plate. In those animals distracted
at 2 mm/day, it was clear that at the end of the distraction phase, separation
through the zone of hypertrophic chondrocytes had occurred, i.e., distraction epiphysiolysis (Fig. 7). Six months later the growth plate was still
disorganized. Similar results were obtained at a rate of 1 mm/day. At
distraction of 0.5 mm/day there was a mixture of hyperplasia and separation. Some areas showed extreme hyperplasia with total disorganization of
the cartilage columns (Fig. 8). In other areas there was a clear separation
of the plate as seen at the faster rates of distraction. Thus we agree with De
Pablos *et al.* (1986) in that our results did not confirm that at this slower
rate of 0.5 mm/day in lambs, hyperplasia, rather than separation of the
plate, regularly occurred.

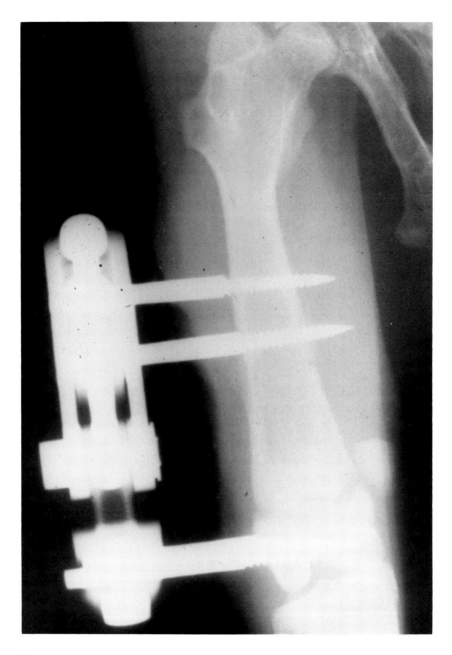

Fig. 6 Radiograph showing application of prototype distractor to the lower femoral growth plate in the sheep.

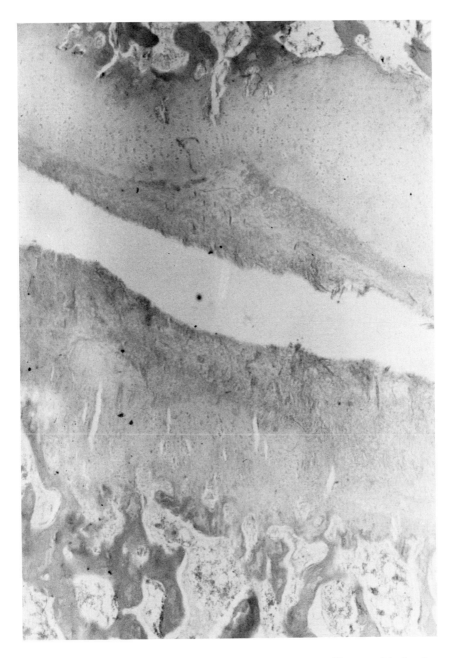

Fig. 7 Photomicrograph showing clear separation through the zone of hypertrophic chondrocytes in the sheep growth plate following rapid distraction.

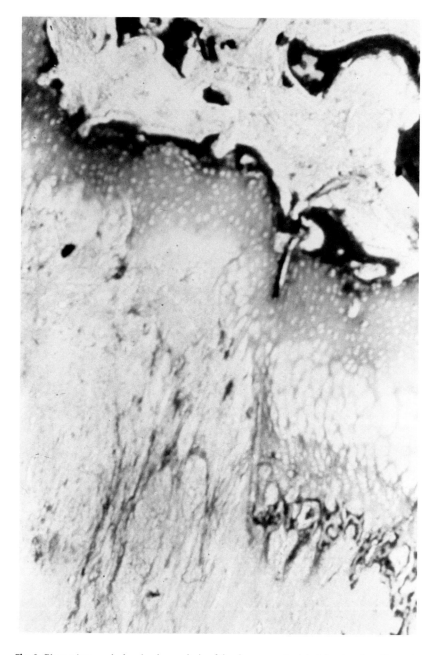

Fig. 8 Photomicrograph showing hyperplasia of the sheep growth plate following slow distraction.

The vascular studies showed that both the epiphyseal and metaphyseal blood vessels were well preserved at all speeds and that no evidence of gross disorganization of either circulation was found. The epiphyseal blood supply maintained its relationship to the epiphyseal bone plate and first layer of cells. Likewise, the metaphyseal circulation maintained its columnar relationship with the cartilage columns, although the two circulations were separated on either side of the distraction gap as might be expected. Following these experiments we used a further sample of New Zealand white rabbits to investigate the same phenomenon, using the same speeds of distraction and the same methods of investigation. Our conclusions have been broadly similar to those of the sheep experiments.

Summary

In conclusion, therefore, chondrodiatasis represents an exciting new concept in the field of limb lengthening. The idea of being able to stimulate growth physiologically has taxed the minds of biologists and surgeons almost since the discovery of the growth plate itself. All methods so far have failed to stimulate growth reliably, despite the fact that many methods, e.g., periosteal stripping, formation of arteriovenous fistulae, medullary drilling, and the insertion of foreign material and bone blocks into the medullary cavity, are known to stimulate growth to some extent. What at present is lacking is a method to reliably accelerate long bone growth at the physis.

Chondrodiatasis probably represents a way forward, but the exact mechanism of its application (i.e., constant or intermittent distraction) and the nature of its action upon the physis remain to be determined as does its long-term effect upon physeal function.

Acknowledgments

We would like to thank Miss Tracey Butler for typing the manuscript and also the Photographic Department, Royal Hospital, Wolverhampton, United Kingdom for providing the illustrations.

References

Aldegheri, R., Trivella, G., and Lavini, F. (1989). Epiphyseal distraction. Chondrodiatasis. *Clin. Orthop. Rel. Res.*, **241**: 117–127.

Bassett, C. A. L. (1971). Biophysical principles affecting bone structure. In: *The Biochemistry and Physiology of Bone*. Bourne, G. H., Ed., Academic Press, New York.

Bensahel, H., Huguenin, P., and Briard, J. L. (1983). L'allongement trans-épiphysaire du tibia. A propos d'uncas. *Rev. Chir. Orthop.*, **69**: 245–247.

Berchiche, R. and Wittek, F. (1983). Allongement du squelette jambier par épiphysiolyse distraction. Traitement des inegalites des membres inférieurs. *Acta. Orthop. Belg.*, **49**: 321–323.

Bourret, L. A. and Rodan, G. A. (1975). The role of calcium in the inhibition of cAMP accumulation in epiphyseal cartilage cell exposed to physiological pressure. *J. Cell Physiol.*, **88**: 353–362.

Brighton, C. T. (1984). The growth plate. *Orthop. Clin. North Am.*, **15**: 571–595.

De Bastiani, G., Aldegheri, R., Renzi-Brivio, L., and Trivella, G. (1984). Controlled symmetrical distraction of the growth plate (chondrodiatasis) to achieve limb lengthening in children. In: *Leg Length Inequality. International Orthopaedic Symposium.* Jaabeurs. Congrescentrum. Utrecht, Netherlands, 13a–b.

De Bastiani, G., Aldegheri, R., Renzi-Brivio, L., and Trivella, G. (1986a). Chondrodiatasis — controlled symmetrical distraction of the epiphyseal plate. *J. Bone Jt. Surg.*, **68B**: 550–556.

De Bastiani, G., Aldegheri, R., Renzi-Brivio, L., and Trivella, G. (1986b). Limb lengthening by distraction of the epiphyseal plate. A comparison of two techniques in the rabbit. *J. Bone Jt. Surg.*, **68B**: 545–549.

De Pablos, J., Villas, C., and Canadell, J. (1986). Bone lengthening by physeal distraction. An experimental study. *Int. Orthop.*, **10**: 163–170.

Ehrlick, M. G., Mankin, H. J., and Treadwell, B. V. (1972). Biochemical and physiological events during closure of the stapled distal femoral epiphyseal plate in rats. *J. Bone Jt. Surg.*, **54A**: 309–322.

Eydelshteyn, B. M., Udalova, N. F., and Bochkarev, G. F. (1973). Dynamics of reparative regeneration after lengthening by the method of distraction epiphysiolysis. *Acta Chir. Plast. (Prague)*, **15**: 149–154.

Fishbane, B. M. and Riley, L. H. (1978). Continuous transphyseal traction. *Clin. Orthop. Rel. Res.*, **136**: 120–124.

Fischenko, P. J., Karimova, L. F., and Pilipenko, N. P. (1976). Distraction epiphysiolysis in congenital shortening of lower extremities. *Ortop. Traumatol. Protez.*, **37**: 44–49.

Franke, J., Hein, G., and Schuh, W. (1984). Limb lengthening by distraction epiphysiolysis method of Ilizarov. In: *Leg Length Inequality. International Orthopaedic Symposium.* Jaabeurs Congrescentrum. Utrecht, Netherlands, 14a–b.

Gelbke, H. (1951). The influence of pressure and tension on growing bone in experiments with animals. *J. Bone Jt. Surg.*, **33A**: 947–954.

Grill, F. and Altenhuber, J. (1984). The Ilizarov method. Early results. In: *Leg Length Inequality. International Orthopaedic Symposium.* Jaabeurs Congrescentrum. Utrecht, Netherlands, 15a.

Grill, F. (1984). Distraction of the epiphyseal cartilage as a method of limb lengthening. *J. Paediat. Orthop.*, **4**: 105–108.

Harris, W. R. and Hobson, K. W. (1956). Histological changes in experimentally displaced upper femoral epiphyses in rabbits. *J. Bone Jt. Surg.*, **38B**: 914–921.

Harsha, W. N. (1962). Distracting effects placed across the epiphyses of long bones. *JAMA*, **179**: 132–136.

Hert, J. (1969). Acceleration of the growth after decrease of load on epiphyseal plates by means of spring distractors. *Folia Morphol. (Warsaw)*, **17**: 194–203.

Hert, J. and Liskova, M. (1964). The growth of bone after experimental overloading or unloading of the epiphyseal cartilages. *Cesk. Morfol.*, **12**: 104–115.

Hinrichsen, G. J. and Storey, E. (1968). The effect of force on bone and bones. *Angle Orthodont.*, **38**: 155–165.

Houghton, G. R. (1982). Distraction epiphysiolysis. An experimental study in the rabbit. *Iowa Orthop. J.*, **3**: 57–61.

Houghton, G. R. and Dekel, S. (1979). The periosteal control of long bone growth. *Acta Orthop. Scand.*, **50**: 635–637.

Hueter, C. (1862). Anatomische Studien an den Extremitatengelenken Neugeborener und Erwachsener. *Virchows Arch. Pathol. Anat.*, **25**: 572–599.

Ilizarow, G. A. and Soybelman, L. M. (1969). Some clinical and experimental data concerning bloodless lengthening of the lower extremities. *Eksp. Khir. Anesteziol.*, **14**: 27–32.

Ilizarow, G. A. and Soybelman, L. M. (1970). Some roentgenographic and morphological data on bone tissue regeneration in experimental distraction epiphysiolysis. *Ortop. Travmatol. Protez.*, **31**: 26–30.

Jani, J. (1984). An experimental study of tibial lengthening in rabbits. In: *Leg Length Inequality. International Orthopaedic Symposium.* Jaabeurs. Congrescentrum. Utrecht, Netherlands, 12a–b.

Janovec, M. and Fait, M. (1981). Prolongation of the leg by distraction of the proximal growth cartilages. *Acta Chir. Orthop. Traumatol. Cech.*, **48**: 150–158.

Kenwright, J. and Spriggins, A. J. (1986). Effects of distraction on the growth plate of the tibia — an experimental study. In: *Recent Advances in External Fixation.* Sept. 28–30. 1986. Conference Centre, Riva del Garda, Italy, 166.

Letts, R. M. and Meadows, L. (1978). Epiphysiolysis as a method of limb lengthening. *Clin. Orthop. Rel. Res.*, **133**: 230–237.

Li, W. H., Wu, J. M., and Xu, M. Q. (1985). Epiphyseal distraction for leg lengthening: report of 55 cases. *Chung Hua Wai Ko Tsa Chih*, **23**: 106–109.

Moen, C. T. and Pelker, R. R. (1984). Biomechanical and histological correlations in growth plate failure. *J. Pediatr. Orthop.*, **4**: 180–184.

Monticelli, G. and Spinelli, R. (1981a). Distraction epiphysiolysis as a method of limb lengthening. I. Experimental study. *Clin. Orthop. Rel. Res.*, **154**: 254–261.

Monticelli, G. and Spinelli, R. (1981b). Distraction epiphysiolysis as a method of limb lengthening. III. Clinical applications. *Clin. Orthop. Rel. Res.*, **154**: 274–285.

Noble, J., Diamond, R., Stirrat, C. R., and Sledge, C. B. (1982). Breaking force of the rabbit growth plate and its application to epiphyseal distraction. *Acta Orthop. Scand.*, **53**: 13–16.

Noble, J., Sledge, C. B., Walker, P. S., Diamond, R., Stirrat, C., and Sosman, J. L. (1978). Limb lengthening by epiphyseal distraction. *J. Bone Jt. Surg.*, **60B**: 139–140.

Peltonen, J., Alitalo, I., Karaharju, E., and Helio, H. (1984). Distraction of the growth plate. Experiments in pigs and sheep. *Acta Orthop. Scand.*, **55**: 359–362.

Ring, P. A. (1958). Experimental bone lengthening by epiphyseal distraction. *Br. J. Surg.*, **196**: 169–173.

Salter, R. B. and Harris, W. R. (1963). Injuries involving the epiphyseal plate. *J. Bone Jt. Surg.*, **45A**: 587–622.

Sledge, C. B. and Noble, J. (1978). Experimental limb lengthening by epiphyseal distraction. *Clin. Orthop. Rel. Res.*, **136**: 111–119.

Smith, W. S. and Cunningham, J. B. (1957). The effect of alternating distracting forces on the epiphyseal plates of calves: a preliminary report. *Clin. Orthop. Rel. Res.*, **10**: 125–130.

Speer, D. P. (1982). Collagenous architecture of the growth plate and perichondrial ossification groove. *J. Bone Jt. Surg.*, **64A**: 399–405.

Startseva, I. A. and Gorbunova, Z. I. (1982). Effect of distraction epiphysiolysis on the growth of lengthened bone. (An experimental study). *Ortop. Travmatol. Protez.* **6**: 36–41.

Trueta, J. and Amato, V. P. (1960). The vascular contribution to osteogenesis. III. Changes in the growth cartilage caused by experimentally induced ischaemia. *J. Bone Jt. Surg.*, **42B**: 571–587.

Turner, A. and Anderson, J. (1986). Mechanical distraction of the growth plate in the experimental animal, using an orthofix prototype distractor. A histological and vascular study using varying distraction rates. In: *Recent Advances in External Fixation* (Abstracts). Sept. 28–30, 1986. Conference Centre, Riva del Garda, Italy, 164.

8

Prospects for Regeneration of Growth Plates in Mammals

RICHARD M. LIBBIN
Veterans Administration Medical Center, Brooklyn
and Department of Anatomy and Cell Biology
SUNY - Health Science Center at Brooklyn
New York

Introduction

Epiphyseal fractures account for 15 to 20% of long bone fractures in children (Rogers, 1970; Worlock and Stower, 1986; Mizuta *et al.*, 1987). An even higher incidence of epiphyseal injury has been reported in hand fractures (Hastings and Simmons, 1984). Despite the development of many innovative approaches to the treatment of injuries involving growth plates in the 20th century, including transplantation of physes and even entire joints, the results have often been quite variable, and the challenge posed by the repair of a severely damaged growth plate has not been entirely met. Early descriptions of the effects of experimentally created physeal injuries have been provided by Ollier (1867) who demonstrated that partial excision of growth plate cartilage resulted in shortening and angular deformation of the bone, while total excision produces complete arrest of growth. Several years later Bidder (1873) provided a histological analysis of experimental physeal injury, demonstrating that after partial extirpation of growth plate cartilage from the end of a long bone, an osseous bridge formed between the epiphysis and metaphysis at the site of injury. Haas, in 1919, and many others subsequently, have shared the view that physeal injuries exert their effect on bone growth by interfering with the blood supply to the growth plate. In such instances the osseous bridge is thought to result from com-munication between epiphyseal and metaphyseal circulations coincident with translocation of osteoprogenitor cells to the site (Shapiro, 1982).

In children the prepotent cause of physeal injury is a fracture occurring at the end of a long bone, with myeloproliferative disease, septic osteomye-litis, tubercular lesions, Blount's disease and therapeutic radiation, chemo-therapy, and accidental electrocution injuries representing additional etiol-ogies (Langenskiöld, 1981; Ogden, 1988). Salter and Harris (1963) indicate that the type of injury most likely to produce partial damage to a physis is a longitudinal transepiphyseal fracture. In a combined analysis reviewing several previously published series, and excluding the hand, Shapiro (1987) reported that 46% of long bone epiphyseal fractures involved the distal radius, with the distal humerus, distal tibia, distal fibula, distal ulna, prox-imal radius, and proximal humerus appearing in decreasing order of frequency.

Attempts to prevent partial growth plate closure at sites of physeal injury have emphasized surgical resection of the skeletal bridge followed by inter-position of usually inert materials as barriers to hinder its regrowth. Early experimental studies by Vogt (1878) demonstrated that the growth of cap-illaries between epiphysis and metaphysis could be prevented by interposing a layer of gold leaf or rubber (cited by Österman, 1972). Later, other natural and synthetic substances more suitable for surgical implantation were used in this way, including bone wax (Key and Ford, 1958; Österman, 1972), beeswax (Friedenberg, 1957), methyl methacrylate (Kleiger and Mankin, 1964), siliconized Dacron (Schneider and Leyva, 1964), silicone rubber (Speirs and Blocksma, 1963) and free grafts of fat (Österman, 1972; Lan-genskiöld, 1981, 1988; Langenskiöld et al., 1987), skeletal muscle (Seräfin, 1970) and cartilage, the latter used either en bloc or an an autogenous graft obtained through in vitro growth of a cartilage biopsy specimen (Kawabe et al., 1987; Ehrlich et al., 1988). While each of these materials provided limited protection against regrowth of the osseous bridge, autologous fat and car-tilage were particularly useful.

For almost 100 years attempts have been made to transplant growth plates. The design and results of the early experiments have been summa-rized by Hoffman et al. (1972). Following transplantation to ectopic sites such as the anterior ocular chamber (Urist and McLean, 1952), or beneath the renal capsule (Lacroix, 1951), only temporary graft survival was ob-served. More impressive results were obtained when physes were relocated to skeletal sites as indicated by the report of Harris et al. (1965). While bone-to-bone transplants survived with variable success, those implanted within muscle were reabsorbed within 6 to 8 weeks. The results of these and many related studies have been interpreted as indicating that the du-ration and degree of physeal ischemia in the interval preceding revascular-ization are the critical determinants of graft survival, and that free physeal grafts are not likely to retain sustained viability. However, a survey con-

ducted by Freeman (1965), reviewing a large series of free autologous physeal cartilage transplantations in humans, indicated that approximately
40% of the transplants displayed continuous growth, some for up to 10
years. A less encouraging result was reported by Wilson (1966) who transplanted a small number of epiphyses to various locations in the limbs of
children; only in a single instance did a proximal phalanx of a little finger
transplanted to the site of a first metacarpal sustain normal growth of the
digit. Eight years later the growth plate remained open, and the phalanx
equaled its contralateral counterpart in length. Thus, despite reports of a
relatively small number of satisfactory results following growth plate transplantation, early attempts were unpredictable in outcome and generally
rather disappointing.

The clinical history of joint transplantation also reveals a pattern of
variable success. A report by Lexer (1908), presenting details of the transplantation of large weight-bearing joints, describes useful, functional results
in some patients followed for up to 10 years despite radiographic evidence
of joint degeneration. A more recent account of autologous transplantation
of a child's interphalangeal joint and proximal interphalangeal epiphysis by
Eades and Peacock (1966) also describes early degeneration of the joint
surfaces with subsequent regeneration; when examined 10 years later their
original contours had been restored. Subsequent reports have indicated that
joints may be transplanted on a vascularized pedicle with considerable
improvement in outcome (Zaleske et al., 1982; Goldberg et al., 1980; Reeves,
1969). Advances in the technique of microvascular anastomosis have reduced, but not obviated, the unpredictable outcome of such procedures.

It is against this background of limited prior success in the treatment of
severe growth plate injuries that the phenomenon of growth plate cartilage
regeneration is presently examined. The author proposes that fuller appre-
ciation of the capacity of this tissue for innate regrowth, in combination
with additional strategies for inducing it, will lead to improved management
of such injuries.

Regeneration of Growth Plate Cartilage

More than 50 years have passed since Selye (1934) provided the first
account of growth plate regeneration in the distal femur of the neonatal rat
following amputation of the limb. He directed attention to the age of the
animal and the angle of bone transection as important determinants of the
regeneration process. Several years later Nunnemacher (1939) re-examined
this process, attempting to determine whether Selye had described *de novo*
regeneration, or if the physis had regrown from growth plate cartilage left
at the femoral transection surface following its incomplete removal at surgery. His communication documents not only the regeneration of distal
femoral physes, often reappearing as hemiphyses restricted to the skeletal

surface beneath a single femoral condyle, but also upon occasion, the re-growth of a hemiepiphysis. Through his examination of physeal regrowth Nunnemacher identified several elements of the process which he believed influenced a successful outcome. The most elaborate physeal regenerates arose at the ends of femurs enclosed within a mass of vital skeletal muscle which had overgrown the plane of amputation. The distance between the transection plane and the growth plate being ablated influenced the likeli-hood of its regrowth, and Nunnemacher directed attention to the matura-tional history of the physis as a determinant of its replacement. In support of the latter concept it is noted that low transhumeral amputations carried out in Nunnemacher's laboratory resulted only in repair of the skeletal defect and healing of soft tissues; innate physeal regeneration did not occur. Given his concept relating the schedule of physeal maturation to regenera-tive capacity, such a result might have been predicted; in the rat the distal humeral growth plate is quite precocial in comparison with most of the other physes of the extremities, beginning to disappear by the end of the third week of life (Dawson, 1925). Person *et al.* (1979) have confirmed the observation that physeal regeneration does not occur innately in the distal humerus of the rat.

Several additional studies have examined growth plate regeneration at hindlimb amputation sites of neonatal rodents. Banks and Compere (1941) performed amputations through the midfemurs of neonatal rats and rabbits and observed only healing of the transected skeletal tissues. Failure of growth plates to regenerate in their series was not accounted for. (The location of the amputation in the middiaphysis is unlikely to provide a plausible explanation, for Libbin and Weinstein (1986, 1987) have obtained physeal regenerates after amputations through the tibiofibular diaphysis). Several years later Teucq (1948), working in Lacroix's laboratory, reported frequent spontaneous growth plate regeneration in neonatal rats 1 month after low femoral amputations. However, when animals were killed at later postoperative intervals physeal regenerates were encountered less fre-quently. Teucq concluded that regenerated physeal cartilage was ephem-eral, but Libbin and Weinstein (1986) have identified regenerated growth plates which retained typical morphology even after several months.

The latter investigators have conducted a detailed examination of several factors believed to promote or constrain growth plate regeneration (Libbin and Weinstein, 1986). They emphasized precise identification of the level and angle of the amputation relative to the location of the physes being excised. This was accomplished by *en bloc* staining of the entire distal am-putated segment of the limb with methyl green which selectively stains cartilage, and then clearing it to transparency in methyl salicylate (Mc-Cann, 1971). When such preparations were examined with a stereomicro-scope, the level of amputation relative to the position of the distal growth plates was readily determined, and the transection angle accurately mea-sured. However, Libbin and Weinstein (1986) observed that in a small number of amputations the transection had passed within 1 mm of the growth plate, but proximal to it. To verify the completeness of growth plate ablation in such specimens — to ascertain that no physeal cartilage had remained at the amputation surface following its inadvertant division during surgery — they passed these distal femoral or tibiofibular segments back to water, and sectioned them serially in a longitudinal plane after decalcification. On the basis of microscopic examination of the sections, and of the stained-and-cleared preparations described above, Libbin and Weinstein established that each femoral and tibiofibular amputation procedure had completely removed the distal growth plates, leaving no physeal cartilage behind at the amputation surface. This was the objective which Nunnemacher (1939) had sought to accomplish, but which he verified only by observing the trajectory of his scalpel as the limb was amputated. In this brief discussion of methods it is also noteworthy that in all experimental studies of growth plate regeneration in rodents carried out in the author's laboratory, skin wounds were routinely sutured closed following amputation. This practice merits consideration because a number of reports of limb regeneration in amphibians have demonstrated that the regrowth of the limb by the epimorphic process commonly observed in newts and salamanders generally requires initial retention of an open wound. In fact, Illingworth (1974) and Douglas (1972) have described an identical requirement for the regeneration of the finger tips of children. However, Ogo (1987) has shown that regeneration of severed adult human finger tips occurs even if the wound surface is covered by a full-thickness skin graft.

In his analysis of growth plate regeneration Selye (1934) observed that neonatal rat femurs divided obliquely via a sharply angulated transection ceased to grow in length, and that continued growth and physeal regeneration did not commence until the pointed skeletal end had been blunted by osteoclastic resorption of distal bone. To test this finding, Libbin and Weinstein (1986) measured levels and angles of transection, and the lengths of the femurs after various intervals of postoperative recovery. They reasoned that, according to Selye's view, angulated transections would produce a subset of amputees with short femoral stumps, while amputations more perpendicular to the long axis of the bone would result in longer stumps. Examination of distal limb segments after *en bloc* staining and clearing disclosed that 14 of 17 femoral amputations had divided the hindlimb at the level of the distal femoral diaphysis, with three passing through the proximal metaphysis. Transection angles ranged between 90 and 125°. Among the limb stumps measured at postmortem, three were less than 13 mm, with one rat (femoral stump length, 11.5 mm; transection angle 113°) surviving for 73 days. Since the femur of the 10- to 12-day-old rat is about 11 to 12 mm in length, it is evident that slowing or cessation of longitudinal growth had occurred. But at the other end of the scale were two rats with femoral stump lengths of 13.7 and 14.1 mm which had survived for 28 days. In these specimens the angles of transection were 120 and 118°, respectively, indicating no strong correlation between the rate of the longitudinal growth of the femur after amputation and the angle at which it was divided.

When the results of the femoral amputations carried out by Libbin and Weinstein (1986) were compared with those of Nunnemacher (1939), several provocative similarities were noted. First, in approximately two thirds of the amputees in each series, only skeletal and soft tissue healing had occurred. Physeal cartilage regeneration was not observed, the defect at the end of the skeletal shaft being closed with a plug of newly formed cancellous bone (Fig. 1). Among the majority of the remaining rats in each series the skeletal terminus was capped with a plate of newly formed cartilage. Libbin and Weinstein (1986) examined this cartilage histologically, and found that in two of five rats it was entirely nonphyseal, while in three the cartilage plate contained regions of growth plate cell organization. In a single specimen the regrown femoral terminus was distinctly bifid, one side having regrown an elaborately regenerated hemiphysis surmounted by a well-formed hemiepiphysis (Fig. 2a,b). However, the other half of the femoral surface lay beneath a plate of fibrocartilage and displayed little regenerative growth beyond its participation in the restoration of the shape of the femoral extremity. The regeneration of a complete, discoid growth plate covering all or most of the femoral amputation surface was encountered only rarely, appearing twice in Libbin and Weinstein's series and once in Nunnemacher's.

Tibiofibular amputations carried out in another group of neonatal rats enabled Libbin and Weinstein (1986) to examine Nunnemacher's hypothesis relating the probability of growth plate regeneration to the distance separating the amputation site from the excised growth plates. In the rat a body of secondary cartilage unites the lower tibia and fibula early in postnatal life (Moss, 1977). In order to avoid division of this junctional cartilage during amputations through the shank, Libbin and Weinstein (1986) located their limb transection plane in the central tibiofibular diaphyses proximal to it. Among ten rats in this series, eight amputations passed through diaphyseal bone; in two, the junctional cartilage was inadvertently divided. The results of this surgery were comparable to those obtained in the distal femoral amputations previously described, with a slight decrease in numbers of limb stumps displaying only skeletal healing, and a corresponding increase in those forming cartilage plates. In this series a single specimen produced three distinct regions of regenerated growth plate cartilage (Fig. 3a and b), two in contact with the amputated surface of the tibia, and one complete physis ectopically located between the distal tibia and fibula. Although not recognized by the authors at the time, it appears plausible now that the latter physeal regeneration site had formed via chondrocyte reorganization within the junctional cartilage. A similar process has since been observed in other mid-shank amputees, and will be discussed below. The incidence of growth plate cartilage regeneration observed in the tibiofibular group, and its similarity to those results already described for the femoral series, demonstrate that amputations distant from growth plates

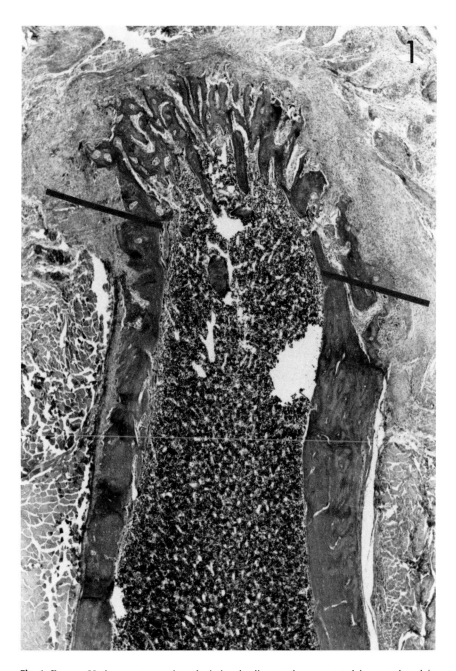

Fig. 1 Femur, 30 days postoperative, depicting healing at the amputated bone end and in adjacent soft tissues in the absence of regeneration. In this frequently observed response to hindlimb transection the skeletal defect has been closed with a plug of newly formed cancellous bone. The interrupted line passing through the femoral shaft identifies the approximate level of amputation. (H and E; ×49.) [From Libbin and Weinstein (1986) and reproduced with the permission of Wiley-Liss.]

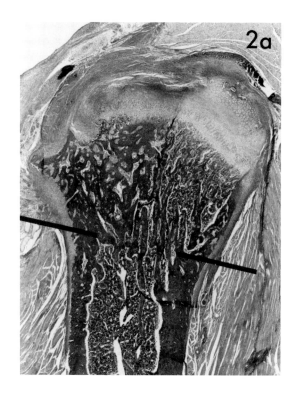

(central tibiofibula) are essentially as effective in inducing physeal cartilage regeneration as those located considerably closer to the growth plate (distal femur).

Quite recently Langenskiöld *et al.* (1989) have summarized the results of their investigation of physeal cartilage regeneration following formation of discrete experimental lesions in the growth plates of several nonprimate mammals. Their observations indicate that growth plate cartilage regrows from the surface of intact cartilage remaining at the site of injury, and that repair of the physes occurs following injuries within the forelimb skeleton. From the latter it is suspected that the failure of the rat to regrow forelimb physeal cartilage may represent a difference peculiar to this species, or common among rodents. Of particular interest is the view held by Langenskiöld and co-workers, based on radiographic evidence, that a similar repair process occurs in children.

Histological Analysis of Growth Plate Cartilage Regeneration

Previous studies from this laboratory and elsewhere have demonstrated that the regeneration of growth plate cartilage, and of entire growth plates, are relatively rare occurrences, unlike regeneration in many salamanders

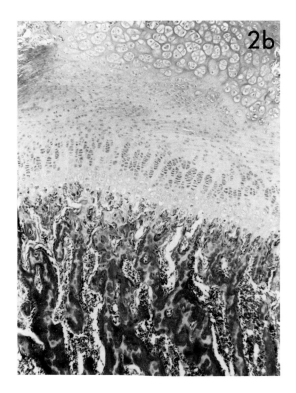

Fig. 2 Femur, 28 days postoperative. (**a**) The femoral terminus distal to the amputation plane (interrupted line) has expanded and now appears bifid, resembling the contour of the intact distal femoral condyle observed in the neonatal rat. Note that a regrown hemiepiphysis has formed on the left side, separated from the underlying metaphysis by a zone of regenerated growth plate cartilage. (H and E; ×22.) (**b**) A detail from (**a**) showing the organization of the regenerated hemiphysis, and of the hemiepiphyseal cartilage distal to it. (H and E; ×61.) [From Libbin and Weinstein (1986) and reproduced with the permission of Wiley-Liss.]

and newts where loss of a limb or other body part is regularly followed by its regrowth. In an attempt to identify critical milestones in the mammalian physeal regeneration process which might be experimentally manipulated to increase the frequency of its occurrence, Libbin and Weinstein (1987) carried out a detailed histological analysis of the growth plate regeneration process. Neonatal rats sustained low femoral or central tibifibular amputations following which the skin wounds were sutured closed. They were killed after 0, 1, 2, 4, 7, 14, 22, or 29 days, and their limb stumps prepared for microscopic examination. The precise location of the amputation was determined as described in the preceding section. Review of distal limb segments stained *en bloc* established that each amputation had completely excised the distal femoral or tibiofibular growth plates. During gross specimen review it was determined that among 53 femoral amputations, 46 were located within the distal diaphysis, two at the diaphyseo-metaphyseal junc-

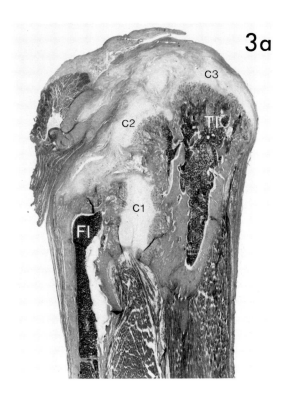

tion, and 3 within the proximal metaphysis. Of the six rats comprising the
tibiofibular group, all amputations divided the central diaphysis, but in one
the transection split the junctional cartilage.

Among animals of the 0-time control group it was noted that the periosteum had been denuded distally for a length of several millimeters during
division of the bone, and that pooled blood occupied the dead space of the
wound, with clot and serous exudate covering skeletal and muscle transection surfaces. Muscle necrosis was evident 24 h postoperatively. The distal
periosteum had become considerably thickened; in half of the animals in
this group it displayed intense metachromasia after staining with toluidine
blue O. Within the zone of distal periosteal hyperplasia irregular bodies of
newly forming hyaline cartilage were observed after 48 h in two thirds of
the specimens (Fig. 4a and b). At this interval mitotic figures and ^{3}H-
thymidine-labeled nuclei were frequently identified in the distal periosteum
and the interfascicular connective tissue of adjacent striated muscle. These
sites adjacent to the amputation surface uniquely displayed high levels of
hyaluronate (Libbin, 1988).

Each of the 96-h postoperative specimens possessed an expanded, grossly
bulbous terminus formed by the continued accretion of periosteal cartilage
which was now beginning to form a compact mass enclosing the skeletal
stump. Within this cartilage mass endochondral ossification was in progress,

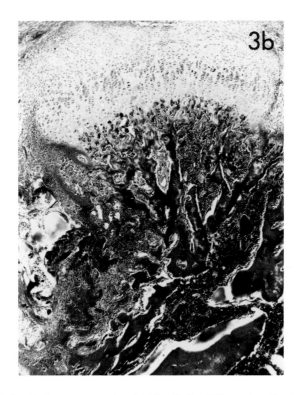

Fig. 3 Tibiofibula, 28 days postoperative. (**a**) The fibular (FI) terminus lies in contact with the side of the tibia (TI), separated only by a body of cartilage (c1) enclosing two laterally adjacent physeal regions (not illustrated), and possibly representing transformed tibiofibular junctional cartilage (see text). Distal to this region of tibiofibular conjunction, a projection of new bone arises from the severed end of the tibia and is capped by a second cartilage body (c2) enclosing a discoid growth plate. An area of cartilage plate devoid of physeal organization (c3) covers the remainder of the tibial transection surface. (H and E; ×7.) (**b**) Detail from (**a**) illustrating the appearance of the regenerated growth plate region identified within cartilage c2. The level of amputation cannot be precisely identified in this section, but lies proximal to cartilage c1. (H and E; ×50.) [From Libbin and Weinstein (1986) and reproduced with the permission of Wiley-Liss.]

forming delicate trabeculae of new bone. In the interval between postoperative weeks one and two, periosteal cartilage and new bone increased considerably in volume, extending beyond the level of amputation (Fig. 5). At postmortem, the ends of the femoral shafts were cartilaginous and, in a number of specimens, resembled regrown distal epiphyses. Within this mass of terminal hyaline cartilage of periosteal origin regenerated growth plate cell architecture was first identified, becoming recognizable by the end of the second postoperative week. One tibiofibular growth plate cartilage regenerate was located to the side of the fibular shaft, rather than at its end, and adjacent to the terminus. Although its hypertrophic zone and primary spongiosa were somewhat disorganized, physeal chondrocytes were arranged in ordered columns and nests.

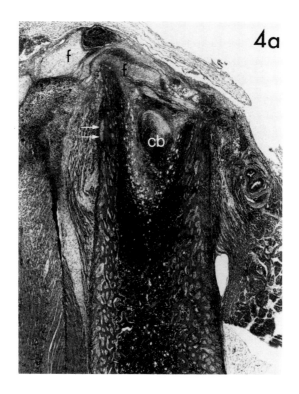

By the end of the third postoperative week, three of seven femoral and both tibiofibular bone ends remained enclosed within masses of newly formed periosteal cartilage, but in no specimen in either group was physeal cartilage organization encountered. However, among specimens of the 4-week postoperative group, five of nine femoral and both tibiofibular skeletal ends were cartilaginous, and within three and two distal cartilage regions, respectively, growth plate cell architecture was identified (Fig. 6a). Chondrocytes were now arranged in closely spaced rows and nests underlain by a hypertrophic zone and a primary spongiosa. Bands of collagen fibers, identified by Sirius red staining, formed septations between rows of cartilage cells, frequently traversing the breadth of the growth plate (Fig. 6b).

In a single specimen of the 4-week postoperative tibiofibular group the skeletal shaft had been divided close to the junctional cartilage uniting the bones of the lower shank. In this unusual foreleg unossified cartilage persisted in the distal tibia and fibula and obscured the plane of amputation. However, despite this developmental irregularity, regions of physeal regrowth were observed in the cartilage which had formed distal to the skeletal transection surfaces, and also within the junctional cartilage proximal to them. Histological review of the structure of this cartilage in intact (unamputated) shanks of neonatal rats revealed that it was of characteristic hyaline type, and nonphyseal throughout. Yet in the present instance, and in several

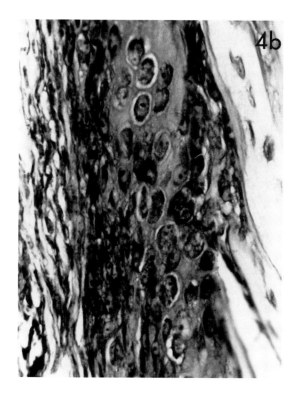

Fig. 4 Femur, 2 days postoperative. (**a**) At this interval the amputation surface is overlain by a projection of subcutaneous connective tissue, beneath which accumulations of fibrin (f) and clotted blood (cb) seal the exposed medullary cavity. Muscle necrosis is now evident, and the distal periosteum appears thickened. Along the right side of the distal femoral shaft a small, elongate nodule of newly formed cartilage has appeared (arrows). (H and E; ×21.) (**b**) Detail from (**a**) after restaining, illustrating the appearance of the intraperiosteal cartilage nodule at greater magnification. Note that its chondrocytes are located within lacunae. The extracellular cartilage matrix is intensely metachromatic. (Toluidine blue O; ×480.) [From Libbin and Weinstein (1987) and reproduced with the permission of Wiley-Liss.]

other tibiofibular amputation specimens examined to date, growth plate cell architecture was encountered, raising the possibility that when appropriately stimulated by adjacent trauma, junctional cartilage may be able to become physislike, and suggesting that the growth plate cartilage phenotype is not as restricted as had been previously supposed.

From the foregoing description of the regenerative histology of the growth plate it is apparent that proliferation of periosteal cartilage similar in morphology to fracture callus is the starting point for physeal regeneration. It is this detail of the process which best explains why regeneration of growth plate cartilage does not occur at forelimb amputation sites of rats, for while exuberant periosteal chondrogenesis rapidly encloses the hindlimb bone ends within a mass of hyaline cartilage, in the forelimb the equivalent

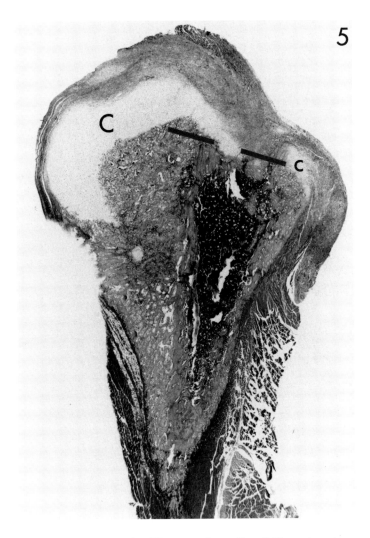

Fig. 5 Femur, 14 days postoperative. The transection surface of this specimen is covered with cartilage (c) of periosteal origin extending beyond the plane of amputation indicated by the interrupted line. Newly formed bone encloses the femoral shaft throughout most of its length. (H and E; ×16.) [From Libbin and Weinstein (1987) and reproduced with the permission of Wiley-Liss.]

process occurs less frequently and is less vigorous, newly formed cartilage rarely extending beyond the plane of amputation. The failure of rat forelimb growth plate cartilage to regenerate may reflect a deficiency in the chondrogenic potential of its periosteum. However, Langenskiöld and Edgren (1950) described the regeneration of growth plate cartilage in the forelimb skeleton of neonatal and juvenile rabbits, suggesting that the proposed defect in the rat's forelimb periosteum may be species- and limb-specific.

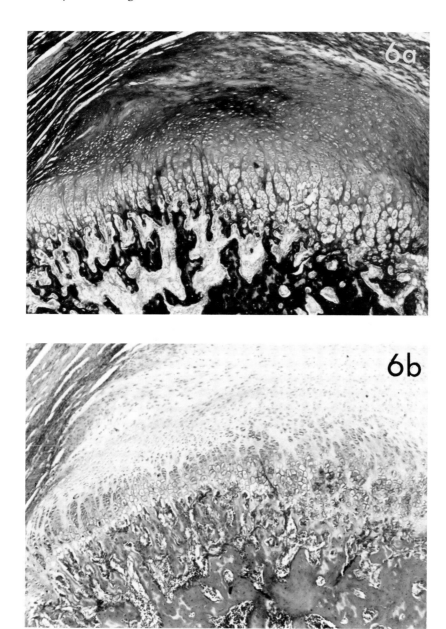

Fig. 6 Tibiofibula, 28 days postoperative. (**a**) Regenerated growth plate cartilage formed of columns of chondrocytes separated by bands of collagen, possessing a distinct hypertrophic zone and a well-formed primary spongiosa. Note that the terminus distal to the growth plate is capped with fibrocartilage. (Sirius red, fast green; ×54.) (**b**) A serial section adjacent to the one depicted in (**a**), stained to illustrate the general appearance of the chondrocyte columns forming the regenerated growth plate region. (H and E; ×54.) [From Libbin and Weinstein (1987) and reproduced with the permission of Wiley-Liss.]

It is also apparent that an innate regrowth frequency of about 30% for growth plate cartilage, if sustained in human long bones, would provide the orthopedist with a therapeutic strategy no more likely to succeed in treatment of severe physeal injuries than growth plate or whole joint transplantation. Thus, it was essential to examine experimental procedures having the potential to stimulate physeal regrowth to a clinically relevant level.

Stimulation of Growth Plate Cartilage Regeneration by Trauma

Although an extensive literature documents the limited capacity of birds and mammals to regrow portions of missing extremities, Polezhaev (1946, 1972) and others have persuasively argued that regenerative capacity is never completely lost in higher vertebrates, and may be restored by resorting to appropriate means. One of the classical experimental challenges in research of this type has been to induce regrowth in the frog's limb, for while the limbs of tadpoles are readily replaced, this capacity is lost during metamorphosis. In comparing regenerating limb tissues of newts and salamanders with nonregenerating stump tissues in frogs, Polezhaev concluded that the defect in the latter resided in the failure of injured tissues to dedifferentiate. Consequently, undifferentiated cells did not form an aggregated cohort at the wound surface, and a regeneration blastema was not assembled. To stimulate dedifferentiation Polezhaev applied various types of trauma to the limbs of frogs and nonregenerating reptiles, intending to enhance tissue breakdown. In many instances, regardless of the nature of the stimulus, limited regeneration was obtained, frequently in the form of a pattern-deficient outgrowth or a spike of cartilage.

Approaching this problem from a different direction, Rose (1944, 1945) recognized that in frogs the wound epidermis covering the amputation site (considered by some experimenters of the period to be an important source of undifferentiated blastemal cells), was soon replaced by normal limb skin thought to lack the capacity to participate in blastema formation. Rose exploited several experimental regimens in an attempt to frustrate the replacement of the wound epidermis by normal skin, including exposure of amputated limbs to hypertonic NaCl solution, and surgical excision of the encroaching integument. Following each of these procedures, and after a number of others reported in the literature, including electrical stimulation (Borgens et al., 1979; Smith, 1967), nerve translocation (Singer, 1954; Tomlinson et al., 1985) and implantation (Mizell, 1968), enhanced regenerative growth was reported. Of interest presently are the observations that a number of seemingly unrelated forms of trauma have elicited some regrowth, and that in most instances the regenerates were primarily cartilaginous.

It was against this experimental background that Libbin and Rivera (1989) examined means of stimulating growth plate regeneration in neonatal rodents, which regrow physeal cartilage only infrequently and, like frog tadpoles, appear to lose this capacity as they mature (Selye, 1934; Nunnemacher, 1939).

In experiments examining enhanced physeal regeneration induced by trauma, the stimulus for regrowth was provided by one or two reamputations through the hindlimb stump (Libbin and Rivera, 1989). These serial amputation sequences removed a small length of the stump terminus (about 2 to 3 mm), the knife passing through the bone end and the mass of periosteal cartilage surrounding it. In practice, the soft tissues enclosing the bone were also resected, and the skin wound then closed with sutures. Following each primary amputation the resected segment of the limb was inspected to precisely identify the level of amputation, in order to establish that complete physeal excision had been achieved. During this examination the total excision of the junctional cartilage was also verified in tibiofibular amputation specimens.

First reamputation surgery was carried out 1 week after primary hindlimb amputation, with second reamputations following 1 week later. In each group a postoperative recovery interval of 2 weeks intervened between last reamputation and the death of the rat (it was known that 2 weeks are required for regenerating growth plate cartilage to become histologically identifiable in tissue sections). In this reamputation series regeneration of growth plate cartilage was scored as having occurred when physeal cartilage organization was recognized microscopically in at least 25 consecutive longitudinal serial sections. In the brief 2-week postoperative interval between final reamputation and sacrifice of the rat it was not expected that the regenerating physis would cover the entire skeletal stump and, in fact, the growth plate cartilage which regrew extended over the transection surface of the bone somewhat variably. In a few specimens the regenerated physeal region had an approximate diameter of only about 150 μm, but in most it appeared as a hemiphysis, restricted to one side of the femoral shaft or, in the tibiofibular group, applied to the end of only one shank bone. In some it was present as an essentially complete growth plate with a diameter of 2.5 to 3.0 mm.

Following first reamputation the incidence of physeal cartilage regeneration increased approximately threefold, from about 25 to over 80%. First reamputations dividing the central tibiofibula evoked an increase in physeal regeneration of similar magnitude. However, following second tibiofibular reamputations carried out on five rats, the frequency of growth plate cartilage regeneration further increased, closely approximating that scored for femurs following first reamputation. Improvement in the quality of the regenerate was also noted. In three femoral reamputation specimens epiphysis-like outgrowths arose distal to and in direct contact with the regenerated growth plate region (Figs. 7a and b). They lacked articular cartilage at their extremities and were located either at the severed end of the long bone (two specimens) or along the shaft (one specimen). Among two spec-

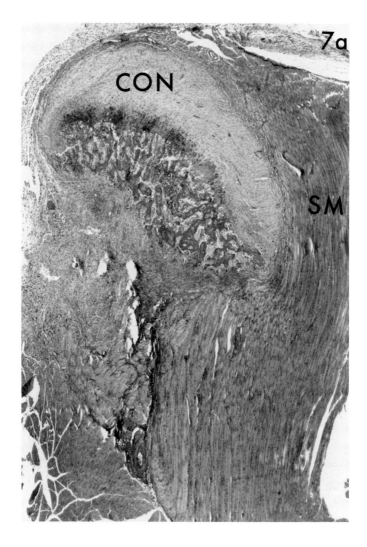

imens a broad physeal regenerate intervened between the transection surface
of the bone and the outgrowth. In a similar response to femoral reamputation an irregular conical extension of periosteal cartilage arose from the side
of the femoral shaft, adjacent to the plane of primary amputation (Fig. 8a).
Among two of three regenerates of this type, the cartilage had formed
regions of growth plate cell architecture (Fig. 8b).

Although examination of amputation specimens confirmed that each tibiofibular primary amputation in the reamputation series had completely
ablated the junctional cartilage of the lower shank, its regrowth was noted
in three second reamputation specimens. In each instance the regrown
junctional cartilage now contained extended regions of growth plate cytoar-
chitecture, suggesting that physeal organization is not restricted to the ends

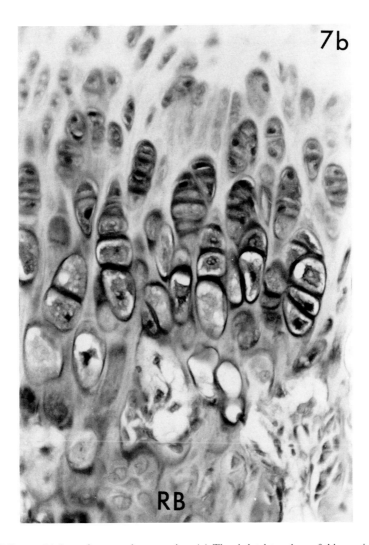

Fig. 7 Femur, 14 days after second amputation. (**a**) The skeletal terminus of this specimen is surmounted by a condyle-like mass of cartilage (CON), with deeply staining regenerated growth plate intervening. Most of the femoral shaft lies outside the plane of the section, but the skeletal parts illustrated have arisen distal to the level of second amputation. Note that part of the condylar outgrowth is enclosed within a covering of regional skeletal muscle (SM). (H and E; ×34.) (**b**) Detail of an area of the regenerated growth plate illustrated in (**a**), but from a serial section approximately 150 μm distant. (H and E; ×397.) [From Libbin and Rivera (1989) and reproduced with the permission of Raven Press.]

of long bones, but may be provoked to occur at other sites as well.

Via application of the serial amputation procedure it has been possible to increase the frequency of growth plate cartilage regeneration considerably beyond the likelihood of its unstimulated occurrence following primary limb amputations. The author presently believes that additional trauma might

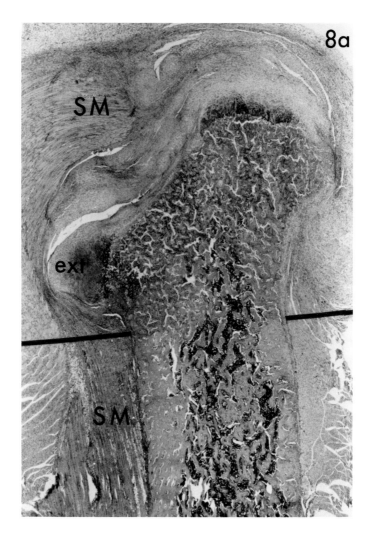

increase this type of regeneration further, perhaps to a value approaching 100%, and notes that excision of a physis by limb amputation challenges the regenerative potential of the skeleton far more rigorously than even the severest injuries sustained by children and adolescents. Induction of physeal regeneration employing surgical trauma equivalent to serial amputation is not, however, readily applicable to the treatment of human growth plate injuries.

Physeal Ectopia

Growth plate cell organization represents a unique tissue design in nature.

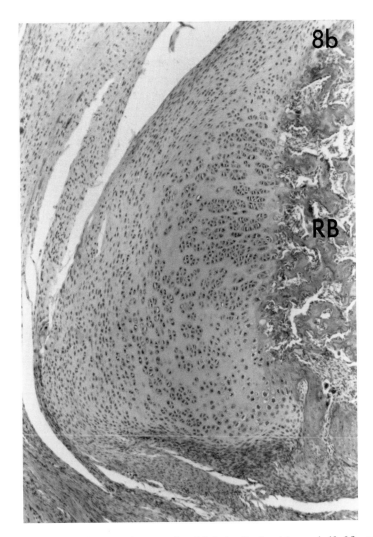

Fig. 8 Femur, 14 days after second amputation. (**a**) At its distal end (upper half of figure) the skeletal shaft terminates in a deeply stained regenerated growth plate. From the side of the shaft a cartilaginous extension (ext) projects into adjacent skeletal muscle (SM) which surrounds the terminus on that side. The interrupted line indicates the approximate level of primary amputation. The level of second amputation cannot be identified, but lies distal to the extension. (H and E; × 18.) (**b**) Detail of a region of the cartilaginous outgrowth illustrated in (**a**) from a serial section approximately 100 μm distant, depicting the formation of ectopic growth plate cartilage within it. Proximal to this physislike region other areas of less organized cartilage cell arrangement are present. Note that the outgrowth is applied directly to underlying regenerated bone (RB), in the absence of a hypertrophic zone. (H and E; × 85.) [From Libbin and Rivera (1989) and reproduced with the permission of Raven Press.]

Neither the cell layers of the cerebral cortex, nor the retina, nor even the palisade mesophyll of the leaves of plants closely duplicate it, and none of these storiform cell arrangements make provision for a process similar to the one by which physeal chondrocyte matrix is incorporated into endochondral bone. Yet despite the singularity of this pattern of tissue organization, and its restriction primarily to cartilage retained at the ends of growing bones, it may be duplicated in nonphyseal hyaline cartilage from adjacent sites following regional trauma, and frequently appears in a less organized state within rodent skeletal muscle which had been excised, minced, and then reimplanted (Carlson, 1978). Thus, a small body of evidence indicates that nonphyseal cartilage, and perhaps skeletal muscle as well, may be able to replace damaged regions of the physis or even entire growth plates. As noted previously, physeal ectopia was described by Libbin and Weinstein (1987) within cartilage uniting the lower tibia and fibula of the neonatal rat. Tibiofibular skeletal conjunction is encountered frequently among rodents which employ a skipping or hopping gait (Romer, 1966), and Moss (1977) has demonstrated that osseous union is preceded by secondary cartilage in the junction region as early as the seventh day of life. Calcification of this cartilage is evident by day 11; it is eventually replaced by bone. The observation that junctional cartilage which becomes physislike later fails to rapidly ossify is of some interest, for it suggests that as growth plate-like morphology is acquired subsequent to adjacent surgical trauma, it also becomes resistant to rapid, progressive osseous replacement. This is a detail of some importance for considering transplantation of permanent hyaline cartilage to a site of physeal injury with the expectation that the graft will replace the damaged physeal region both structurally and functionally.

It has also been noted that periosteum adjacent to sites of hindlimb reamputation forms outgrowths of cartilage which often closely resemble the long bone physis in details of cellular organization. Taken together with observations of physeal cell architecture in junctional cartilage, this indicates that any cartilage or cartilage-forming tissue may be able to form growth plate. It further suggests that physeal cartilage may be provoked to form anywhere along the length of a long bone, or elsewhere in the skeleton, and that autogenous cartilage modified in this way may represent the material of choice for repairing parts of the damaged physis.

Information obtained through the exploitation of several different animal model systems indicates that physeal cartilage regeneration occurs spontaneously following ablation or localized injury, and that its regrowth may be stimulated by a procedure which also increases the level and duration of tissue damage. Because human growth plate injuries occur with greatest frequency in the long bones of the upper extremity, it is of particular importance to establish the capacity of physeal cartilage of the forelimb for innate and induced regrowth. Attempts to demonstrate growth plate regeneration in the forelimb skeleton of the rat have been unsuccessful (Nunnemacher, 1939; Person *et al.*, 1979), but in rabbits it appears to occur readily following localized experimental X-ray damage (Langenskiöld and Edgren, 1950). It is also notable that the most morphologically detailed studies of physeal regeneration exploited the use of limb amputation models, while the reports of Langenskiöld and colleagues described the repair of relatively circumscribed lesions created within intact growth plates. This observed variation in physeal regrowth capacity may reflect not only species- and limb-specific differences, but also the properties of the model system itself. The *de novo* organization of growth plate cartilage at the end of a severed bone, and the regrowth of this cartilage from remaining physis left at the injury site represent accomplishments of very different magnitude, particularly in the former system where the germinal cells were entirely excised.

Another potential source of observed difference between the capacity of the upper and lower extremities to regenerate growth plate cartilage may relate to the chondrogenic potential of the periosteal covering of the skeletal parts involved. However, the observations which presently support this conjecture are casual, and require verification through transplantation and *in vitro* studies. The author speculates that in the amputated rat hindlimb, locally acting growth factors produced by damaged tissues may be required for successful growth plate cartilage regeneration, and that levels of these growth regulating substances may be increased by repeated tissue injury and interrupted healing resulting from serial surgery. O'Keefe *et al.* (1989) have reported that basic fibroblast growth factor and transforming growth factor-β are potent mitogens for growth plate chondrocytes in cell culture, and it is likely that in the near future related studies will further define their growth factor requirements. Fuller understanding of the importance of these factors for successful repair of experimental injuries may make it possible to effectively stimulate growth plate regeneration without resort to repeated surgical trauma. Their direct application to sites of human physeal injury may hasten or otherwise beneficially affect the repair process.

While rodent amputation models have been useful in identifying and examining details of growth plate regeneration, in virtually no important respects do they resemble the types of physeal injuries encountered in children and adolescents, and so will have limited use in future investigations designed to improve their treatment. The localized physeal defects exploited by Langenskiöld and co-workers more closely satisfy this requirement, but they also possess only slight resemblance to the range of growth plate fractures and fracture-separations seen by the orthopedist. In order to accurately define the requirements for regeneration of human growth plate cartilage it may be essential to develop additional animal models which more closely duplicate epiphyseal and metaphyseal fracture patterns, including periosteal and neurovascular injury and possibly even related muscle and joint trauma. To explore the full potential of the growth plate for self-repair it would be useful to have access to a model in which its germinal cells are cleanly excised or selectively destroyed. The ability to recover normal structure and function following such an insult would represent an experimental *tour de force* particularly relevant to the treatment of growth plate injuries consequent to therapeutic irradiation of a limb or medication with some of the chemotherapeutic agents currently used in the treatment of malignant disease.

Among the metazoa a variety of cellular mechanisms has evolved for the repair or replacement of tissues, organs, and members. In some lower organisms undifferentiated cells circulating in the hemolymph or blood, or scattered among the tissues of the body as reserve cells, migrate to sites of tissue damage or loss, there reorganizing to form a replica of the missing part. From observations of replacement of portions of growth plate cartilage Langenskiöld *et al.* (1989) have demonstrated that physeal cartilage is regenerated by interstitial growth of uninjured cartilage remaining at the injury site. However, after complete physeal ablation following division of the limb, it is periosteal cartilage which forms the regenerate, the characteristic ordered arrangement of growth plate chondrocytes appearing within an expanse of nonphyseal, hyaline cartilage as had occurred during the development of the bone in fetal and neonatal life. Viewed together with previously presented observations on physeal ectopia, these facts suggest that the growth plate cartilage tissue phenotype may be readily expressed wherever cartilage is present, and that some exostoses and exchondroses may begin with the formation of physeal nodules within cartilage or periosteum. They further suggest that the most useful material for prevention of skeletal bridging and use in growth plate reconstruction may be cartilage obtained from any location, or periosteum capable of rapidly forming cartilage. While Langenskiöld's group has documented the utility of fat as an innocuous and clinically effective interposition material, its use precludes the opportunity to implant a material which appears capable of participating directly in the repair of the injury. That material is cartilage. Whether it is applied as a block, as an autograft preparation of cells grown in culture, or as a strip of periosteum capable of forming cartilage may be inconsequential.

Nunnemacher (1939) and Libbin and Weinstein (1986) described the occasionally observed innate regrowth of hemiepiphyses resembling regenerated condyles at femoral amputation sites. In each instance the regrown part lay in contact with a regenerated hemiphysis proximally, but was deficient distally, lacking an articular cartilage surface layer. Such observations suggest that the signals required for regrowth of the physis and epiphysis may be closely catenated, while those required for completion of the articulating surface of the bone may be of a different type. These investigators have also noted that hemiphyseal regrowth occurred within an enclosure of regional voluntary muscle surrounding the skeletal end, raising the question of a possible role for muscle in physeal regrowth, perhaps as a transmitter of contractile forces to the bone end, or as a physical barrier blunting biomechanical stimuli produced during weight bearing and progression.

References

Banks, S. W. and Compere, E. L. (1941). Regeneration of epiphyseal cartilage. *Ann. Surg.*, **114**: 1076–1084.

Bidder, A. (1873). Experimente über die kunstliche Hemmung des Längenwachsthums von Röhrenknochen durch Reizung und Zerstörung de Epiphysenknorpels. *Naunyn-Schmeideberg's Arch. Exp. Pathol. Pharmakol.*, **1**: 248–263.

Borgens, R. B., Vanable, J. W., Jr., and Jaffe, L. F. (1977). Bioelectricity and regeneration. I. Initiation of frog limb regeneration by minute currents. *J. Exp. Zool.*, **200**: 403–416.

Carlson, B. M. (1978). Types of morphogenetic phenomena in vertebrate regenerating systems. *Am. Zool.*, **18**: 869–882.

Dawson, A. B. (1925). The age order of epiphyseal union in the long bones of the albino rat. *Anat. Rec.*, **31**: 1–17.

Douglas, B. S. (1972). Conservative management of guillotine amputation of the fingers in children. *Aust. Paediatr. J.*, **8**: 86–88.

Eades, J. W. and Peacock, E. E., Jr. (1966). Autogenous transplantation of an interphalangeal joint and proximal phalangeal epiphysis. Case report and ten-year follow-up. *J. Bone Jt. Surg.*, **48**: 775–778.

Ehrlich, M. G., Zaleske, D. J., Lalanandham, T., and Mankin, H. J. (1988). Biology of growth plate transfers. In: *Behavior of the Growth Plate*, Uhthoff, H. K. and Wiley, J. J., Eds., Raven Press, New York, 61–64.

Freeman, B. S. (1965). The result of epiphyseal transplant by flap and by free graft: a brief survey. *Plast. Reconstr. Surg.*, **36**: 227–230.

Friedenberg, Z. B. (1957). Reaction of the epiphysis to partial surgical resection. *J. Bone Jt. Surg.*, **39**: 332–340.

Goldberg, V. M., Porter, B. B., and Lance, E. M. (1980). Transplantation of the canine knee joint on a vascular pedicle. A preliminary study. *J. Bone Jt. Surg.*, **62**: 414–424.

Haas, S. L. (1919). The changes produced in the growing bone after injury to the epiphyseal cartilage plate. *J. Orthop. Surg.*, **1**: 67–99; 166–179; 226–239.

Harris, W. R., Martin, R., and Tile, M. (1965). Transplantation of epiphyseal plates. *J. Bone Jt. Surg.*, **47**: 897–914.

Hastings, H., II and Simmons, B. P. (1984). Hand fractures in children: a statistical analysis. *Clin. Orthop.*, **188**: 120–130.

Hoffman, S., Siffert, R. S., and Simon, B. E. (1972). Experimental and clinical experiences in epiphyseal transplantation. *Plast. Reconstr. Surg.*, **50**: 58–65.

Illingworth, C. M. (1974). Trapped fingers and amputated finger tips in children. *J. Pediatr. Surg.*, **9**: 853–858.

Kawabe, N., Ehrlich, M. G., and Mankin, H. J. (1987). Growth plate reconstruction using chondrocyte allograft transplants. *J. Pediatr. Orthop.*, **7**: 381–388.

Key, J. A. and Ford, L. T. (1958). A study of experimental trauma to the distal femoral epiphysis in rabbits. *J. Bone Jt. Surg.*, **40**: 887–896.

Kleiger, B. and Mankin, H. J. (1964). Fracture of the lateral portion of the distal tibial epiphysis. *J. Bone Jt. Surg.*, **46**: 25–32.

Lacroix, P. (1951). *The Organization of Bones*, (translated from the amended French edition by S. Gilder), Blakiston, Philadelphia.

Langenskiöld, A. (1981). Surgical treatment of partial closure of the growth plate. *J. Pediatr. Orthop.*, **1**: 3–11.

Langenskiöld, A. (1988). Growth plate regeneration. In: *Behavior of the Growth Plate*, Uhthoff, H. K. and Wiley, J. J., Eds., Raven Press, New York, 47–50.

Langenskiöld, A. (1988). Osseous bridging of the growth plate. In: *Behavior of the Growth Plate,* Uhthoff, H. K. and Wiley, J. J., Eds., Raven Press, New York, 259–261.

Langenskiöld, A. and Edgren, W. (1950). Imitation of chondrodysplasia by localized roentgen ray injury — an experimental study of bone growth. *Acta Orthop. Scand.,* **99**: 353–373.

Langenskiöld, A., Heikel, H. V. A., Nevalainen, T., Österman, K., and Videman, T. (1989). Regeneration of the growth plate. *Acta Anat.,* **134**: 113–123.

Langenskiöld, A., Österman, K., and Valle, M. (1987). Growth of fat grafts after operation for partial bone growth arrest: demonstration by computed tomography scanning. *J. Pediatr. Orthop.,* **7**: 389–394.

Lexer, E. (1908). Substitution of whole or half joints from freshly amputated extremities by free plastic operation. *Surg. Gynecol. Obstet.,* **6**: 601–607.

Libbin, R. M. (1988). Hyaluronate at rat hindlimb amputation sites: preliminary histochemical observations. *Anat. Rec.,* **220**: 58A.

Libbin, R. M. and Rivera, M. E. (1989). Regeneration of growth plate cartilage induced in the neonatal rat hindlimb by reamputation. *J. Orthop. Res.,* **7**: 674–682.

Libbin, R. M. and Weinstein, M. (1986). Regeneration of growth plates in the long bones of the neonatal rat hindlimb. *Am. J. Anat.,* **177**: 369–383.

Libbin, R. M. and Weinstein, M. (1987). Sequence of development of innately regenerated growth-plate cartilage in the hindlimb of the neonatal rat. *Am. J. Anat.,* **180**: 255–265.

McCann, J. A. (1971). Methyl green as a cartilage stain. Human embryos. *Stain Technol.,* **46**: 263–265.

Mizell, M. (1968). Limb regeneration: induction in the newborn opossum. *Science,* **161**: 283–285.

Mizuta, T., Benson, W. M., Foster, B. K., Paterson, D. C., and Morris, L. L. (1987). Statistical analysis of the incidence of physeal fractures. *J. Pediatr. Othrop.,* **7**: 518–523.

Moss, M. L. (1977). A functional analysis of fusion of the tibia and the fibula in the rat and mouse. *Acta Anat.,* **97**: 321–332.

Nunnemacher, R. F. (1939). Experimental studies on the cartilage plates in the long bones of the rat. *Am. J. Anat.,* **65**: 253–289.

Ogden, J. A. (1988). Skeletal growth mechanisms injury patterns. In: *Behavior of the Growth Plate,* Uhthoff, H. K. and Wiley, J. J., Eds., Raven Press, New York, 85–96.

Ogo, K. (1987). Does the nail bed really regenerate?. *Plast. Reconstr. Surg.,* **80**: 445–447.

O'Keefe, R. J., Crabb, I. D., Puzas, J. E., and Rozier, R. N. (1989). Synergistic effects of IGF-I with TGF-β and FGF are specific for DNA synthesis in growth plate chondrocytes. *Proc. 35th Annu. Meet. Orthop. Res. Soc.,* Feb. 6–9, Las Vegas, NV, 258.

Ollier, L. (1867). *Traité Expérimentale et Clinique de la Régéneration des Os et de la Production Artificielle du Tissu Osseux,* Vols. 1–2. Masson, Paris.

Österman, K. (1972). Operative elimination of partial premature epiphyseal closure. *Acta Orthop. Scand. Suppl.,* **147**: 1–79.

Person, P., Libbin, R. M., Shah, D., and Papierman, S. (1979). Partial regeneration of the above-elbow amputated rat forelimb. I. Innate responses. *J. Morphol.,* **159**: 427–438.

Polezhaev, L. W. (1946). Morphological data on regenerative capacity in tadpole limbs as restored by chemical agents. *C. R. Dokl. Acad. Sci. URSS,* **54**: 281–284.

Polezhaev, L. W. (1972). *Loss and Restoration of Regenereative Capacity in Tissues and Organs of Animals,* Harvard University Press, Cambridge, MA, 84–119.

Reeves, B. (1969). Orthotopic transplantation of vascularized whole knee joints in dogs. *Lancet,* **1**: 500–502.

Rogers, L. F. (1970). The radiography of epiphyseal injuries. *Radiology,* **96**: 289–299.

Romer, A. S. (1966). *Vertebrate Paleontology,* 3rd ed. University of Chicago Press, Chicago, 302–310.

Rose, S. M. (1944). Methods for initiating limb regeneration in adult anura. *J. Exp. Zool.,* **95**: 149–170.

Rose, S. M. (1945). The effect of NaCl in stimulating regeneration of limbs of frogs. *J. Morphol.,* **77**: 119–139.

Salter, R. B. and Harris, W. R. (1963). Injuries involving the epiphyseal plate. *J. Bone Jt. Surg.*, **45**: 587–622.

Schneider, C. and Leyva, S. (1964). Siliconized Dacron interposition for traumatic radio-ulnar synostosis. *J. Med. Assoc. State Ala.*, **33**: 185–188.

Selye, H. (1934). On the mechanism controlling the growth in length of the long bones. *J. Anat.*, **68**: 289–292.

Seräfin, J. (1970). Effect of longitudinal transection of the epiphysis and metaphysis on cartilaginous growth. *Am. Dig. Foreign Orthop. Lit. Third Q.*, 17–21.

Shapiro, F. (1982). Epiphyseal growth plate fracture-separations: a pathophysiologic approach. *Orthopedics*, **5**: 720–736.

Shapiro, F. (1987). Epiphyseal disorders. *N. Engl. J. Med.*, **317**: 1702–1710.

Singer, M. (1954). Induction of regeneration of the forelimb of the frog by augmentation of the nerve supply. *J. Exp. Zool.*, **126**: 419–471.

Smith, S. D. (1967). Induction of partial limb regeneration in *Rana pipiens* by galvanic stimulation. *Anat. Rec.*, **158**: 89–98.

Speirs, A. C. and Blocksma, R. (1963). New implantable silicone rubbers. An experimental evaluation of tissue response. *Plast. Reconstr. Surg.*, **31**: 166–175.

Teucq, E. (1948). Reconstruction d'un cartilage de croissance apres amputation. *Arch. Biol.*, **59**: 1–6.

Tomlinson, B. L., Tomlinson, D. E., and Tassava, R. A. (1985). Pattern-deficient forelimb regeneration in adult bullfrogs. *J. Exp. Zool.*, **236**: 313–326.

Urist, M. R. and McLean, F. C. (1952). Osteogenic potency and new bone formation by induction in transplants to the anterior chamber of the eye. *J. Bone Jt. Surg.*, **34A**: 443–476.

Vogt, P. (1878). Die traumatische Epiphysentrennung und deren Einfluss auf das Längenwachsthum der Röhrenknochen. *Langenbecks Arch. Klin. Chir.*, **22**: 343–373.

Wilson, J. N. (1966). Epiphyseal transplantation. *J. Bone Jt. Surg.*, **48**: 245–256.

Worlock, P. and Stower, M. (1986). Fracture patterns in Nottingham children. *J. Pediatr. Orthop.*, **6**: 656–660.

Zaleske, D. J., Ehrlich, M. G., Piliero, C., May, J. W., Jr., and Mankin, H. J. (1982). Growth plate behavior in whole joint replantation in the rabbit. *J. Bone Jt. Surg.*, **64**: 249–258.

9

Digital Regeneration in Mammals

DANIEL A. NEUFELD

Department of Anatomy
University of South Dakota
School of Medicine
Vermillion, South Dakota

Introduction

As a generality, mammals do not regenerate digits, although a compelling case can be made for regeneration of digit tips. Certain non-mammalian vertebrates regularly demonstrate a dramatic degree of appendage regeneration. Manipulation of mammalian amputation sites has produced a degree of plasticity which suggests that mammals possess a latent capability for growth after amputation, the extent of which is unknown. This review attempts to synthesize information from clinical observations, basic research of digit-tip regrowth, limb regeneration in amphibians, postamputational healing, and attempted induction of outgrowths in mammals to define a series of questions which outline what is known about digital regeneration in mammals.

Because this volume focuses on skeletal biology, this review emphasizes skeletal tissues, but when dealing with entire digits the other tissues cannot be ignored. The term "regeneration" will be used to denote replacement of removed tissue by tissue which is structurally and functionally similar to the original.

Observations of Human Digit-Tip Regeneration

The digit-tip is an anatomically distinct subunit of the digit containing a nail plate, nail bed, nail matrix, pulp space, volar pad, profusion of special sensory organs, and unique structure of the distal end of the terminal phalanx. The regenerative properties of the tip are descriptively and functionally related to these special structures and are appropriately considered separately from those of the remainder of the digit.

What can be gained from case studies of human digit-tip regrowth? Although detailed documentation of the mechanism of digit-tip regeneration cannot be obtained, a number of studies have provided empirical evidence from which generalities can be abstracted. Particularly informative data have resulted from comparison of treatment strategies employed following amputation through the terminal phalanx. Considerations of the functional, economic, and cosmetic outcome influence the treatment strategy. There are generally six approaches that can be taken following digit-tip amputation (Webster, 1950): no treatment (or conservative treatment), replantation of the amputated part, reamputation at a more proximal level, split-thickness graft, full-thickness graft, or pedicle graft. With few exceptions those studies in which digit-tip regeneration has been reported have employed a conservative strategy following amputation (Fig. 1).

What is the clinical significance of a conservative strategy? Several studies have compared results of surgical intervention with those from conservative treatment after traumatic amputation (Bojsen-Moller *et al.*, 1961; Scott, 1974, Holm and Zachariae, 1974; Das and Brown, 1978; Koderberg *et al.*, 1983). These studies have unanimously advocated conservative treatment, citing the advantages of reduced surgical morbidity, simplicity of treatment, retained digit length, and results which are at least comparable if not better than surgical results in terms of digit function, sensibility, and cosmetic appearance. The study of 134 cases by Bojsen-Moller et al. (1961) cited earlier studies (in German) which dated at least to 1934 advocating conservative treatment of finger-tip injuries. Other studies that used exclusively conservative treatment reached similar conclusions (Virgin *et al.*, 1971; Douglas, 1972; Illingworth, 1974; Bossley, 1975; Chow and Ho, 1977; Fox *et al.*, 1977; Farrell *et al.*, 1977; King, 1979; Rosenthal *et al.*, 1979; Allen, 1980; and DeBoer and Collinson, 1981). All of these studies also strongly advocated conservative treatment of digit-tip amputations. Although conservative treatment appears to be the treatment of choice in most terminal phalangeal amputations, separate consideration must be given to each case. The precise level of amputation, angle of amputation, amount and location of nail matrix, amount of volar pad loss, and degree of maceration of stump tissue all influence the final contour deformity, nail deformity, and general appearance of the terminal phalanx. Various surgical strategies have been and continue to be proposed (Sturman and Duran, 1963; Fisher, 1967; Beasley, 1969; Sandzen, 1974; Atasoy *et al.*, 1979; Rosenthal, 1983; Shepard,

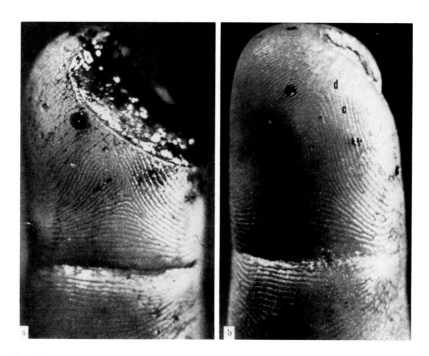

Fig. 1 Digit-tip regrowth following partial tip amputation. Conservative treatment permits natural regrowth to approximate original digit contours. Note that within the growth distal to the three tattoo marks, which designate the amputation plane, volar ridges have been reestablished in region "c". Region "d" is primarily scar tissue with overlying nail plate. (From Soderberg *et al.*, 1983. With permission.)

1983; Zacher, 1984; Anderson, 1987; Robbins, 1988; and Evans and Martin, 1988), but with the possible occasional exception of digital tip replantation (see Goldner *et al.*, 1989; Rose *et al.*, 1989) results of these procedures have not surpassed those of conservative treatment. Regeneration is, however, rarely perfect and occasional "beaked" or splintered nails may be corrected by grafting or cosmetic surgery (see Beasley, 1969; Shepard, 1990).

Which structures regenerate? The term "regeneration" was used by 15 of the 17 studies cited above that employed conservative strategies, and at least three other studies (Polezhaev, 1980; Khonovets, 1983; and Ogo, 1987) to describe results in patients. Expressions such as, "finger appears to lengthen" (Farrell *et al.*, 1977) or, "remodeling of the pulp" (DeBoer and Collinson, 1981) were commonly used. The clinical presentation of results, however, generally concentrated on cosmetic appearance (especially of nails), and return of sensation, particularly that related to tactile or gripping functions. Evidence of volar pad reconstitution is anecdotal and contradictory, perhaps because of variability in patient age, volar angle of amputation, and time elapsed prior to evaluation. It has been established that the nail will regenerate if the nail matrix is left intact (Illingworth, 1974), and that the nail bed is also capable of regenerating (Ogo, 1987). Recent studies have demonstrated the extraordinary plasticity of the nail as an organ and the degree to which surgical manipulation can restore a mutilated nail to normal or near normal appearance and function (see Keyser *et al.*, 1990; Shepard, 1990; and Van Beek *et al.*, 1990). Nail matrix is also transplantable (Kligman, 1961). Of central interest to this review, however, none of these studies of human digit-tip regeneration has presented radiographic findings or evidence to indicate whether bone did or did not regrow.

Is age a factor in the outcome? Although tip regeneration in children has been emphasized, especially in studies evaluating children exclusively (Douglas, 1972; Illingworth, 1974; Das and Brown, 1978; Rosenthal *et al.*, 1979; King, 1979; Polezhaev, 1980; and Khonovets, 1983), it is clear from other studies (Soderberg *et al.*, 1983; Ogo, 1987) that at least to some degree these generalities hold for adults as well. As above, however, these are descriptive results that relate to cosmetic and functional repair.

It is evident from these case studies that functional soft tissues can reform distal to the amputation plane, and that a conservative or "open wound" protocol maximizes this regrowth. Questions that immediately arise are related to the ubiquity of the phenomenon in mammals, how the process occurs, whether bone regenerates, why conservative treatment may be more conducive to outgrowth, and whether this process is appropriately termed "true regeneration".

Animal Studies of Digit-Tip Regeneration

Is digit-tip regrowth widespread in mammals? Although digit tip re-growth after amputation has been repeatedly reported in the clinical liter-ature, only recently have studies examined the phenomenon in other mam-mals (Fig. 2). It was not until 1982 that Borgens documented digit-tip regrowth in young adult mice, and in 1987 that similar observations were made for young Rhesus monkeys (Singer *et al.*, 1987). Very recently, digit-tip regeneration was also reported in neonatal rats and mice (Atherley and Neufeld, 1989), and it has also been found in adult rats (Neufeld, unpub-lished observations). Following the publication by Borgens (1982) several investigators commented anecdotally that they had observed digit-tip re-growth when animals that had been "toe clipped" through the terminal phalanx for identification could no longer be identified after several months because tips had regenerated.

Does the phenomenon appear grossly similar in experimental animals and humans? In all of the studies using rodents, the correlation between level of amputation and regenerative response has been addressed. In his study of 20 mice, Borgens (1982) confirmed for adult mice Illingworth's (1974) observation in humans that digit-tips regrow if amputations were distal to the nail matrix. As in humans there was no regrowth at more

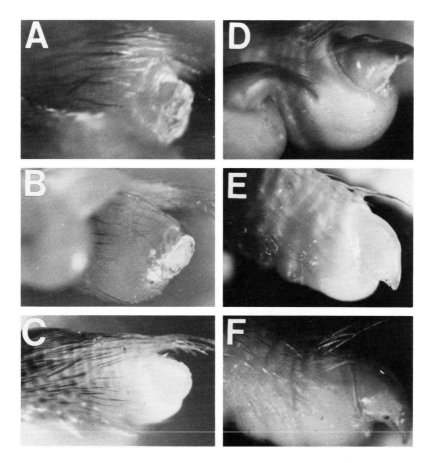

Fig. 2 Gross appearance of digit-tip regeneration in neonatal rodents. Figures A through C are stages of regrowth from one mouse amputated at 7 days of age. Figures D through F are representative examples from other animals at approximately 4 weeks postamputation. Although tips are functionally complete they are slightly misshapen compared to control digit (D, lower left), being flattened (D) or beaked (E,F). Contouring of both nail and volar pad continues for several weeks. (Submitted for publication to *J. Exp. Zool.*)

proximal levels. Atherley and Neufeld (1989) have also confirmed this observation for neonatal rats and mice (Fig. 3, and see below). A recent study of adult mouse digit-tip regeneration (Revardel and Chebouki, 1987), however, suggested that the terminal phalanx did not always regenerate. These authors reported that if the angle of the amputation plane passed proximally through the proximal one half of the terminal phalanx, skeletal tissue formed in only two digits out of ten at 21 days. This finding apparently contradicts that of Borgens in which his plane of amputation as indicated schematically passed through the base of the proximal phalanx. Several possibilities may reconcile this discrepancy. The amount of tissue visible in the section of the removed tip (Fig. 3B of Borgens, 1982a) indicates that perhaps the plane

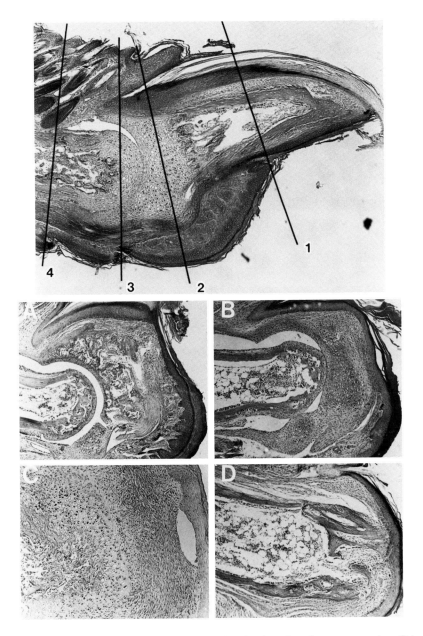

Fig. 3 Histological appearance of tissues from various levels at 2 weeks postamputation. Orientation photomicrograph (top) illustrates that in 7-day-old mice amputation planes may pass through either cartilage or bone. Level 1 amputations (anywhere through the osseous part of the terminal phalanx) consistently regenerated an appearance similar to A. Amputations through levels 2 or 3 provoked cartilage hypertrophy, but no new osseous growth (B and C). Amputation through the bone of the second phalanx produced woven bone remodeling, but no distal growth of bone or cartilage (D).

of amputation was slightly further distal than schematically illustrated, indicating amputation through the more distal portion of the distal phalanx. Also, because Revardel and Chebouki do not illustrate their digit tips at 21 days several possibilities remain: (1) they may have accurately described failure of regrowth, (2) they may have misinterpreted their observations, or (3) they may not have waited long enough, Borgens having waited 34 days prior to his observations. It is apparent from both studies that there has been growth distal to the amputation plane, but, with the possible exception of Revardel and Chebouki, Fig. 10, precisely what has regrown is not clear since markers of the original amputation plane have been obliterated.

Does bone regenerate? Failure to demonstrate a definitive marker of the amputation plane is a common problem of most studies of mammalian postamputational events. Recently, I administered Calcein, an autofluorescent marker which is deposited at sites of calcium deposition (Suzuki and Matthews, 1966), to newborn mice at 8 days postamputation and killed animals 24 days later. When so administered, a fluorescent line indicates areas of calcium deposition at that time (i.e., at 8 days postamputation), and any bone deposited in the intervening 24 days will appear as unlabeled bone distal to that line. Results are seen in Fig. 4. At least two thirds of the bulk of the terminal phalanx was regenerated during the 24 days after label injection. This rapid bone growth occurred from the second to the fifth week postamputation when most digit regrowth was also seen grossly (Fig. 2). It can be seen that the regenerated bone forms a semi-dense woven bone of approximately appropriate dimensions but without a single central marrow cavity.

How do bone and soft tissues regrow? Conflicting observations again characterize the initial explanations of the mechanism of bone regrowth. Borgens, who presented no pictorial evidence of stages of regrowth, stated that there was " . . . no evidence of a classical blastema comprised of stellate, mesenchymatous cells". The opposite conclusion was reached in a different study which presented both micrographs and a schematic summary of stages of regeneration. Revardel and Chebouki (1987, p. 3168) state that during the second week postamputation "Ce blasteme est analogue a celui des Urodeles et se caracterise par des cellules mesenchymateuses a longs prolongements cytoplasmiques . . . " Although three micrographs contain the label "blasteme", the strict use of the term to represent a structure functionally analogous to the multipotential blastema which precedes newt limb regeneration may be questioned. Lacking additional evidence of the fate of these cells, it might be more appropriate to term the highly vascular mass of multiply oriented cells, "blastema-like". Atherley and Neufeld (1989) report a similar, although typically less extensive, mass of blastema-like cells between amputation surface and epithelium during the rapid growth phase of neonatal rodents. The issue raised by the presence of such cells is whether or not they are a vehicle for the reexpression of genetically pro-

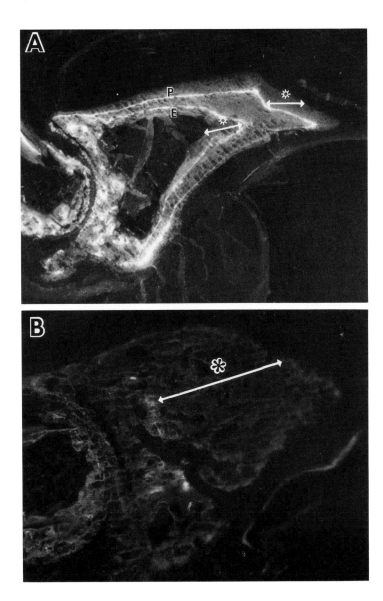

Fig. 4 Calcein distribution in intact and regenerating digits of neonatal mice. Midsaggital section through the terminal phalanx of intact (A) third digit of left hind foot of 40-day-old mouse, injected with calcein on day 16. Lines indicate sites of bone synthesis in endosteum (E) and periosteum (P) on day 16. Unlabeled bone superficial to P and deep to E (bars/asterisks) was synthesized between day 16 and day 40. The terminal phalanx of the right hind foot (B) of the same animal was amputated on day 8. Regenerated bone is indicated by bar/asterisk. The central marrow cavity has not been regenerated. (Submitted for publication to *J. Exp. Zool.*)

grammed morphogenetic information necessary for the reconstruction of missing bone and soft tissues.

If regeneration of mammalian digit-tips were strictly analogous to limb regeneration in amphibians, one would expect to see the mesenchyme cells condense into a prechondrogenic mass which would produce a cartilaginous template and would subsequently be replaced by the definitive bone. This does not appear to occur. Despite several references to neocartilage and chondrogenesis by Revardel and Chebouki, their pictorial evidence does not support the concept of cartilage template formation. Atherley and Neufeld (1989) examined histologically more than 40 digit tips and found no evidence of a cartilage template preceding bone formation. If bone does not form by template formation and endochondral ossification, how does it form and does it represent a type of regeneration?

Recent work in my laboratory indicates that the new bone most likely arises by apposition of woven bone onto the existing bone surface, but other mechanisms may also be involved. If a digit from an 8-day-old mouse is amputated, the level of amputation may be selected to pass through either bone or cartilage (Fig. 3). If the cut is through bone and digits are examined histologically approximately 2 weeks later, the apicodorsal tip immediately beneath the end of the regenerating nail is consistently seen to be an area of active bone deposition onto the stump bone (Fig. 5A). Perhaps because it grows so rapidly, the tissue may resemble a form of chondroid initially, but it never is frankly cartilaginous and rapidly assumes the structure and staining properties of woven bone. If the cut is through cartilage, a different process ensues and we are less certain of the outcome. When examined as late as 14 days postamputation, although the cartilage block often had hypertrophied slightly, these digit stumps displayed no bone at the amputation site. Because we have not examined such tissues at later times, we do not know whether and how bone develops. In one fortuitous example the amputation plane passed precisely through the interface between cartilage and bone (see Fig. 5B). In that example at 2 weeks postamputation woven bone appeared to be developing *de novo* in the mesenchyme distal to the persistent cartilage of the stump. Closer examination of serial sections revealed that this island of bone was continuous with a small block of bone at the amputation plane which apparently had begun ossification prior to amputation and served as a scaffold onto which new bone could be apposed. Amputation through cartilage obviously needs to be investigated further as results have implications for prognosis of proximal level amputations in very young children.

Interpretation of the reconstituted digit-tip is problematic. Because the process is grossly similar in humans and experimental animals, we can assume as a working hypothesis that the mechanisms of regrowth are similar. The process resembles "true epimorphic regeneration" as seen during the reconstruction of newt limbs in that bone appears to develop from an adjacent mesenchyme-like mass which is found immediately beneath a mod-

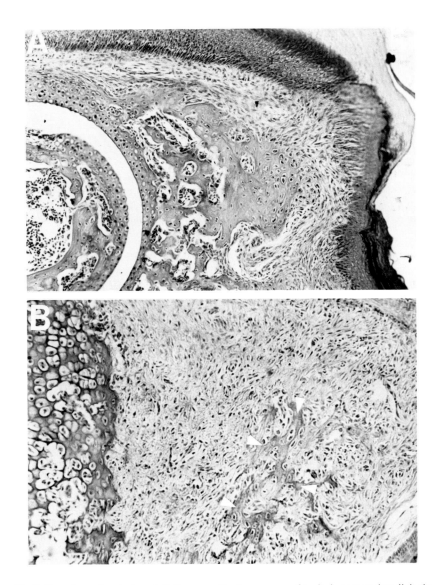

Fig. 5 Bone formation during digit-tip regrowth. Appearance of typical regenerating digit-tip (Figure A). The cartilaginous base of the terminal phalanx has been replaced by bone (a normal developmental occurrence). The phalanx is elongating by vigorous bone growth distally, especially in the vicinity of the epithelium at the tip of the elongating nail bed. Exuberant growth may superficially resemble a form of cartilage, but matrix is eosinophilic indicating a form of woven bone. Note the collection of elongate or stellate cells between bone and epithelium (A) and surrounding spicules of forming bone (white arrowheads, B). Amputation through the cartilage-bone interface preserves cartilage proximally (B) while generating new woven bone distally. (From Atherley and Neufeld, 1989.)

ified overlying epithelium (see below). The completed bone, which represents the endpoint of the process, also resembles the original bone at least in outline. However, the process is different from true regeneration in that the blastema-like tissue is not as extensive and a cartilaginous template does not form. Perhaps, provisionally, digit-tip regrowth might be termed a unique form of regeneration.

If digit-tips regenerate, is it possible that proximal level amputations might also regenerate? To examine prospects for true regeneration it is necessary to look more closely at how limb regeneration occurs in amphibians, to compare that process with events of healing after amputation in mammals, and to examine results of studies that have attempted to induce growth by modifying postamputational healing in mammals.

Animal Studies of Proximal Level Amputations

There is no report that digits amputated proximal to the nail matrix can regenerate, but several studies have investigated postamputational healing at proximal levels. Investigations underway are attempting to understand why mammals fail to regenerate and how postamputational growth might be enhanced. It is encouraging that many of the characteristics seen during limb regeneration in amphibians can be seen or can be made to appear during postamputational events in mammals.

What are the principles of true appendage regeneration? Aspects of true and complete regeneration of limbs in amphibians have been investigated in more than 1000 studies spanning more than 250 years. Several books have reviewed this information (Schmidt, 1968; Goss, 1969; Rose, 1970; Polezhaev, 1972; Thornton and Bromley, 1973; and Wallace, 1981), and a number of generalities have emerged. A modified epithelium must cover the amputation site and must persist for several weeks while the cells of the growth bud (blastema) accumulate. Formation of the bud is concurrent with, and apparently dependent upon, dedifferentiation and remodeling of tissues in the adjacent stump. Growth of the bud and limb requires an abundant local nerve supply and a variety of humoral factors. Differentiation of blastemal mesenchyme parallels that of ontogenetic development, including condensation into pretissue primordia with subsequent expression of phenotype and matrix constituents. Growth continues until the amputated segment has been duplicated. To the degree that true mammalian regeneration, if it could be induced, would parallel these processes it is helpful to examine how those tenets of limb regeneration are related to mammalian postamputational healing.

Does the epithelium covering the mammalian amputation site resemble that covering regenerating limbs? As is true for developing limbs, regenerating appendages must be covered by modified epithelium. Unique features of this "modified" epithelium are not well characterized biochemically, and morphological details are also sparse. Histologically, it is typically at least slightly thickened and cells appear irregularly oriented (Rose, 1948). Ultrastructurally, the most active zones lack a full-thickness basement membrane (Aulthouse and Neufeld, 1985a; Neufeld and Aulthouse, 1986). During normal postamputational healing in mice, a thickened apical epithelium also initially lacks an underlying basement membrane (Neufeld and Aulthouse, 1987; and Neufeld, 1989) but the basement membrane rapidly reappears as contracture and wound repair seal the end of the digit at the end of the first week postamputation. By surgically removing contracted skin and reinjuring the site physically or with sodium chloride baths it has been possible to experimentally prolong zones lacking basement membrane as evidenced by the distribution of Alcian blue stained basement membrane materials (Neufeld, 1983). Whether such basement membrane-free regions assume all of the functions of "inductive epithelia" seen during limb regeneration is unknown, but it is encouraging that more subjacent cells are frequently seen in proximity to such areas.

Do mesenchyme-like cells appear after amputation in mammals? The accumulated mesenchymal cells of the blastema are the source of skeletal and other tissues which subsequently differentiate internally. In mice, after amputation a small pool of relatively undifferentiated-appearing cells can be found surrounding the periosteum proximal to the amputation plane (Neufeld, 1989), but few such cells can be seen distally. Those which appear initially mixed with inflammatory cells are rapidly replaced by ingrowing endothelium and large migrating fibroblasts which appear under the reestablished basement membrane and are almost exclusively present by 10 days postamputation. Surgical removal of skin combined with trauma not only prolongs "modified epithelium" (see above), but also increases the number of irregularly oriented mesenchyme-like cells distal to the amputation plane (Neufeld, 1983; and see Fig. 6). As in the newt blastema, distal cells of treated mouse digits are mitotically active as evidenced by ^{3}H-thymidine incorporation and autoradiographic visualization (Neufeld, 1980a). We have also removed mesenchyme-like cells from treated mouse tips, grown the cells in three-dimensional agarose gels, and found that a few stain positively with Alcian blue at low pH, indicating that they have synthesized cartilage matrix (Neufeld and Johnson, unpublished observations). If these preliminary data are substantiated, it would mean that blastema-like cells capable of chondrogenesis can be found under experimental conditions distal to the amputation plane of mammals.

Why is cartilage distal to the amputation plane significant? Chondrogenesis distal to the amputation plane may be highly significant because cartilage is normally not seen distally in adult mammals (Schotte and Smith, 1959; and Neufeld, 1985; and see Fig. 7), but in newt limb regeneration formation of the cartilage template distally is the hallmark of true regeneration. Although bony overgrowth may be a common complication following amputation in humans (Christie et al., 1979; Speer, 1981), the phenomenon

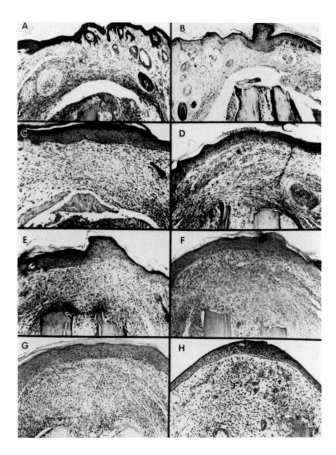

Fig. 6 Generation of mesenchyme-like cells in digits of adult mice. Amputations were through the mid-diaphysis of the proximal phalanx, and digits (A–G) are arranged in sequence of increasing treatment intensity as seen at 14 to 16 days PA. Control digits (A, B) heal by skin contracture and scar tissue formation. Additional non-inflammatory cells can be recruited by surgical removal of skin once (C) or twice (D, E). When skin removal is combined with mechanical teasing of local tissues the resultant amputation sites (F,G) resemble the blastema of a regenerating newt limb (H). Cartilage occurs distal to the amputation plane in some digits of maximally treated adult mice. (From Neufeld, 1983. With permission.)

has been carefully examined in rabbits (Speer, 1981), and there is no evidence that such growth is preceded by cartilage. In mice, too, such growth can be demonstrated, but it arises directly as woven bone usually derived from the endosteum of the open marrow cavity (Neufeld, 1985). On oblique fracture surfaces lacking either periosteum or endosteum, a chondroid form of tissue has been noted. It was neither woven bone nor hyaline-type cartilage in appearance and had staining properties intermediate to the two (Fig. 8). One study of rats (Bunch *et al.*, 1977) has reported cartilage on the distal end of amputated tibias, but animals were 5 days old at the time of amputation and original amputated segments were not preserved. As has

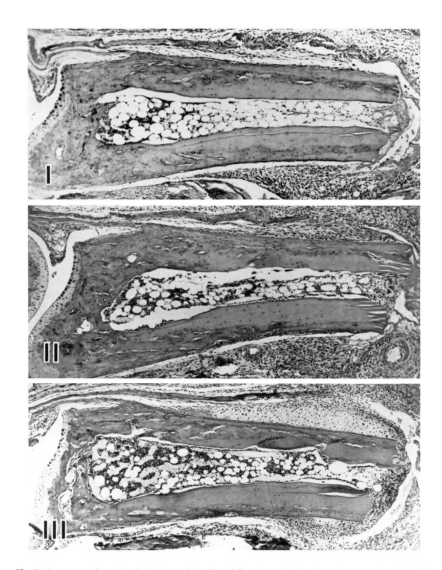

Fig. 7 Sequence of proximal phalangeal healing following mid-diaphyseal amputation in adult mice. Avascular necrosis distally (I) is followed peripherally by periosteal activation (II), chondrogenesis (III), partial calcification (IV), vascular bud invasion of matrix (V), and replacement by bone (VI). Although the marrow becomes effectively sealed by woven bone (IV–VI), hyaline cartilage does not extend beyond the periosteum proximal to the amputation plane. (From Neufeld, 1985. With permission.)

been pointed out above (Atherley and Neufeld, 1989), if the amputation plane has passed through cartilage in the neonate the cartilage will be preserved for some time, which may explain the presence of distal cartilage at the time of sacrifice (see below for further discussion of studies of neonatal animals). Ignoring for the moment the significance of cartilage at the am-

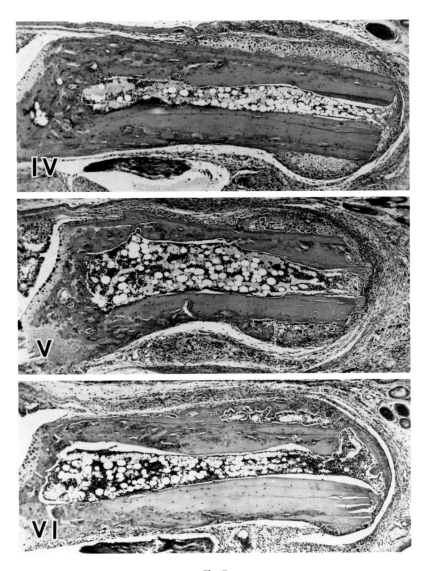

Fig. 7

putation site of neonates, cartilage at the site in adult mice would demonstrate that another of the hallmarks of limb regeneration could be found in adult mammals.

Have studies attempted to induce digit regeneration in adult rodents? Few studies have reported modified postamputational repair following proximal level amputation of mammalian digits. Schotte and Smith (1959) initially described the postamputational events in adult mouse digits and subsequently (Schotte and Smith, 1961) unsuccessfully attempted to generate a blastema or distal growth by hormonal injections. Another unsuccessful attempt (Neufeld, 1980b) was based upon the principle that an

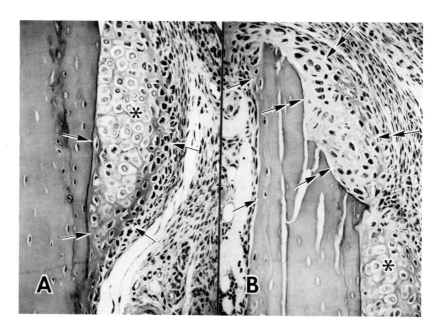

Fig. 8 Occasional occurrence of chondroid bone on oblique amputation surfaces. Typical periosteal growth (A) was hyaline-type cartilage (asterisk) capped by woven bone (arrows). In (B) the marrow cavity (left) is also lined distally by newly formed endosteal woven bone (arrows). Peripherally, hyaline cartilage (asterisk) has formed from periosteum proximally, but a different form of chondroid tissue (double arrows) has formed across the oblique amputation plane which obviously was covered with neither endosteum nor periosteum prior to amputation. (From Neufeld, 1985. With permission.)

augmented nerve supply can induce skeletal outgrowth at the amputation site of nonregenerating adult anurans (Singer, 1951). Although regenerative growth was not induced in digits of adult mice, the added nerve at the amputation site was associated with local soft tissue proliferation. In several of the animals treated as described above (Neufeld, 1983; 1985) hyaline cartilage could be found on the distal amputation surface, and when $CaCl_2$ baths were added to the protocol an exaggerated growth of hyaline-type cartilage was produced on one animal (Fig. 9). The cartilage occurred not only distal to bone but also distal to the marrow cavity, a relationship which also is seen in regenerating newt limbs (Aulthouse and Neufeld, 1985b). Recently, Revardel and Chebouki (1987) suggested that distal chondrogenesis could be induced, following proximal amputation of adult mouse digits, by injections of growth hormone or wound epithelial extract prepared at the time of injection. Although the micrographs of cartilage are convincing and the data are encouraging, the planes of section illustrated are not midsaggital and the cartilage is not unequivocally seen distal to the amputation plane. This criticism of the plane of section cannot be overemphasized. A parasaggital section through the exuberant periosteal callus which

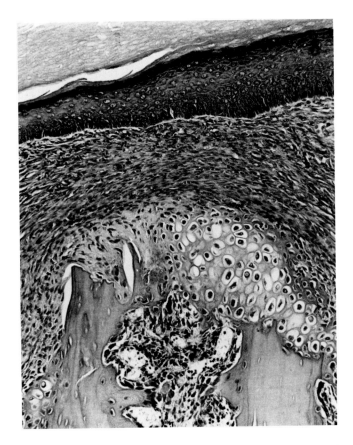

Fig. 9 Induced chondrogenesis distal to the amputation plane in an adult mouse. Amputation through the proximal phalanx was treated by skin removal, mechanical tissue disruption, and CaCl$_2$ baths. Hyaline cartilage is not found distally in untreated animals.

includes a tangential section of underlying bone gives a vivid, but false, impression of distal cartilaginous growth. In this and most other studies of modified mammalian postamputational growth the data are encouraging but not convincing because the amputation plane, as evidenced by the end of the marrow cavity, has not been clearly illustrated in relation to the level of the new growth.

Can regenerative growth be induced in neonates? The several studies of neonates are extremely difficult to interpret but are sufficiently provocative that their results cannot be ignored. Scharf (1961) amputated the 4th and 5th digits through the proximal phalanx of 20 1- or 2-day-old rats. They were divided into a group of 8 controls and 12 experimental animals treated with trypsin and CaCl$_2$ for 40 min 1 day after amputation. When examined 98 days later, the controls had not regenerated (one photomicrograph), but the experimentals (two photomicrographs of one digit) had regenerated the complete proximal phalanx, although no structures distal to the PIP joint were formed. If valid, these data are extremely significant. However, this study like virtually all other claims of induced regeneration is incomplete: in this case, no evidence of the plane of amputation is presented for the digit which is claimed to have "regenerated". An even more provocative finding was published by the same author (Scharf, 1963) subsequently, indicating that proximal level amputations of neonatal rats (as above) occasionally produced "cornified, nail-like outgrowths". Of the 45 amputated animals, 17 produced "projections" (digital outgrowths), and 11 of those 17 produced nail-like outgrowths (5 were treated with trypsin and $CaCl_2$ as above and 6 were untreated). As the author points out, "the level of amputation was at least $2^1/_2$ phalanges proximad to the level of normal nail primordium . . . " indicating that a distal structure had been produced essentially *de novo* following a proximal level amputation. In an earlier study (Rogal, 1951, in Russian) neonates from dams deprived of vitamins A and D regenerated similar, grossly visible nail-like outgrowths, some of which contained histologically visible skeletal elements (see Polezhaev, 1972; and Fig. 10). Neither of these findings has been subsequently investigated.

Are studies of attempted induction of mammalian limb regeneration more enlightening? These latter studies are representative of most studies of attempted induction of mammalian limb regeneration which has been reviewed elsewhere (Neufeld, 1980; Borgens, 1982b), and will receive only brief comment here. Many such studies have produced some evidence of experimentally induced outgrowths, but most have been incompletely documented and findings have not been pursued. They therefore stand as tantalizing but isolated observations of a latent but inducible growth potential following amputation in mammals. Results of two recent studies (Smith, 1981; Sisken and Fowler, 1984) fall into this category. Both used electrical stimulation to induce bone growth in the vicinity of amputation sites, but both studies lack documentation of the level of amputation and both documented only the endpoints of growth. Despite impressive new growth, particularly in the latter study which simultaneously implanted fetal nerve tissue, it is impossible to know how the growths arose and, consequently, what is the meaning of such growth in the context of attempted induction of mammalian regeneration. Because neither study has been pursued, they are perhaps best interpreted as additional isolated observations of electrical stimulation of osteogenesis at amputation sites. A well-documented series of investigations of postamputational growth of rat limbs has recently begun in the laboratory of Libbin (Libbin and Weinstein, 1986; Libbin and Weinstein, 1987; Libbin, 1988; and elsewhere in this volume). The definitive demonstration of amputation level, clear and ample display of data, and continuity of study contribute significantly to an understanding of growth plate regeneration after amputation.

A final miscellaneous category of pertinent observations would include several clinical studies which provide evidence of bone growth following

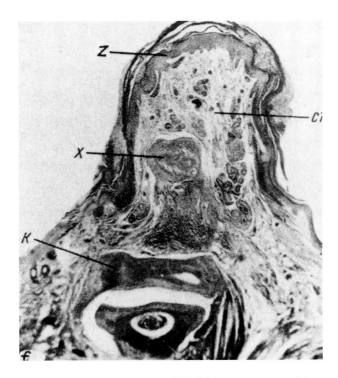

Fig. 10 Induced distal outgrowth on a mouse digit. Digits were amputated from neonates of dams deprived of vitamins A and D. Histological sections revealed new cartilage (X) distal to the amputation plane (K). Because other details of treatment and results are incomplete, and because subsequent studies have not been published, this photomicrograph is a provocative example of an isolated observation of an induced mammalian outgrowth. (From Polezhaev, 1972. With permission.)

removal at proximal levels of digits. The podiatry literature includes several references to spontaneous regeneration of phalangeal heads following surgical resection (Duvries and Shogren, 1962; Franklin, 1968). In a study of 32 amputations (14 of which were followed for only 3 weeks) 11 demonstrated regeneration of at least one half of the head and 5 of these demonstrated complete head regeneration at 3 months postoperatively (Slomsky, 1966). A similar report noted regeneration of a distal phalanx in an otherwise intact digit from which it was avulsed in a lawnmower accident (Neumann, 1988). All of these cases were radiographically confirmed. Most likely they represent periosteal reconstruction of extirpated bone segments as has occasionally been observed in other areas of the body following surgical (Nagase et al., 1985) or traumatic (Varma and Srivastava, 1979) extrusion.

Summary and Prospects

From the foregoing it seems appropriate to conclude that digit-tips may regrow in mammals, that the process resembles, but is not identical to, limb regeneration in newts, that digits do not regenerate when amputated anywhere proximal to the nail matrix, and that some limited growth has been experimentally induced from proximal level amputation sites.

How is growth following conservative treatment of digit-tips in humans related to appendage regeneration in amphibians and mammals? An intact dermis across a wound site is inhibitory to continued outgrowth. At least as early as 1906, Tornier (as cited by Rose, 1970) observed that intact skin across the amputation site blocked amphibian limb regeneration. Variations of this observation have been confirmed many times in studies of amphibian limb regeneration, and observations of mammalian amputational healing also seem consistent. Regrowth of the digit-tip in adults and juveniles is repeatedly seen to be enhanced by preservation of the open wound rather than by rapid skin closure by suture or grafting. Conversely, removal of contracted skin from proximal amputation sites creates a more favorable environment for growth. A singular exception to this principle seems to be the recent work by Ogo (1987), in which sutured digit-tips regenerated beautifully (Fig. 11). Careful examination of his protocol reveals that although volar skin was sutured across the open wound, the intact nail matrix was preserved. It seems plausible that the nailbed, as it grew distally maintained an active epithelium at the apicodorsal tip and provided a growth focus which permitted continued outgrowth as does the active epithelium in the regenerating newt limb. The preliminary data reported here (Figs. 4 and 5) suggest that the apicodorsal epithelium is morphologically unique and perhaps is instrumental in permitting growth of underlying soft and hard tissues during "normal" digit-tip regrowth. Certainly future experiments could address the role of nailbed epithelium in preventing total dermal closure distally. The correlation between nail growth and bone growth should also be explored.

Do other principles of regeneration appear to be valid for mammals? An adequate supply of cells must be present at the amputation site for continued growth to occur. In the 1930s Polezhaev (as reviewed by Polezhaev, 1972) in a series of experiments, demonstrated the importance of dedifferentiation as a source of cells during urodele and anuran regeneration. Using physical trauma (see Polezhaev, 1972) or chemical baths (Rose, 1945), growth could be induced in postmetamorphic frogs. Presumably the treatments were responsible for liberating cells from the local tissues which contributed to the outgrowths. The same principle seems to hold for mammals as well. Trauma treatments of proximal level amputation sites generate partial blastema-like conditions in which numerous mitotically active multiply oriented cells are capable of producing cartilage distal to the amputation plane (Neufeld, 1980a; Neufeld, 1983). A different process appears to occur distally, how-

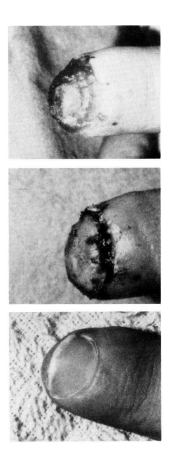

Fig. 11 Regeneration of an amputated digit-tip following suturing of a volar skin flap. Regrowth is usually impeded by a distal skin flap. Note that in this procedure the nail matrix was intact, leading to speculation that digit-tip regeneration was related to nail bed reformation by an "active" epithelium at the distal tip. The digit is illustrated at debriding, following surgery, and 6 months after treatment. (From Ogo, 1987. With permission.)

ever, in that at least to date, no dedifferentiation has been observed in local tissues prior to digit-tip regeneration. Because that system is not well documented, dedifferentiation may have been overlooked, or more likely, appositional bone formation distally may not require the presence of a growth bud. Histologically that process more resembles *de novo* bone formation in the embryo. Nonetheless, regrowth of the distal tip seems to involve reexpression of morphogenetic information in that both bone and soft tissues reestablish more or less original contours when the process is completed. Although dedifferentiation does not appear to be a significant prerequisite to this process, during distal tip regrowth, as in the aborted regrowth proximally and true regeneration in amphibians, mesenchyme-like cells are interposed between regrowing skeletal tissues and overlying modified epithelium. Perhaps such cells, regardless of their source, are involved in the reexpression of morphogenetic information.

Can true mammalian regeneration from proximal levels be induced? Whether a growth bud can be generated at a mammalian amputation site and true regeneration ensues as a recapitulation of ontogenetic development remains conjecture. As has been suggested by others, size of the mammalian amputation sites may be an insurmountable limitation. In the embryo at the time that positional information is established within the limb bud, that bud is only a tiny fraction of the size of a mammalian amputation surface. Given the limitation of distances that information specifying skeletal pattern formation travels in the embryo, one could anticipate that the initial amputation growth bud would be grossly almost invisible. The ensuing growth required to fill out the appendage would be enormous, although not inconceivable given the volumes of tissue formed during liver regeneration. Although work continues in this area, it does not seem likely that true regeneration of entire appendages in mammals from a growth bud is likely to occur in the immediate future.

Are there alternatives which present a more favorable prognosis for digital amputations? Accessible technology can be applied to enhance elongation or growth of digits or appendages at amputation sites. As an experimental strategy this would almost certainly involve working with open rather than closed amputation sites. Local application of lytic agents such as trypsin or collagenase might liberate cells for the reconstruction process in mammals, as has been suggested above. Local application of growth-promoting agents for both hard and soft tissues is immediately feasible. For soft tissues platelet-derived growth factor (PDGF), nerve growth factor (NGF), epidermal growth factor (EGF), and particularly fibroblast growth factor (FGF) are all commercially available (see Volume 1, Chapter 4). For stimulation of skeletal tissue growth bone morphogenetic protein (BMP), implantation of demineralized bone matrix, and prechondrogenic tissues such as periosteum could be used to enhance distal bone growth. An interesting study suggested simple distraction as a mechanism for elongation of amputated digits (Yankov, 1986). Another study demonstrated that nail matrix is transplantable (Kligman, 1961). Toe to hand transfer has been feasible for some time (Gobbel, 1913), but a recent variation which includes digital distraction plus vascularized transplantation has created a long, stable digit with a wide range of motion (Singer et al., 1989). When the strategy of amputation treatment changes from one of immediate wound closure to one of growth enhancement, combinations of above approaches could use both surgical and chemical intervention to produce a different prognosis following proximal level digit amputation. Certainly much basic research is necessary before any treatment regime becomes routine clinical protocol, but a concerted research effort might produce impressive results in the forseeable future using available technology. The use of body tissues, growth enhancement, and surgical innovation to bioengineer a cosmetically and functionally acceptable replacement is feasible.

Acknowledgments

I thank Mike Atherley, Angel Patten, and Russ Husby for technical assistance, Dr. Harry Settles and Mike Atherley for helpful discussion, and Dr. S. M. Rose for fostering my interest in this subject.

References

Allen, M. (1980). Conservative management of finger tip injuries in adults. *Hand*, **12**: 57–265.

Anderson, M. G. (1987). Fingertip amputations and injuries. *Ethiop. Med. J.*,**25**: 147–152.

Atasoy, E., Ioakimidis, E., Kasdan, M. L., Kutz, J. E., and Kleinert, H. E. (1979). Reconstruction of the amputated finger tip with a triangular volar flap. *J. Bone Jt. Surg.*, **52A**: 21–926.

Atherley, M. and Neufeld, D. (1989). Tissue regeneration in neonatal rodents following distal phalangeal digit amputations. *Anat. Rec.*, **233**: 9A.

Aulthouse, A. and Neufeld, D. (1985a). Variations in basement membrane structures at the epithelial-mesenchymal interface during blastemal morphogenesis in regenerating newt limbs. *Anat. Rec.*, **211**: 3A.

Aulthouse, A. and Neufeld, D. (1985b). Chondrogenesis and skeletal morphogenesis occur despite intervening adipocytes in regenerating newt limbs. *J. Exp. Zool.*, **233**: 117–120.

Beasley, R. W. (1969). Reconstruction of amputated fingertips. *Plast. Reconstr. Surg.*, **44**: 349–352.

Bojsen-Moller, J., Pers, M., and Schmidt, A. (1961). Finger-tip injuries: late results. *Acta Chir. Scand.*, **122**: 177–183.

Borgens, R. B. (1982a). Mice regrow the tips of their foretoes. *Science*, **217**: 747–750.

Borgens, R. B. (1982b). What is the role of naturally produced electrical current in vertebrate regeneration and healing?, *Int. Rev. Cytol.*, **76**: 245–298.

Bossley, C. (1975). Conservative treatment of digit amputations. *N. Z. Med. J.*, **82**: 379–380.

Bunch, W. H., Deck, J. D., and Romer, J. (1977). The effect of denervation on bony overgrowth after below knee amputation in rats. *Clin. Orthop. Rel. Res.*, **122**: 333–339.

Chow, S. P. and Ho, E. (1977). Open treatment of fingertip injuries in adults. *J. Hand Surg.*, **7**: 470–476.

Christie, J., Lamb, D. W., McDonald, J. M., and Britten, S. (1979). A study of stump growth in children with below-knee amputations. *J. Bone Jt. Surg.*, **61B**: 464–465.

Das, S. K. and Brown, H. G. (1978). Management of lost finger tips in children. *Hand*, **10**: 16–27.

DeBoer, P. and Collinson, P. O. (1981). The use of silver sulphadiazine occlusive dressings for finger-tip injuries. *J. Bone Jt. Surg.*, **63B**: 545–547.

Douglas, B. (1972). Conservative management of guillotine amputation of the finger in children. *Aust. Paediatr. J.*, **8**: 86–89.

Duvries, H. and Shogren, C. (1962). Spontaneous restoration of the head of a proximal phalanx following amputation — a case report. *J. Am. Podiatr. Assoc.*, **52**: 126–127.

Evans, D. M. and Martin, D. L. (1988). Step-advancement island flap for fingertip reconstruction. *Br. J. Surg.*, **41**: 105–111.

Farrell, R. G., Disher, W. A., Nesland, R. S., Palmatier, T. H., and Truhler, T. D. (1977). Conservative management of fingertip amputations. *JACEP*, **6**: 243–246.

Fisher, R. H. (1967). The Kutler method of repair of finger-tip amputations. *J. Bone Jt. Surg.*, **49A**: 317–320.

Franklin, L. (1968). Regeneration of resected phalangeal heads. *J. Am. Podiatr. Assoc.*, **58**: 511–513.

Fox, J. W., Golden, G. T., Rodeheaver, G., Edgerton, M. T., and Edlich, R. F. (1977). Nonoperative management of fingertip pulp amputation by occlusive dressings. *Am. J. Surg.*, **133**: 255–256.

Gobbel, T. (1913). Erstaz von Fingergelenken Durch Zehengelenke. *Munchen Med. Wochenschr.*, **60**: 1598–1599.

Goldner, R. D., Stevanovic, M., Nunley, J., and Urbaniak, J. (1989). Digital replantation at the level of the distal interphalangeal joint and the distal phalanx. *J. Hand Surg.*, **14A**: 214–220.

Goss, R. (1969). *Principles of Regeneration.* Academic Press, New York.

Holm, A. and Zachariae, L. (1974). Fingertip lesions: an evaluation of conservative treatment versus free skin grafting. *Acta Orthop. Scand.*, **45**: 382–392.

Illingworth, C. M. (1974). Trapped fingers and amputated finger tips in children. *J. Pediatr. Surg.*, **9**: 853–858.

Keyser, J., Littler, W., and Eaton, R. (1990). Surgical treatment of infections and lesions of the perionychium. *Hand Clin.*, **6**: 137–157.

Khonovets, I. A. (1983). Cases of regeneration of the fingers. *Feldsher Akush.*, **48**: 54–55.

King, P. A. (1979). Trapped finger injury. *Med. J. Aust.*, **2**: 580–582.

Kligman, A. M. (1961). Why do nails grow out instead of up?. *Arch. Dermatol.*, **84**: 181–183.

Koderberg, T., Nystrom, A., Hallmans, G., and Hulten, J. (1983). Treatment of fingertip amputations with bone exposure. A comparative study between surgical and conservative treatment methods. *Scand. J. Plast. Reconstr. Surg.*, **17**: 147–152.

Libbin, R. (1988). Hyaluronate at rat hindlimb amputation sites: preliminary histochemical observations. *Anat. Rec.*, **220**: 58A.

Libbin, R. and Weinstein, M. (1986). Regeneration of growth plates in the long bones of the neonatal rat hindlimb. *Am. J. Anat.*, **177**: 369–383.

Libbin, R. and Weinstein, M. (1987). Sequence of development of innately regenerated growth-plate cartilage in the hindlimb of the neonatal rat. *Am. J. Anat.*, **180**: 1–11.

Nagase, M., Ueda, K., Suzuki, I., and Nakajima, T. (1985). Spontaneous regeneration of the condyle following hemimandibulectomy by disarticulation. *J. Oral Maxillofac. Surg.*, **43**: 218–220.

Neufeld, D. (1980a). Partial blastema formation after amputation in adult mice. *J. Exp. Zool.*, **212**: 31–36.

Neufeld, D. (1980b). Nerve augmentation fails to induce a regenerative outgrowth in adult mice after amputation. *Anat. Rec.*, **196**: 136–137A.

Neufeld, D. (1983). Postamputational healing of mouse digits modified by trauma. In: *Limb Development and Regeneration*, Part A, Fallon, J. and Caplan, A., Eds., Alan R. Liss, New York, 407–412.

Neufeld, D. (1985). Bone healing after amputation of mouse digits and newt limbs: implications for induced regeneration in mammals. *Anat. Rec.*, **211**: 156–165.

Neufeld, D. (1989). Epidermis, basement membrane, and connective-tissue healing after amputation of mouse digits: implications for mammalian appendage regeneration. *Anat. Rec.*, **233**: 425–432.

Neufeld, D. and Aulthouse, A. (1986). Association of mesenchyme with attenuated basement membranes during morphogenetic stages of newt lamb regeneration. *Am. J. Anat.*, **176**: 411–422.

Neufeld, D. and Aulthouse, A. (1987). Basal lamina reestablishment following amputation of newt limbs and mouse toes. *Anat. Rec.*, **218**: 97–98A.

Neumann, L. (1988). Post-traumatic bony regeneration in a toe. *J. Trauma*, **28**: 717–718.

Ogo, K. (1987). Does the nail bed really regenerate?. *Plast. Reconstr. Surg.*, **80**: 445–447.

Polezhaev, L. (1972). *Loss and Restoration of Regenerative Capacity in Tissues and Organs of Animals.* Harvard University Press, Cambridge, MA.

Polezhaev, L. V. (1980). Regeneration of the fingers in children. *Khirurgiia*, **12**: 76–77.

Revardel, J.-L. and Chebouki, F. (1987). Etude de la reponse a l'amputation des phalanges chez la souris: role morphogenetique des epitheliums, stimulation de la chondrogenase. *Can. J. Zool.*, **65**: 3166–3176.

Robbins, T. H. (1988). The "jam roll" flap for fingertip reconstruction. *Plast. Reconstr. Surg.*, **81**: 109–111.

Rogal, I. (1951). Contribution to the study of regeneration capacity of extremities in rats (in Russian). *Dokl. Akad. Nauk. SSSR*, **78**: 161–164.

Rose, E. H., Norris, M., Kowalski, T., Lucas, A., and Fleegler, E. (1989). The "cap" technique: nonmicrosurgical reattachment of fingertip amputations. *J. Hand Surg.*, **14A**: 513–518.

Rose, S. (1948). Epidermal dedifferentiation during blastema formation in regenerating limbs of *Triturus viridescens*. *J. Exp. Zool.*, **108**: 337–361.

Rose, S. (1970). In: *Regeneration*. Appleton Century-Crofts, New York, 264.

Rose, S. M. (1945). The effect of NaCl in stimulating regeneration of limbs of frogs. *J. Morphol.*, **77**: 119–139.

Rosenthal, E. A. (1983). Treatment of fingertip and nail bed injuries. *Orthop. Clin. North Am.*, **14**: 675–697.

Rosenthal, L. J., Reiner, M. A., and Bleicher, M. A. (1979). Nonoperative management of distal fingertip amputations in children. *Pediatrics*, **64**: 1–3.

Sandzen, S. C. (1974). Management of the acute fingertip injury in the child. *Hand*, **6**: 190–197.

Sharf, A. (1961). Experiments on regenerating rat digits. *Growth*, **25**: 7–23.

Sharf, A. (1963). Reorganization of cornified nail-like out-growths related with the wound healing process of the amputation sites of young rat digits. *Growth*, **27**: 255–269.

Schmidt, A. (1968). *Cellular Biology of Vertebrate Regeneration and Repair*. University of Chicago Press, Chicago.

Schotte, O. E. and Smith, C. B. (1959). Wound healing processes in amputated mouse digits. *Biol. Bull.*, **117**: 546–561.

Schotte, O. E. and Smith, C. B. (1961). Effects of ACTH and of cortisone upon amputational wound healing processes in mice digits. *J. Exp. Zool.*, **146**—: 209–229.

Scott, J. E. (1974). Amputation of the finger. *Br. J. Surg.*, **61**: 574–576.

Shepard, G. H. (1983). Treatment of nail bed avulsions with split-thickness nail bed grafts. *J. Hand Surg.*, **8**: 49–54.

Shepard, G. H. (1990). Nail grafts for reconstruction. *Hand Clin.*, **6**: 79–102.

Singer, D. I., McC O'Brien, B., Angel, M., and Gumley, G. (1989). Digital distraction lengthening followed by free vascularized epiphyseal joint transfer. *J. Hand Surg.*, **14A**: 508–512.

Singer, M. (1951). Induction of regeneration of forelimb of the postmetamorphic frog by augmentation of the nerve supply. *Proc. Soc. Exp. Biol. Med.*, **76**: 413–416.

Singer, M., Weckesser, E. C., Geraudie, J., Maier, C. E., and Singer, J. (1987). Open finger tip healing and replacement after distal amputation in rhesus monkey with comparison to limb regeneration in lower vertebrates. *Anat. Embryol.*, **177**: 29–36.

Sisken, B. F. and Fowler, I. (1984). Response of amputated rat limbs to fetal nerve tissue implants and direct current. *J. Orthop. Res.*, **2**: 177–189.

Slomsky, M. (1966). Spontaneous bony regeneration in the hemiphalangectomy. *J. Am. Podiatr. Assoc.*, **10**: 445–449.

Smith, S. D. (1981). The role of electrode position in the electrical induction of limb regeneration in subadult rats. *Bioelectrochem. Bioenerg.*, **8**: 661–670.

Speer, D. P. (1981). The pathogenesis of amputation stump overgrowth. *Clin. Orthop.*, **159**: 294–307.

Soderberg, T., Nystrom, A., Hallmans, G., and Hulten, J. (1983). Treatment of fingertip amputations with bone exposure. *Scand. J. Plast. Reconstr. Surg.*, **17**: 147–152.

Sturman, M. J. and Duran, R. J. (1963). Late results of finger-tip injuries. *J. Bone Jt. Surg.*, **45A**: 289–298.

Suzuki, H. and Matthews, A. (1966). Two-color fluorescent labeling of mineralizing tissues with tetracycline and 2,4-bis[n,n'-di-(carbomethyl) aminomethyl] fluorescein. *Stain Technol.*, **41**: 57–60.

Thornton, C. and Bromley, S. (1973). *Vertebrate Regeneration*. Dowden, Hutchingson, and Ross, Stroudsburg, PA.

Van Beek, A., Kassan, M., Adson, H., and Dale, V. (1990). Management of acute fingernail injuries. *Hand Clin.*, **6**: 23–25.

Varma, B. P. and Srivastava, M. S. (1979). Successful regeneration of large extruded diaphyseal segments of the human radius. *J. Bone Jt. Surg.*, **61A**: 290–292.

Virgin, C., Fahey, J., Raisbeck, C., and Maylahn, D. (1971). Finger-tip amputations — a short cut to success. *J. Bone Jt. Surg. Proc.*, **53**: 1244.

Wallace, H. (1981). *Vertebrate Limb Regeneration*. John Wiley & Sons, New York.

Webster, G. V. (1950). Treatment of fingertip amputation. *Postgrad. Med.*, **8**: 416–419.

Yankov, E. (1986). Elongation of fingers after post-tramatic amputations in children and adolescents. *Acta Chir. Plast.*, **28**: 220–231.

Zacher, J. B. (1984). Management of injuries of the distal phalanx. *Surg. Clin. North Am.*, **64**: 747–760.

10

Bone Formation in Soft Tissues

KRZYSZTOF H. WLODARSKI
Department of Histology and Embryology
Institute of Biostructure
Medical Academy
Warsaw, Poland

Introduction

The phenomenon of bone formation in postnatal life outside the skeletal system, i.e., in soft tissues, called "induction of heterotopic (or ectopic) osteogenesis", has been known since the last century. It remains not fully understood.

Embryonic Models of Tissue Induction

The term "tissue induction" means cell differentiation by contact with other cells or their products. A number of embryonic systems of induction, including cartilage and bone differentiation, have been described (Holtzer, 1968; Lash *et al.*, 1957; 1960). In chicken embryos membrane bone formation depends upon tissue interaction between mesenchyme and epithelium (Tyler, 1989) or its basement membrane component (Hall and Van Exan, 1982; Hall *et al.*, 1983). Chondrogenesis, however, is not dependent upon the same epithelium (Tyler, 1983) and can be inhibited by it (Coffin-Collins and Hall, 1989).

The inducing system is composed of at least two components: inducing tissue (or its products) and undifferentiated, responding tissue, which under the influence of the former are stimulated to differentiate.

Holfreter's (1948) observation that induction can be mediated not only by living cells, but also by devitalized cells or even by their extracts, has opened up new perspectives of understanding the mechanisms of tissue induction. It became evident that inductor information must be translated into chemical language, which can be read by the undifferentiated, "instructed" cells. Thus the attempts to define chemically the nature of "inductors" began, and in recent years we have learned a lot about the chemistry of some bone-inducing agents.

It is generally accepted that inductors repress or derepress genes of the responding cells initiating the chain of events known as differentiation processes. Although the nature of such actions remains mysterious as yet, there are some speculations on the mechanisms of cell recognition. Roth (1973), for example, postulated that the early events of embryonal development comprise an interaction of enzymes glycosyltransferases, present on the cell surface, with the substrate — glycosyl, also present on the surface of other cells or in the extracellular matrix. The close physical contact between two cells provides the binding of a substrate by the enzyme and the formation of the complex consists, according to this hypothesis, of cell recognition. On the other hand, transferases can react with sugars of the extracellular matrix, thus modifying them and creating a different milieu for other cell generations. The extracellular components containing a substrate for enzymes anchored to the cell surface can thus work as morphogenetic substances. Reddi (1976) considered collagen, a highly heterogeneous protein produced by connective and epithelial tissues and detected in embryos long before the specialized connective tissue cells can be identified, as the extracellular component with inductive potency. He bases such an assumption on the fact that collagen occurs mainly in solid form and the high heterogeneity of molecular structure warrants the required specificity. Also, a number of physical features of collagen, especially its piezoelectric properties can play a key role in modulation of the cell surface and triggering of differentiation processes.

Similarly, *in vitro* studies indicate that the proteinous component of the epithelial basement membrane is an inductive stimulus for bone differentiation within the mandibular ectomesenchyme (Hall and Exan, 1982). Although it is difficult to extrapolate from results obtained in tissue culture to the *in vivo* situation, there is considerable evidence indicating that the epithelium adjacent to the developing mesenchymal cells influences the type of their differentiation. Solursh (1989) suggested that actin cytoskeleton-extracellular matrix interactions play a fundamental role in connective tissue differentiation. Extracellular matrix receptors might be developmentally regulated and modify the epithelial effects upon mesenchymal cells.

For a long time the concept of tissue induction was rather simple: the inducing cells release a specific substance ("inductor") which teaches the undifferentiated, "naive" cells how to differentiate. Now it is assumed that the induction phenomenon is not limited merely to the instructive function of the inducing agent, but more frequently is permissive for new traits expression hitherto masked. In other words, the present concept of tissue induction points to the competent cells as a target for inductive stimuli (Holtzer, 1968). Thus, in the model of embryonal cartilage induction in the mesoderm of somites by the notochord and neural tube (Lash *et al.*, 1957; 1960; Minor, 1973) the mesodermal cells should not be considered as "naive", undifferentiated ones, but as determined, "secretly differentiated", competent cells in which the "inductor" reveals or permits new traits.

Epithelial Heterotopic Bone Induction in Postnatal Life

A link of the urinary tract epithelium (transitional epithelium) with bone induction was observed as early as 1859 (cited by Huggins, 1931), when Blessing reported the presence of bone ossicles in the rabbit kidney calix following renal artery ligation. This observation was soon confirmed in the beginning of this century by numerous authors in rabbits (Asami and Dock, 1920; Liek, 1908; Sacerdotti and Frattin, 1902) and dogs (Pearce and Notes, 1909).

Soon it was established that in dogs surgical intervention on the urinary tract mucosa initiates local bone formation (Neuhoff, 1917; Strauss, 1914). In the 1920s clinical reports appeared pointing to a link between surgical injury of human urinary bladder and the appearance of bone tissue in the adjacent musculature (Keith, 1927; Kretschmar, 1928: Lewis, 1923). The turning point in the investigations on induced ectopic osteogenesis is the year 1931, when C. B. Huggins published a now classic paper "The formation of bone under the influence of epithelium of the urinary tract". He demonstrated that autologous grafts of urinary tract mucosa into the muscles produced within a few days a cyst completely lined with epithelium, and in the proximity of this newly formed epithelium, in the recipient part of the cyst, bone and occasionally hyaline cartilage appeared 8 to 10 days later. These data were soon confirmed by others (Abbot and Goodwin, 1932; Copher, 1938; Marshall and Spellman, 1957; Ostrowski *et al.*, 1957; for reviews see Ostrowski and Wlodarski, 1971; Wlodarski, 1984). The phenomenon of bone induction by implantation of transitional epithelium is not species specific; however, its dynamics vary in different species: guinea pigs (Abbot *et al.*, 1938; Beresford and Hancox, 1967; Cankovic *et al.*, 1967;

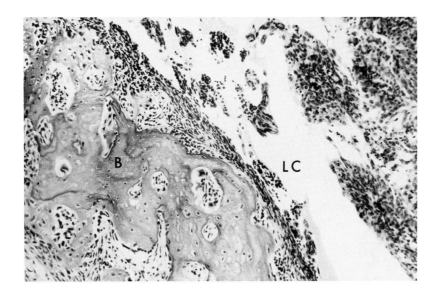

Fig. 1 Bone (B) induced by allogeneic implants of guinea-pig urinary bladder wall; 3 weeks after implantation. On the right, remnants of epithelial cells lining the lumen of a cyst (LC). (H and E; × 100.)

Dziedzic-Goclawska *et al.*, 1971; Fahrer *et al.*, 1970; Friedenstein, 1961, 1962, 1968; Loewi, 1954; Makin, 1962; Mestel and Spain, 1967; Moskalewski, 1963; Zaleski, 1961, 1963; Zaleski *et al.*, 1963) and cats (Abbot *et al.*, 1938; Johnson and McMinn, 1956; Marmor, 1963) are good responders, while in rats (Blumel and Piza, 1958; Huggins, 1931; Huggins *et al.*, 1936; Roberts *et al.*, 1974), gerbils (Wlodarski *et al.*, 1973), hamsters (Zaleski, 1961), and rabbits (Huggins, 1931; Wlodarski *et al.*, 1973) the incidence and yield of induced bone by allogeneic uroepithelium are low.

By all criteria applied it was established that, up to about the 30th day post grafting of allogeneic urinary bladder mucosa in guinea pigs or hamsters, the induced bone exhibited typical features of young woven bone (Fig. 1). This bone was remodeled into lamellar one in about 3 to 4 months; by this time the transitional epithelium was damaged due to the histoincompatibility reaction. Moreover, a typical bone marrow developed inside the induced bone trabeculae (Czerski and Zaleski, 1962). Allogeneic grafts, however, evidently had a weaker potency to induce bone as compared with autogenic ones, and in dogs, for example, such grafts did not induce bone formation.

In the mouse induction of bone by auto- and allogeneic implants of bladder mucosa is observed very rarely (in about 10% of cases) (Wlodarski *et al.*, 1971c; Zaleski and Moskalewski, 1963). The mouse, however, is a very good respondent to transitional epithelium grafts from other species, such as dog, guinea pig, or sheep (Wlodarski *et al.*, 1971c; Wlodarski, 1984;

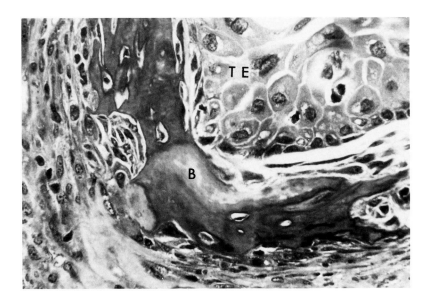

Fig. 2 Bone (B) induced around an island of xenogeneic urinary bladder epithelium of guinea pig (TE) grafted intramuscularly into cortisone-treated mice. (Toluidine-blue; × 200.)

1989; Solarczyk and Moskalewski, 1989). Thus the extremely weak bone induction by murine transitional epithelium can be explained by the very low inductive potency of this particular uroepithelium (Wlodarski *et al.*, 1971c).

The host immune response against allogeneic grafts of transitional epithelium may destroy the implant before it can reveal its osteoinductive potency. This is why xenogeneic grafts of transitional epithelium failed to induce bone (Lorenzi and Batacchi, 1951; Zaleski *et al.*, 1963). The imunosuppressive treatment of recipients enables bone induction by xenogeneic grafts of the urinary bladder wall (Wlodarski *et al.*, 1971c; Fig. 2).

Auto- and allogeneic implants of urinary bladder mucosa of all but murine species have induced bone primarily (Friedenstein, 1968; Zaleski, 1962), while cartilage formation in such a system is a rarity (Huggins, 1931). In the case of xenogeneic grafts of transitional epithelium, hyaline cartilage is induced, which is later substituted by or transdifferentiated into bone (Wlodarski *et al.*, 1971c). The difference is possibly due to the relatively large quantity of implanted xenogeneic epithelium into the mouse recipient muscles and its rapid proliferation resulting in oxygen consumption increase, followed by local hypoxia — a factor known to switch the differentiation of osteoprogenitor cells toward chondrogenesis (Thorogood and Hall, 1976).

Heterotopic Bone Induction by Epithelial Established Cell Lines

Another, simpler model of heterotopic osteogenesis in postnatal life by an epithelial established cell line grown *in vitro* was introduced by Anderson (1967, 1976) and Anderson et al. (1964). They noted hyaline cartilage and bone development in the vicinity of FL cells (human amnion established cell line) implanted intramuscularly into cortisone-treated mice. Electron microscopic and autoradiographic studies showed that grafted FL cells did not transform into either fibroblasts or chondroblasts (Anderson, 1976).

This novel model of cartilage/bone induction by human transformed cells has been studied intensively in our laboratory (Ostrowski *et al.*, 1975; Wlodarski, 1969; Wlodarski and Jakobisiak, 1978a; Wlodarski and Ostrowski, 1975, 1979; Wlodarski *et al.*, 1971a,b). Established and primary cell lines of various origin and sources have been tested for their osteoinductive properties: various species of host animals and various immunosuppressive procedures have been applied to learn the limitations of this novel system of skeletal tissue induction. The panel of cells examined, their characteristics, and the results obtained are given in Table 1.

It was demonstrated that, besides FL cells, other epithelial *in vitro* established cell lines such as K, KB, HeLa, Hep-2, WISH, as well as vaccinia- and varicella-virus transformed fibroblasts, which following transformation acquire an epithelial status, were also able to induce cartilage and bone (Figs. 3 and 4). It was found, moreover, that primary as well as established fibroblast cell lines of various origin did not exhibit osteoinductive properties.

The sequence of events in this model of induction is always the same: in cortisone-treated mice the xenogeneic epithelial cells survived up to 14 days and then were destroyed by mononuclear cell infiltration. Similar results are observed when cortisone is substituted by antilymphocytic serum (Wlodarski and Hancox, 1972). Six to eight days post cell inoculation a young hyaline cartilage appears in the young connective tissue surrounding the grafted cells. The cartilage proliferate and from the 10th day onward, the marginal zone of cartilage becomes acidophilic and cells resemble osteocytes; no sharp border line is seen between cartilage and newly formed bone. One has the impression that chondrocytes transdifferentiate into osteoblasts (Wlodarski and Ostrowski, 1975) as was recently postulated for another system (Moskalewski and Malejczyk, 1989). The central part of the cartilage becomes hypertrophic and is invaded by blood vessels, resorbed, and substituted by bone. The process of bone formation is very similar, if not identical, to the endochondral osteogenesis in long bones development. Gradually the cartilage decreased in amount, in favor of bone tissue, although sometimes cartilage can be detected as late as the 5th week. After 3 weeks bone tissue predominates; the bone trabeculae are covered with osteoblasts and osteoclasts appear and begin to resorb the induced bone. Among bone ossicles true bone marrow appears (Wlodarski and Jakobisiak, 1978b; Wlodarski *et al.*, 1980) (Table 2). The induced bone is completely resorbed within a few months.

Table 1.

Expression of Osteoinductive Competence in Various Cell Lines as Revealed by
Intramuscular Grafting into Cortisone-immunosuppressed Mice

Designation and Origin of Cell Line		Incidence of Bone Induction	References
Cells Expressing Strong Osteoinductive Properties			
CLV-X	Vaccinia virus transformed	14/16	Wlodarski, 1969
CLV-4	mouse embryo fibroblasts	8/8	
CLV-Var	Human fibroblasts transformed by varicella virus	20/22	Wlodarski and Ostrowski, 1975
FL	Human amnion	39/42	Wlodarski, 1969 Wlodarski and Jakóbisiak, 1978a,b Wlodarski *et al.*, 1970
HeLa	Cervix cancer	36/42	Ostrowski *et al.*, 1975 Wlodarski, 1969
D-98/AM2	Derivate of HeLa	18/20	Ostrowski *et al.*,1975
HEp-2	Larynx carcinoma	18/18	Wlodarski, 1969 Wlodarski and Jakóbisiak, 1978b
HT-40	Human tumor	13/13	Wlodarski and Ostrowski, 1979
K	Human amnion	16/29	Hancox and Wlodarski, 1972 Wlodarski and Hancox, 1972
KB	Human oral cancer	25/26	Wlodarski, 1969
WISH	Human amnion	97/119	Wlodarski, 1969, 1978 Wlodarski *et al.*, 1970, 1971a,b, 1976a,b Wlodarski and Jakóbisiak, 1978b
Cells Expressing Moderate Osteoinductive Activity			
CLV-J3	Human fibroblasts transformed by vaccinia virus	5/16	Wlodarski *et al.*, 1971b
GMK	Monkey kidney	1/21	Wlodarski and Ostrowski, 1975

320 Krzysztof H. Wlodarski

Table 1. (continued)
Expression of Osteoinductive Competence in Various Cell Lines as Revealed by
Intramuscular Grafting into Cortisone-immunosuppressed Mice

Designation and Origin of Cell Line		Incidence of Bone Induction	References
Cells With No Osteoinductive Competence			
Ameloblasts of rat		0/7	Wlodarski and Reddi, 1986a
Ehrlich ascites carcinoma		0/15	Wlodarski and Ostrowski, 1975
HF-1510	Human fibroblasts	0/8	Wlodarski and Reddi, 1986a
HT-29	Human epithelial tumor	0/6	Wlodarski and Reddi, 1986a
L-929	Mouse fibroblasts	0/46	Wlodarski, 1969
LNSV	SV-40-virus transformed human fibroblasts	0/22	Ostrowski *et al.*, 1975
MK 2	Monkey kidney	0/13	Wlodarski and Reddi, 1986a
MSVC	Moloney sarcoma cell line	0/90	Wlodarski, 1985 Wlodarski and Reddi, 1986a
Primary cultures of mouse fibroblasts		0/36	Wlodarski, 1969
Primary cultures of human fibroblasts		0/18	Wlodarski, 1969
SV3T3	SV-40-virus transformed 3T3 fibroblasts	0/13	Wlodarski *et al.*, 1974
3T3	Mouse embryo fibroblasts	0/14	Wlodarski and Ostrowski, 1979
T-24	Human bladder cancer	0/42	Wlodarski and Ostrowski, 1975
Vero	Monkey kidney	0/22	Wlodarski and Ostrowski, 1979
WAMIB	Mouse carcinoma	0/100	Wlodarski, 1985

The same pattern of induction by established epithelial cell lines is observed in species other than mice, viz., in rats and hamsters (Hancox and Wlodarski, 1972; Wlodarski *et al.*, 1971b).

Ectopic Bone Formation by Demineralized Bone and Dentin

The most common method for obtaining heterotopic bone induction, which has found application clinically, is implantation of demineralized bone matrix.

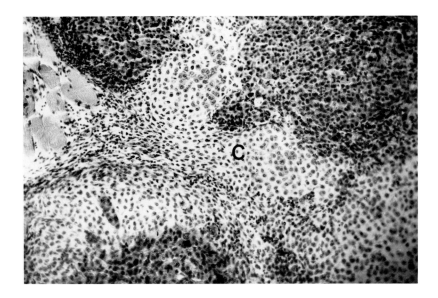

Fig. 3 Young hyaline cartilage (C) in the vicinity of human HeLa cells grafted intramuscularly into cortisone-treated mice; 8 days post HeLa cell inoculation. (H and E; × 100.)

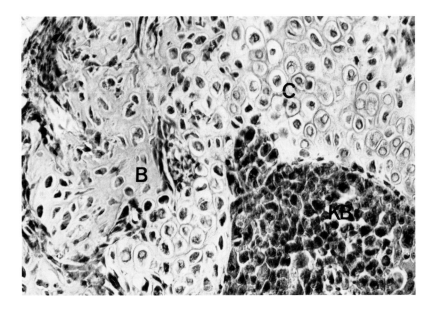

Fig. 4 Cartilage (C) and bone (B) formation in the vicinity of human KB cells (KB) grafted intramuscularly into cortisone-treated mice; 10 days post cell inoculation. (H and E; × 200.)

Table 2.

Myelograms of the Marrow from Bone Induced by FL Cell Grafting and of Host Femur Bor Marrow, Recovered 3 (n = 4) and 4 (n = 10) Weeks Post Cell and Cortisone Administration

Cell Type	Weeks After FL Cell Inoculation	Induced Bone Marrow		Host Femur Bone Marrow	
		Mean %	S.E.	Mean %	S.E
Erythropoietic	3	0.8	0.8	5.9	0.9
	4	3.7	0.6	13.7	2.9
Granulopoietic	3	47.1	14.6	71.0	4.6
	4	55.2	2.6	64.7	2.7
Lymphocytes	3	50.1	14.5	17.9	4.8
	4	36.3	2.8	17.0	2.4
Reticular	3	2.2	0.4	5.1	1.3
	4	4.2	0.7	4.2	0.4
Other	4	0.5	0.3	0.4	0.3

This model of skeletal tissue induction was introduced in 1965 by Urist and group (van de Putte and Urist, 1965; Urist, 1965). Bone demineralized by mild HCl hydrolysis, when implanted intramuscularly into allogeneic rabbits, rats, and mice, stimulated mesenchymal cells to proliferate and differentiate into chondroblasts and osteoblasts. The initially formed hyaline cartilage was gradually substituted by bone and about 3 weeks after implantation of bone matrix true bone marrow appeared among bone trabeculae (Reddi and Anderson, 1976; Bernick et al., 1989; Wlodarski, 1982).

Demineralized enamel and dentin are equally good inducers of chondro/osteogenesis (Bang, 1972, 1973; Nilsen, 1980; Urist, 1971). A comprehensive review on cartilage/bone induction by demineralized bone matrix implantation has recently been published (Harakas, 1984).

Other Means of Heterotopic Osteogenesis

Beside the three main modes for ectopic bone formation, their is a vast literature on spontaneous heterotopic osteogenesis and on osteogenesis mediated by other, more or less, unspecific factors.

Osteoinductive properties of gallbladder epithelium were reported (Huggins and Sammet, 1933; Moskalewski, 1963; Shipton, 1957); however, the bone-inducing potency is much weaker than that of transitional epithelium.

The attempts to induce bone by transplantation of digestive and reproductive tracts mucosa in general gave negative results (for review see Ostrowski and Wlodarski, 1971). However, there are separate reports on osteoinduction by gastric (Myirani, 1956) and seminal vesicle mucosa (Huggins, 1969).

In humans, chronic inflammation (Joines and Roggli, 1989) and some neoplasms might produce in their stroma bone ossicles (Battendorf *et al.*, 1976; Flanagan *et al.*, 1965; Kinney and Kovarik, 1965).

Devitalized tissues other than bone, as whole embryos or osteosarcoma, also induced heterotopic osteogenesis (Amitami and Nakata, 1975; Bridges and Pritchard, 1958).

In humans and birds foci of cartilage and bone are occasionally seen in the lungs. They do not originate from pathologic processes but probably are abnormal embryonic induction of mesenchyme or cartilaginous stem cells displaced from the adjacent bronchi (Asley, 1970; Wight and Duff, 1985). Heterotopic bone formation in postoperative abdominal scars is also explained by the accidental implantation of cells from the injured xiphoid process (Lohela *et al.*, 1983).

A bone-inducing capacity of saline cell-free extract of allogeneic thyroid was reported in guinea pig (Zarrin, 1977). Reports on bone induction by alcoholic extracts of bone should be taken with caution as in rabbits alcohol itself can stimulate bone formation unspecifically (Heinen *et al.*, 1949).

Heterotopic Bone Formation Following Total Hip Replacement or Neurologic Insult

In man, heterotopic bone formation (known as *myositis ossificans*) is a frequent disorder characterized by an initial inflammatory lesion of muscles and deposition of bone ossicles among them (Brokker *et al.*, 1973; Orzel and Rudd, 1985; Hierton *et al.*, 1983; Bundrick *et al.*, 1985), and complicates total hip arthroplasty in up to 50% of cases. It can occur as a complication of paralysis from spinal cord or brain trauma (Garland, 1987). It sometimes mimics thrombophlebitis (Yarkony *et al.*, 1989). In man, myositis ossificans can also develop without history of significant trauma (Spencer and Missen, 1989).

The pathogenesis of ectopic bone formation in these conditions is unclear. The basic mechanism is perhaps the transformation of the inducible osteo-progenitor cells (IOPC) resident in the musculature in response to the BMP-like protein released from the injured and immobilized muscles (Urist *et al.*, 1978).

Genetic predisposition to heterotopic osteogenesis is suspected, but not proved (Garland, 1987; Ritter and Vaughan, 1977). Postoperative radiation therapy is effective in preventing heterotopic osteogenesis (Ayres *et al.*, 1986; Sylvester *et al.*, 1988; Lo *et al.*, 1988). It has been suggested that radiation interferes with differentiation of IOPC into osteoblasts. It was shown on an animal model that heterotopic bone induction was reduced or abolished when the animals were irradiated prior to implantation of decalcified bone matrix or of transitional epithelium grafts (Wlodarski and Jakóbisiak, 1981).

Nonsteroidal anti-inflammatory therapy with indomethacin or ibuprofen is also effective in preventing heterotopic ossification in total hip arthroplasty patients (Elmsted *et al.*, 1985; Ritter and Gioe, 1982), but diphos-phonate therapy is not effective (Thomas and Amstutz, 1985).

Heterotopic Bone Formation by Bone Marrow Transplants

Since Bruns reported, in 1881, the presence of bone ossicles at the sites of heterotopic autografts of bone marrow, the osteogenic competence of bone marrow has been repeatedly demonstrated (Ashton *et al.*, 1984; Burwell, 1966; Conoly *et al.*, 1989; Friedenstein *et al.*, 1966; Harada *et al.*, 1988; Johnson *et al.*, 1988; Ohgushi *et al.*, 1989; Pfeifer, 1948; Tavassoli, 1971; Urist and McLean, 1952). Osteoprogenitor cells of bone marrow belong to the stromal, not to the hemopoietic, compartment of the marrow. Stromal cells form a scaffolding for the hemopoietic cells and provide a microenvi-ronment for their development and differentiation (Quesenberry *et al.*, 1985). The stromal compartment of bone marrow extends into the endosteal sur-face (endosteum) and Haversian canals of bone and into the cambial layer of the periosteum (Ashton *et al.*, 1984; Owen, 1980).

In tissue culture bone marrow stromal cells adhere to the glass. The cells of the adherent layer of marrow stroma are fibroblasts, eipthelioid cells, fat cells, reticular cells, and macrophages. Precursor stromal cells which *in vitro* form fibroblastic colonies are designated CFU-F (fibroblastic colony forming units).

Colonies of bone marrow stroma on transplantation under the kidney capsule or implantation into diffusion chambers produce fibrous tissue, cartilage, and bone (Ashton *et al.*, 1980; Harada *et al.*, 1988; Mardon *et al.*, 1986; Miskarova *et al.*, 1970; Tabuci *et al.*, 1986). Friedenstein has named such cells determined osteoprogenitor cells (DOPC). DOPC form osteogenic tissue spontaneously, without participation of an inducing agent. Another subpopulation of bone marrow stroma and stromal cells of other than bone marrow lymphopoietic organs (thymus, spleen, peritoneal cavity) are ca-pable of producing cartilage and bone when exposed to bone inducing factors (Harada *et al.*, 1988; Friedenstein, 1976; Owen, 1980; Takagi and Urist, 1982). Such cells were designated as inducible osteoprogenitor cells (IOPC, Friedenstein, 1976). These cells are a target for BMP (Bentz *et al.*, 1989; Harada *et al.*, 1988; Takagi and Urist, 1982).

Thus, in the bone marrow stroma, two classes of cells with osteogenic competence are present: DOPC and IOPC. This rich source of osteocom-petent cells in the marrow stroma was used to stimulate osteogenesis in conjunction with bone-inducing agents such as decalcified bone matrix or autologous bone (so-called "composite grafts") (Lindholm and Urist, 1980; Nade and Burwell, 1977; Takagi and Urist, 1982).

What is the Nature of the "Bone Inductor"?

The reason why some epithelial cells on contact with mesenchymal cells induce bone formation is as yet an open question.

Ectopic transitional epithelium which lines the cyst formed following urinary bladder mucosa transplantation differs from the original one. Its morphology and histochemical characteristic indicate a high secretory and proliferative activity (Abdin and Friedenstein, 1972; Friedenstein, 1962, 1968; Fahrer et al., 1970; Ioseliani, 1972; Makin, 1962; Williams et al., 1970). According to Friedenstein (1968) proliferating transitional epithelium releases into connective tissue polysaccharides which are stimulators of osteogenesis. The secretion by transitional epithelium of substances with osteoinductive properties was confirmed by experiments with diffusion chambers filled with transitional epithelium. Bone was formed outside the chamber (Friedenstein, 1962). Others, however, were unable to confirm these data (Ostrowski and Moskalewski, 1962).

As it is necessary that the epithelial cells be living for bone induction to occur, it has been suggested that bone induction by epithelial cells might be triggered by contact of inducing cells with host mesenchymal ones. The importance of specific cell surface receptors characteristic for all osteoinductive cells has been discussed, but so far no specific ligand receptors on the cell membrane of the osteoinductive cells have been detected (Wlodarski et al., 1974; Wlodarski and Ostrowski, 1979). All osteoinductive cells, however, possess receptors for Concanavalin A.

Recently a biochemical marker for osteoinductive cells, which is the high activity of alkaline phosphatase has been found (Wlodarski and Reddi, 1986a). When a wide spectrum of bone-inducing and non-inducing cells was examined for alkaline and acid phosphatase activity, it was noted that in cells devoid of osteoinductive competence (of both epithelial and fibroblastic origin) the alkaline isoenzyme activity was extremely low, in contrast to the osteoinductive cells which were characterized by high alkaline phosphatase activity. The activity of acid isoenzyme was similar in both categories of cells. The different pattern of phosphatase isoenzymes in the bone-inducing and in non-inducing cells could be attributed to the different surface properties (alkaline phosphatase is a cell membrane bound enzyme), and consequently, to different biological activity as expressed by inductive vs. noninductive properties.

It is also postulated that glycoprotein Ca (Oxford) antigen expressed by human malignant cells and by uroepithelium is an inductor of ectopic bone (Beresford, 1984).

These data speak in favor of the concept, stressing the importance of surface contacts between grafted cells and host mesenchymal ones for the bone induction process.

In contrast to living epithelia, the nature of the bone inductor present in bone (and dentin) has been established independently by several groups.

Urist and group (1984) isolated bone morphogenetic protein (BMP) from bovine bones. It is an 18.5 kDa acidic polypeptide with no carbohydrate detected, binding to hydroxyapatite, sensitive to trypsin but resistant to many other hydrolases. Administration of this protein evoked bone formation. Bentz et al. (1989) isolated from a similar source and characterized an osteoinductive factor, which is a 22 to 28 kDa glycoprotein. Its enzymatic or chemical deglycosylation abolished inductive activity. The osteoinductive activity of this molecule is greatly enhanced by transforming growth factor β, which most likely recruits or stimulates to proliferate precursor cells.

Sampath et al. (1987) isolated a bone-inducing protein of 22 kDa from rat bone osteogenin.

Isolated by Wang and colleagues (Wozney et al., 1988) bovine BMP is composed of three glycosylated 30, 18, and 16 kDa polypeptides whose amino acid sequences were established. The same group isolated human complementary DNA clones corresponding to these polypeptides and obtain expression of the recombinant human proteins. Each of the three appears to be independently capable of inducing bone formation in vivo. Two of the encoded proteins are members of the transforming growth factor β family (Wozney et al., 1989).

The relationship of the bone-inducing factor of epithelial and neoplastic cells (Ca antigens?) to the BMP remains to be elucidated; however, the similarity of their effects might indicate that they are similar or closely related proteins.

Biology of Heterotopically Induced Bone

The common opinion is that bone induced heterotopically by transitional epithelium is stable and that its fate does not depend on the fate of the transplant (Czerski and Zaleski, 1962; Huggins, 1931; Zaleski, 1962), although some reported a link of induced bone resorption with the destruction of the grafted epithelium (Friedenstein, 1961).

Basically, the ectopic bone shows the same biological properties as orthotopic bone does (Bridges, 1958; Friedenstein, 1961; Huggins, 1931). The metabolism of bone induced heterotopically in dogs and guinea pigs by transplantation of urinary bladder mucosa has been intensively examined (Blumel and Piza, 1958; Ostrowski and Wilczyński, 1958; Ostrowski et al., 1967; Zaleski, 1962). Induced bone vigorously incorporates radioactive phosphate, sulfur, and collagen precursors (Ostrowski and Wilczyński, 1958; Zaleski, 1962). The mineralization of induced bones as measured by electron spin resonance technique is similar to that in the orthotopic bones (Dziedzic-Goclawska et al., 1971). Neither does enzyme histochemistry of bones induced by transitional epithelium differ from that of orthotopic ones (Kagawa, 1965; Nielsen and Magnusson, 1981).

The composition of bone marrow in ectopically induced bone and in the host's orthotopic bone marrow are alike (Wlodarski, 1982; Wlodarski *et al.*, 1980). The only claimed difference between ectopic and orthotopic bone was, according to Friedenstein, the lack of DOPC in the former (Friedenstein, 1976).

It has recently been proven on the basis of extensive biochemical and morphological studies with the application of a novel model of stimulation of the periosteal membrane by the Moloney sarcoma virus (Wlodarski *et al.*, 1979) that bone induced heterotopically by demineralized bone matrix does not develop a true, functioning periosteum (Wlodarski and Reddi, 1986b). In contrast, the periosteum of syngeneic costal transplants in response to Moloney sarcoma proliferates and produces new bone in the same manner as orthotopic bones at the sites of Moloney sarcoma do. The author's opinion is that the lack of true periosteum in the foci of heterotopic bone is the main, if not the only, biological difference between them and orthotopic bones.

The lack of a true periosteum (the connective tissue surrounding the foci of ectopic osteogenesis is merely a fibrous capsule) might explain why such bones do not proliferate or regenerate after cessation of inductive stimuli.

Some Factors Affecting Heterotopic Induction of Osteogenesis

The age of the host influences the yield of induced bone in such a way that in old and senescent animals ectopic osteogenesis declines (Irving *et al.*, 1981; Nishimoto *et al.*, 1985; Mimni *et al.*, 1988; Wlodarski and Reddi, 1986c). Genetic defects also influence ectopic ossification. In X-linked hypophosphatemic mice the mineralization of heterotopically induced bone is abnormal; phosphorus supplementation improves their mineralization, as in the human homolog (Tanaka *et al.*, 1988). Inhibition of collagen cross-linking caused by β-dimethylcysteine (penicillamine) administration is associated with a decrease in induced bone formation (Weiss *et al.*, 1984).

Corticosteroids, when administered at an early stage of bone induction, impaired osteogenesis and mineralization, indicating that the action of corticosteroids on differentiation may be mediated primarily through the suppression of progenitor cell proliferation (Rath and Reddi, 1979).

Calcitonin accelerates the rate of induced osteogenesis (Thompson and Urist, 1973; Weiss *et al.*, 1981), while the vitamin D_3 analog — dihydrotachysterol enhances heterotopic bone induction in ovariectomized (quasi postmenopausal) rats by stimulation of osteoprogenitor cell proliferation and osteoblasts maturation (Tabuci *et al.*, 1989). On the other hand, monokine TNF-α administered systematically impairs the ability of osteoprogenitor cells to respond to the bone-inducing substance at an early stage of ectopic bone formation (Yoshikawa *et al.*, 1988).

Wieniawska-Szewczyk (1988) compared the effect of prolonged administration of various immunosuppressive agents on matrix-induced osteogenesis and orthotopic osteogenesis in the epiphysis. Cortisone inhibited both induced and orthotopic osteogenesis: cyclophosphamide markedly inhibited ectopic, but not orthotopic bone formation: methotrexate inhibited more profoundly induced than orthotopic osteogenesis, while a single dose of 600 R was without effect on either. Similar observations on the methotrexate effect on ectopic and orthotopic bone were reported by Nilson et al. (1986).

Systemic administration of aluminium salt prevents precipitation of the mineral phase in the matrix-induced endochondral bone formation, while aluminum salt implanted locally with the matrix was toxic to the cellular processes leading to chondrogenesis and osteogenesis (Talvar *et al.*, 1986). Bisphosphonate C12MBP, but not HEBP, affect collagen fiber arrangement in the organic matrix of heterotopically induced bone (Ostrowski *et al.*, 1988).

The appearance of heterotopic bone induction in rats and mice is limited to permissive sites which are the striated muscle milieau (Chalmers *et al.*, 1975). Epithelial inducers — guinea pig transitional epithelium of WISH cell line — when grafted into the kidney parenchyma of immunosuppressed mice survived and proliferated satisfactorily, but never induced osteogenesis, in contrast to grafts into the muscles (Wlodarski, 1978). In implants of decalcified bone matrix or epithelial cells with osteoinductive capacity into peritoneal cavity or subcutaneous, bone formation was negligible, observed only sporadically. The induction was restricted to the cases when implants were by chance attached to the muscles (Hancox and Wlodarski, 1972; Wlodarski *et al.*, 1973; Wlodarski and Reddi, 1986d).

Cells Involved in Bone Formation

In bone regeneration and fracture healing the osteoblasts resident in the periosteum, endosteum, and in bone marrow stroma (DOPC) are activated and deposit new bone. Moreover, IOPC of the bone marrow stroma can be engaged into this process. Bone morphogenetic protein(s) released from the resorbed bone acting in concert with other local and systemic factors (Triffit, 1987) can trigger differentiation of IOPC into osteoblasts, as many authors suggest (Takagi and Urist, 1982; Harada *et al.*, 1988; Bentz *et al.*, 1989).

Heterotopic bone formation by extramedullar bone marrow transplantation is evoked by osteoblasts (DOPC) and an inductive stimulus is not required.

Ectopic bone induction involves IOPCs — a variety of cells responding to the bone inductor. Among them, undifferentiated mesenchymal cells are most commonly considered as the chondro/osteoinducible cells (for review see Wlodarski, 1990). Beresford (1981) noted, however, that mesenchymal cells *ex definitione* do not exist in postnatal life. So-called "mesenchymal cells" which appear in the area of bone induction are, in fact, young fibro-blasts, which can be modulated toward chondro/osteoblasts by specific stimuli, such as BMP, or products, or contact with some epithelial cells (Abdin and Friedenstein, 1972; Harada *et al.*, 1988). Even more differentiated mesenchyme-derived cells, such as endothelial cells (Burwell, 1964), stromal cells of bone marrow (Bentz *et al.*, 1989), and of other lymphopoietic organs (Friedenstein, 1976), perivascular cells (Trueta, 1963), and lymphocytes (Lalykina and Friedenstein, 1969) are reported to be osteogenic. Recently Wlodarski suggested the possibility that satellite cells of striated muscles might be another source of osteogenic cells. The argument for such a hypothesis is discussed in detail elsewhere (Wlodarski, 1990).

In conclusion, bone formed heterotopically in soft tissues can develop from sources different than orthotopic bone. Ectopic bone, on the whole, is sensitive to the same systemic and local factors which affect normal bones. The only substantial difference between ectopic and orthotopic bone is that the former does not develop periosteal membrane and thus is not capable of regeneration.

References

Abbot, A. C. and Goodwin, A. M. (1932). Observation of bone formation in abdominal wall following transplantation of the mucosa membrane of the urinary bladder. *Can. Med. Assoc. J.* **26**: 393–397.

Abbot, A. C. and Goodwin, A. M. (1938). Heterotopic bone formation produced by epithelial transplants from urogenital tract of dogs, rabbits, guinea-pigs and cats. *J. Urol.*, **40**: 294–311.

Abdin, M. and Friedenstein, A. Y. (1972). Electron microscopic study on bone induction by the transitional epithelium of the bladder in guinea-pig. *Clin. Orthop. Rel. Res.*, **82**: 182–194.

Amitami, K. and Nakata, Y. (1975). Studies on the factors responsible for new bone formation from osteosarcoma in mice. *Calcif. Tissue Res.*, **17**: 139–150.

Amitami, K., Nakata, Y., and Stevens, J. (1974). Bone induction by lyophilized osteosarcoma in mice. *Calcif. Tissue Res.*, **16**: 305–313.

Anderson, H. C. (1967). Electron microscopic studies of induced cartilage development and calcification. *J. Cell Biol.*, **35**: 81–101.

Anderson, H. C. (1976). Osteogenic epithelial-mesenchymal cell interactions. *Clin. Orthop.*, **119**: 211–224.

Anderson, C. H. and Coulter, P. R. (1967). Bone formation induced in mouse thigh by cultured human cells. *J. Cell Biol.*, **33**: 165–177.

Anderson, H. C., Merker, P. C., and Fogh, J. (1964). Formation of tumors containing bone after intramuscular injection of transformed human amnion cells (FL) into cortisone-treated mice. *Am. J. Anat.*, **44**: 507–519.

Asami, G. and Dock, W. (1920). Experimental studies on heteroplastic bone formation. *J. Exp. Med.*, **32**: 745–751.

Ashley, J. B. (1970). Bony metaplasia in trachea and bronchi. *J. Pathol.*, **102**: 186–188.

Ashton, B. A., Allen, T. D., Howlett, C. R., Eagleson, C. C., Hattori, A., and Owen, M. E. (1980). Formation of bone and cartilage by marrow stroma cells in diffusion chambers in vivo. *Clin. Orthop.*, **151**: 294–307.

Ashton, B. A., Eagleson, C. C., Bab, I., and Owen, M. E. (1984). Distribution of fibroblastic colony-forming cells in rabbit bone marrow and assay of their osteogenic potential by an in vivo diffusion chamber method. *Calcif. Tissue Int.*, **36**: 83–86.

Ayres, D. C., Evarts, C. M., and Parkinson, J. R. (1986). The prevention of heterotopic ossification in high-risk patients by low-dose radiation therapy after total hip arthroplasty. *J. Bone Jt. Surg.*, **68A**: 1423–1430.

Bang, G. (1973). Induction of heterotopic bone formation by demineralized dentin in guinea-pigs: relationship to time. *Acta Pathol. Microb. Scand. Sect. A Suppl.* **236**: 60–70.

Bang, G. (1972). Induction of heterotopic bone formation by demineralized dentin in guinea-pigs. Antigenicity of the dentin matrix. *J. Oral Pathol.*, **1**: 172–185.

Battendorf, U., Rommele, W., and Laaf, H. (1976). Bone formation by cancer metastases. *Virchows Arch. A*, **369**: 359–365.

Beresferd, W. A. and Hancox, N. M. (1967). Urinary bladder mucosa and bone regeneration in guinea pig and rats. *Acta Anat.*, **66**: 78–117.

Beresferd, W. A. (1984). Ca (Oxford) antigen: an inducer of ectopic bone?. *Surv. Synth. Pathol. Res.*, **3**: 437–441.

Beresferd, W. A. (1981). Undifferentiated mesenchymal cells. In: *Chondroid Bone. Secondary Cartilage and Metaplasia*. Urban and Schwarzenberg, Baltimore, 113–123.

Bernick, S., Paule, W., Erti, D., Nishimoto, S. K., and Nimni, M. E. (1989). Cellular events associated with the induction of bone by demineralized matrix. *J. Orthop. Res.*, **7**: 1–11.

Blumel, G. and Piza, F. (1958). Ein weiter Beitrag zur problem der heterotopen Kmochenbildung mitteis Radiophosphor. *Burn's Beitr. Klin. Chir.*, **197**: 152–157.

Bridges, J. B. (1958). Heterotopic ossification in the ischemic kidney of the rabbit, rat and guinea-pig. *J. Urol.*, **79**: 903–910.

Bridges, J. B. and Pritchard, J. J. (1958). Bone and cartilage induction in the rabbits. *J. Anat.*, 92: 28.

Brooker, A. F., Bowerman, J. W., Robinson, R. A., and Riley, L. H. (1973). Ectopic ossification following total hip replacement. Incidence and the method of classification. *J. Bone Jt. Surg.*, **55A**: 1629–1632.

Bruns, P. (1881). Uber transplantation von Knochemnark. *Arch. Klin. Chir.*, **26**: 661–668.

Bundrick, T. J., Cook, D. E., and Resnik, C. S. (1985). Heterotopic bone formation in patients with DISH following total hip replacement. *Radiology*, **155**: 595–597.

Burwell, R. G. (1966). Studies in the transplantation of bone. VIII. Treated composite homograft-autograft of cancellous bone. An analysis of inductive mechanisms in bone transplantation. *J. Bone Jt. Surg.*, **48B**: 532–566.

Chalmers, J., Gray, D. H., and Rush, J. (1975). Observations on the induction of bone in soft tissues. *J. Bone Jt. Surg.*, **57B**: 36–45.

Cancovic, J., Piletic, O., Popovic, S., Japundzic, M., and Knezewic, B. (1967). Contribution to the experimental histological study of induction of heterotopic bone in guinea pigs. *Acta Med. Iugosl.*, **21**: 77–88.

Coffin-Collins, P. A. and Hall, B. K. (1989). Chondrogenesis of mandibular mesenchyme from the embryonic chick is inhibited by mandibular epithelium and by epidermal growth factor. *Int. J. Der. Biol.*, **33**: 297–311.

Connolly, J., Guse, R., Lippiello, L., and Dehne, R. (1989). Development of an osteogenic bone-marrow preparation. *J. Bone Jt. Surg.*, **71A**: 684–691.

Copher, G. H. (1938). The effects of urinary bladder transplants and extracts on the formation of bone. *Ann. Surg.*, **108**: 934.

Czerski, P. and Zaleski, M. (1962). Bone marrow formation accompanying induced osteogenesis. *Hematol. Lat.*, **5**: 33–40.

Dziedzic-Goclawska, A., Wlodarski, K. H., Stachowicz, W., Michalik, J., and Ostrowski, K. (1971). Quantitative evaluation of the rate of mineralization of induced skeletal tissues by the electron spin resonance technique. *Experientia*, **27**: 1405–1406.

Elmsted, E., Lindholm, T. S., Nilsson, O. S., and Tornkvist, H. (1985). Effect of ibuprofen on heterotopic ossification after total hip replacement. *Acta Orthop. Scand.*, **56**: 25–27.

Fahrere, M., Rintoul, J. R., and Williams, L. M. (1970). A light, histochemical and ultrastructural study of experimentally induced osteogenesis by autologous bladder mucosal transplants in guinea pigs. *J. Anat.*, **106**: 409.

Flanagan, P., McCracken, A. W., and Cross, R. (1965). Squamous carcinoma of the lung with osteocartilaginous stroma. *J. Clin. Pathol.*, **18**: 403–407.

Friedenstein, A. J. (1961). Osteogenic activity of transplanted transitional epithelium. *Acta. Anat.*, **45**: 31–59.

Friedenstein, A. Y. (1962). Humoral nature of osteogenic activity of transitional epithelium. *Nature*, **194**: 698–699.

Friedenstein, A. Y. (1968). Induction of bone tissue by transitional epithelium. *Clin. Orthop.*, **59**: 21–37.

Friedenstein, A. Y. (1976). Precursor cells of mechanocytes. *Int. Rev. Cytol.*, **47**: 327–359.

Friedenstein, A., Platetzky-Shapiro, J. J., and Petrakova, K. V. (1966). Osteogenesis in transplants of bone marrow cells. *J. Embryol. Exp. Morphol.*, **16**: 381–390.

Garland, D. E. (1988). Clinical observations on fractures and heterotopic ossification in the spinal cord and traumatic brain injured populations. *Clin. Orthop.*, **233**: 86–101.

Hall, B. K. and Van Exan, R. J. (1981). Induction of bone by epithelial cell products. *J. Embryol. Morphol.*, **69**: 37–46.

Hall, B. K., Van Exan, R. J., and Brunt, S. L. (1983). Retention of epithelial basal lamina allows isolated mandibular mesenchyma to form bone. *J. Craniofac. Genet. De. Biol.*, **3**: 253–267.

Hancox, N. M. and Wlodarski, K. (1972). The role of host site in bone induction by transplanted xenogeneic epithelial cells. *Calcif. Tissue Res.*, **8**: 258–261.

Harada, K., Oida, S., and Sasaki, S. (1988). Chondrogenesis and osteogenesis of bone marrow-derived cells by bone-inductive factor. *Bone*, **9**: 177–183.

Harakas, N. K. (1984). Demineralized bone matrix-induced osteogenesis. *Clin. Orthop.*, **188**: 239–251.

Heinen, J. H., Dabbs, G. H., and Mason, H. A. (1948). The experimental production of ectopic cartilage and bone in the muscles of rabbits. *J. Bone Jt. Surg.*, **31A**: 765–775.

Hierton, C., Biomgren, G., and Lindgren, U. (1983). Factors associated with heterotopic bone formation in cemented total hip prosthesis. *Acta Orthop. Scand.*, **54**: 698–702.

Holftreter, J. (1948). Concepts of the mechanism of embryonic induction and its relation to pathogenesis and malignancy. *Symp. Soc. Exp. Biol.*, **2**: 17–48.

Holtzer, H. (1968). Induction of chondrogenesis: a concept in quest of mechanisms. In: *Epithelial-Mesenchymal Interactions*. Fleischmajer, R. and Billingsham, W. E., Eds., Williams & Wilkins, Baltimore, 152–164.

Holtzer, H. and Abbot, J. (1968). Oscillation of the chondrogenic phenotype in vitro. In: *Results and Problems of Cell Differentiation*, Vol. 1. Urspung, H., Ed., Springer, New York, 1–16.

Huggins, C. B. (1931). The formation of bone under the influence of epithelium of the urinary tract. *Arch. Surg.*, **22**: 377–408.

Huggins, C. B. (1969). Epithelial osteogenesis. A biological chain reaction. *Proc. Am. Phil. Soc.*, **113**: 458–463.

Huggins, C. B., McCarrol, H. R., and Blocksom, B. H. (1936). Experiments on the theory of osteogenesis. The influence of local calcium deposits on ossification, the osteogenic stimulus of epithelium. *Arch. Surg.*, **32**: 915–931.

Huggins, C. B. and Sammet, J. F. (1933). Function of the gall bladder epithelium as an osteogenic stimulus and the physiological differentiation of connective tissue. *J. Exp. Med.*, **58**: 393–400.

Ioseliani, D. G. (1972). The use of tritiated thymidine in the study of bone induction by transitional epithelium. *Clin. Orthop.*, **88**: 183–196.

Irving, J. T., LeBoi, S., and Schneider, E. L. (1981). Ectopic bone formation and aging. *Clin. Orthop.*, **154**: 249–253.

Johnson, K. P., Howlett, C. R., Bellenger, C. R., and Armati-Gulson, P. (1988). Osteogenesis by canine and rabbit bone marrow in diffusion chambers. *Calcif. Tissue Int.*, **42**: 113–118.

Johnson, F. R. and McMinn, M. R. (1956). Transitional epithelium and osteogenesis. *J. Anat.*, **90**: 106–116.

Joines, R. W. and Roggli, V. L. (1989). Dendriform pulmonary ossification. Report of two cases with unique findings. *Am. J. Clin. Pathol.*, **91**: 398–402.

Kagawa, S. (1965). Enzyme histochemistry of bone induction by urinary bladder epithelium. *J. Histochem. Cytochem.*, **13**: 255–264.

Keith, A. (1927). Concerning the origin and nature of osteoblasts. *Proc. R. Soc. Med. (Surg.)*, **21**: 301–307.

Kinney, F. J. and Kovarik, J. L. (1965). Bone formation in bronchial adenoma. *Am. J. Clin. Pathol.*, **44**: 52–58.

Kjaersgaard-Andersen, P., Pedersen, P., Kristensen, S. S., Schmidt, S. A., and Pedersen, N. W. (1988). Serum alkaline phosphatase as an inductor of heterotopic bone formation following total hip arthroplasty. *Clin. Orthop.*, **234**: 102–109.

Kretschmar, H. L. (1928). Myositis ossificans following suprapubic prostatectomy. *J. Urol.*, **20**: 477.

Lalykina, K. S. and Friedenstein, A. Y. (1969). Induction of the bone tissue in populations of lymphoid cells in guinea-pigs (in Russian). *Bull. Eksp. Biol. Med.*, **6**: 105–108.

Lash, J., Holtzer, S., and Holtzer, H. (1957). An experimental analysis of the development of the spinal column. Aspects of cartilage induction. *Exp. Cell Res.*, **13**: 292–303.

Lash, J., Holtzer, H., and Whitehouse, M. W. (1960). In vitro studies on chondrogenesis: the uptake of radioactive sulfate during cartilage induction. *Dev. Biol.*, **2**: 76–89.

Lewis, D. (1923). Myositis ossificans. *JAMA*, **80**: 281–286.

Liek, E. (1908). Ein weiterer Beitrag zur heteroplastischen Knochenbuldung in Nieren. *Arch. Klin. Chir.*, **58**: 118–123.

Lindholm, T. S. and Urist, M. R. (1980). A quantitative analysis of new bone formation by induction in composite grafts of bone marrow and bone matrix. *Clin. Orthop.*, **150**: 288–300.

Lo, T. C. M., Heady, W. L., Covall, D. J., Dotter, W. F., Pfeifer, B. A., Torgerson, W. R., and Wasilewski, S. A. (1988). Heterotopic bone formation after hip surgery: prevention with single-dose postoperative hip irradiation. *Radiology*, **168**: 851–854.

Loewl, G. (1954). The stimulation of osteogenesis by urinary bladder tissue. *J. Pathol. Bacteriol.*, **68**: 419–422.

Lohela, P., Orava, S., and Leinonen, A. (1983). Heterotopic bone formation in abdominal midline scars. *Fortsch. Roentgenstr.*, **139**: 412–415.

Lorenzi, B. M. and Batacchi, G. (1951). Ricerche sul comportamento degli etero-innesti di epitello urinario. *Sperimentale*, **101**: 30–36.

Makin, M. (1962). Osteogenesis induced by vesical mucosal transplant in the guinea pig. *J. Bone Jt. Surg.*, **44B**: 165–193.

Mardon, H. J., Bee, J., Von der Mark, K., and Owen, M. (1987). Development of osteogenic tissue in diffusion chambers from early precursor cells in bone marrow of adult rats. *Cell Tissue Res.*, **250**: 157–165.

Marmor, L. (1963). Bladder mucosa in osteogenesis. *Clin. Orthop.*, **40**: 82–91.

Marshal, V. F. and Spellman, R. M. (1957). Free grafts of mucosa of the urinary bladder. I. For construction of a urethra in humans. II. For production of bone in dogs. *Plast. Reconstr. Surg.*, **20**: 423–436.

Mestel, A. L. and Spain, D. M. (1967). Differences in bone formation induced by urinary bladder autografts, homografts and pedicle grafts. *Exp. Mol. Pathol.*, **6**: 118–130.

Minor, R. R. (1973). Somite chondrogenesis. A structural analysis. *J. Cell Biol.*, **56**: 27–50.

Miskarova, E. D., Lalykina, K. S., Kokorin, I. N., and Friedenstein, A. (1970). Osteogenic potencies of prolonged diploid cultures of myeloid cells (in Russian). *Bull. Exp. Biol. Med.*, **9**: 78–81.

Miyral, B. (1956). Experimental bone formation induced by gastric epithelium. *Trans. Jpn. Pathol. Soc.*, **45**: 645–651.

Moskalewski, S. (1963). Studies on the osteogenetic properties of uncultured isolated cells of the transitional epithelium. *Bull. Acad. Pol. Sci. Ser. Sci. Biol.*, **11**: 303–307.

Moskalewski, S. (1963). Studies on the osteogenetic properties of uncultured and cultured gallbladder epithelium. *Bull. Acad. Pol. Sci. Ser. Sci. Biol.*, **11**: 297–301.

Moskalewski, S. and Malejczyk, J. (1989). Bone formation following intrarenal transplantation of isolated murine chondrocytes: chondrocyte — bone cell transdifferentiation?. *Development*, **107**: 473–480.

Nade, S. and Burwell, R. G. (1977). Decalcified bone as a substrate for osteogenesis. An appraisal of the interrelation of bone and marrow in combined graft. *J. Bone Jt. Surg.*, **59B**: 189–196.

Neuhoff, H. (1917). Fascia transplantation into visceral defects. *Surg. Gynecol. Obstet.*, **26**: 383–427.

Nilsen, R. (1980). Electronmicroscopic study on mineralization in induced heterotopic bone formation in guinea-pig. *Scand. J. Dent. Res.*, **88**: 340–347.

Nilsen, R. and Magnusson, B. C. (1981). Enzyme histochemical studies of acid phosphatase isoenzymes in induced heterotopic bone formation in guinea-pigs. *Scand. J. Dent. Res.*, **89**: 485–490.

Nimni, M. E., Bernick, S., Ertl, D., Nishimoto, S. K., Paule, W., Strates, B. S., and Villanueva, J. (1988). Ectopic bone formation is enhanced in senescent animals implanted with embryonic cells. *Clin. Orthop.*, **234**: 249–253.

Nishimoto, S. K., Chang, C. H., Gendler, E., Stryker, W. F., and Nimni, M. E. (1985). The effect of aging on bone formation in rats. Biochemical and histological evidence for decreased bone forming capacity. *Calcif. Tissue Int.*, **37**: 617–624.

Nisson, O. S., Bauer, H. C. F., Brostrom, L. A., and Brosjo, O. (1986). Methotrexate effects on turnover of induced heterotopic and orthotopic bone. *Calcif. Tissue Int. Suppl.*, **39**: 78 (abstr.).

Ohgushi, H., Goldberg, V. H., and Caplan, A. I. (1989). Heterotopic osteogenesis in porous ceramics induced by marrow cells. *J. Orthop. Res.*, **7**: 568–578.

Orzel, J. A. and Rudd, T. G. (1985). Heterotopic bone formation: clinical, laboratory, and imaging correlation. *J. Nucl. Med.*, **26**: 125–132.

Ostrowski, K., Kostek, T., Wilczyński, M., and Orlowski, W. J. (1957). Investigations on the mechanism of induction of osteogenesis by way of grafts of urinary bladder mucosa. *Bull. Acad. Pol. Sci. Ser. Sci. Biol.*, **5**: 131–132.

Ostrowski, K. and Moskalewski, S. (1962). Investigations on the induced osteogenesis by transplants of urinary bladder mucosa and transitional epithelium cultured *in vitro*. In: *Vergleichungen des I Europalschen Anatomen-Kongresses*. Watzka, M. and Voss, H., Eds., Strasbourg, 225–231.

Ostrowski, K., Rymaszewska, T., Moskalewski, S., Wlodarski, K., and Zaleski, M. (1967). Experimental data on bone induction and bone antigenicity. *Symp. Biol. Hung.*, **7**: 227–240.

Ostrowski, K. and Wilczyński, M. (1958). Badania nad szybkoscia przemiany mineralnej tkanki kostnej indukowanej przeszczepami biony sluzowej pecherza moczowego przy pomocy isotopu promieniotworczego P-32. *Folia Morphol. (Warszawa)*, **4**: 343–346.

Ostrowski, K. and Wlodarski, K. (1971). Induction of heterotopic bone formation. In: *Biochemistry and Physiology of Bone*, Vol. 3, 2nd ed. Bourne, G. H., Ed., Academic Press, New York, 299–336.

Ostrowski, K., Wlodarski, K. H., and Aden, D. (1975). Heterotopic chondrogenesis induced by transformed cells. Use of nude mice as a model system. *Somat. Cell Genet.*, **1**: 391–395.

Ostrowski, K. Wojtowicz, A., Dziedzic-Goclawska, A., and Rozycka, M. (1988). Effect of 1-hydroxyethylidene-1,1-bisphosphonate (HEBP) and dichloromethylidene-bisphosphonate (C12MBP) on the structure of the organic matrix of heterotopically induced bone tissue. *Histochemistry*, **88**: 207–212.

Owen, M. (1980). The origin of bone cells in the postnatal organisms. *Arthritis Rheum.*, **23**: 1073–1080.

Pearce, R. M. (1909). Notes on the later stages of the repair of kidney tissue (dog) with special reference to proliferation of the pelvic epithelium and heteroplastic bone formation. *J. Med. Res.*, **20**: 53–58.

Pfeifer, C. A. (1948). Development of bone from transplanted bone marrow in mice. *Anat. Rec.*, **102**: 225–240.

Quesenberry, P., Song, Z., Alberico, T., Gualtieri, R., Stewart, M., Innes, D., McGrath, E., Cranston, S., and Kleeman, E. (1985). Bone marrow adherent cell hemopoietic growth factor production. In: *Hematopoietic Stem Cell Physiology*, Smith, A., Ed., Alan R. Liss, New York, 247–256.

Rath, N. C. and Reddi, A. H. (1979). Influence of adrenalectomy and dexamethasone on matrix-induced endochondral bone differentiation. *Endocrinology*, **104**: 1698–1704.

Reddi, A. H. and Anderson, W. A. (1976). Collagenous bone matrix-induced endochondral ossification and hemopoiesis. *J. Cell Biol.*, **69**: 557–572.

Reddi, A. H. (1976). Collagen and cell differentiation. In: *Biochemistry of Collagen*. Remachandran, G. H. and Reddi, A. H., Eds., Plenum Press, New York, 449–478.

Ritter, M. A. and Gioe, T. J. (1982). The effect of indomethacine on paraarticular ossification following total hip arthroplasty. *Clin. Orthop.*, **167**: 113–117.

Ritter, M. A. and Vaughan, R. B. (1977). Ectopic ossification after total hip arthroplasty: predisposing factors, frequency, and effect on results. *J. Bone Jt. Surg.*, **59A**: 345–351.

Roberts, D., Leighton, J., Abaza, N., and Troll, W. (1974). Heterotopic urinary bladders in rats produced by an issograft inoculum of bladder fragments and air. *Cancer Res.*, **34**: 2773–2778.

Roth, S. (1973). A molecular model for cell interactions. *Q. Rev. Biol.*, **48**: 541–563.

Sampath, T. K., Mutukumaran, N., and Reddi, A. H. (1987). Isolation of osteogenin, an extracellular matrix-associated bone inductive protein by heparin-affinity chromatography. *Proc. Natl. Acad. Sci. U.S.A.*, **84**: 7109–7113.

Shipton, E. A. and Indyk, J. S. (1957). Heterotopic bone formation in the gall-bladder. *Med. J. Aust.*, **44**: 9–11.

Solarczyk, K. and Moskalewski, S. (1989). Bone induction by urinary bladder epithelium from butchered animals. *Bull. Pol. Acad. Sci. Biol. Ser.*, **37**: 85–89.

Solursh, M. (1989). Extracellular matrix and cell surface as determinants of conective tissue differentiation. *Am. J. Med. Genet.*, **34**: 30–34.

Spencer, J. D. and Missen, G. A. K. (1989). Pseudomalignant heterotopic ossification ("myositis ossificans"). Recurrence after excision with subsequent resorption. *J. Bone Jt. Surg.*, **71B**: 317–319.

Strauss, A. A. (1914). An artificial ureter made from the abdominal wall. *Surg. Gynecol. Obstet.*, **18**: 78–84.

Sylvester, J. E., Greenberg, P., Seich, M. T., Thomas, B. J., and Amstutz, H. (1988). The use of postoperative irradiation for the prevention of heterotopic bone formation after total hip replacement. *Int. J. Radiat. Oncol. Biol. Phys.*, **14**: 471–476.

Tabuchi, C., Simmons, D. J., Fausto, A., Binderman, I., and Avioli, L. V. (1989). Effect of dihydrotachysterol on bone induction in ovariectomized rats. *Bone Miner.*, **5**: 359–370.

Tabuci, C., Simmons, D. J., Fausto, A., Russel, J. E., Binderman, I., and Avioli, L. V. (1986). Bone deficit in ovariectomized rats. Functional contribution of the marrow stromal cell population and the effect of oral dihydrotachysterol treatment. *J. Clin. Invest.*, **78**: 637–642.

Takagi, K. and Urist, M. R. (1982). The role of bone marrow in bone morphogenetic protein-induced repair of femoral massive diaphyseal defects. *Clin. Orthop.*, **171**: 224–231.

Talwar, H. S., Reddi, A. H., Menczel, J., Thomas, W. C., Jr., and Meyer, J. L. (1986). Influence of aluminum on mineralization during matrix-induced bone development. *Kidney Int.*, **29**: 1038–1042.

Tanaka, H., Seino, Y., Shima, M., Yamaoka, K., Yabuchi, H., Yoshikawa, H., Masuhara, K., Takaoka, K., and Ono, K. (1988). Effect of phosphorus supplementation on bone formation induced by osteosarcoma-derived bone-inducing substance in X-linked hypophosphatemic mice. *Bone Miner.*, **4**: 237–246.

Thomas, B. J. and Amstutz, H. C. (1985). Results of the administration of diphosphonate for the prevention of heterotopic ossification after total hip arthroplasty. *J. Bone Jt. Surg.*, **67A**: 400–403.

Thompson, J. S. and Urist, M. R. (1973). Opposing actions of calcitonin and cortisone upon osteogenesis in a heterotopic site. *Clin. Orthop.*, **90**: 201–208.

Thorogood, P. V. and Hall, B. K. (1976). The use of variable lactate/malic dehydrogenase ratios to distinguish between progenitor cells of cartilage and bone in the embryonic chick. *J. Embryol. Exp. Morphol.*, **36**: 305–313.

Triffitt, J. T. (1987). Initiation and enhancement of bone formation. *Acta Orthop. Scand.*, **58**: 673–684.

Trueta, J. (1963). The role of the vessels in osteogenesis. *J. Bone Jt. Surg.*, **45B**: 401–418.

Tyler, M. S. (1989). Promotion of osteogenesis by extraembryonic epithelia in maxillary mesenchyma of the embryonic chick. *Arch. Oral Biol.*, **34**: 387–391.

Tyler, M. S. (1983). Development of the frontal bone and cranial meninges in the embryonic chick: an experimental study of tissue interaction. *Anat. Rec.*, **206**: 61–70.

Urist, M. R. (1965). Bone: formation by autoinduction. *Science*, **150**: 893–899.

Urist, M. R. (1971). Bone histogenesis and morphogenesis in implants of demineralized enamel and dentin. *J. Oral Surg.*, **2**: 88–102.

Urist, M. R., Huo, Y. K., Brownell, A. G., Hohl, W. M., Buyske, J., Lietze, A., Tempst, P., Haukapiller, M., and DeLange, R. J. (1984). Purification of bovine bone morphogenetic protein by hydroxyapatite chromatography. *Proc. Natl. Acad. Sci. U.S.A.*, **81**: 371–375.

Urist, M. R. and McLean, F. C. (1952). Osteogenic potency and new bone formation by induction of transplants to the anterior chamber of the eye. *J. Bone Jt. Surg.*, **34A**: 443–470.

Urist, M. R., Nakagawa, M., Nakata, N., and Nogami, H. (1978). Experimental myositis ossificans. Cartilage and bone formation in muscle in response to a diffusible bone-matrix-derived morphogen. *Arch. Pathol. Lab. Med.*, **102**: 312–316.

Van de Putte, K. A. and Urist, M. R. (1965). Osteogenesis in the interior of intramuscular implants of decalcified bone matrix. *Clin. Orthop.*, **43**: 257–270.

Wang, E. A., Rosen, V., Cordes, P., Hewick, R. M., Kriz, M. J., Luxenberg, D. P., Sibley, B. S., and Wozney, J. M. (1988). Purification and characterization of other distinct bone-inducing factors. *Proc. Natl. Acad. Sci. U.S.A.*, **85**: 9484–9488.

Weiss, R. E., Field, L., Gorn, A., Williams, C., Dux, S., Ravichandra, R., Gallo, A. A., Eswarakrishnan, V., and Nimni, M. E. (1984). Influence of penicillamine and various analogs on matrix-induced bone formation in rats. *Biochem. Med.*, **32**: 331–336.

Weiss, R. E., Singer, F. R., Gorn, A. H., and Hofer, D. P. (1981). Calcitonin stimulates bone formation when administered prior to initiation of osteogenesis. *J. Clin. Invest.*, **68**: 815–818.

Wieniawska-Szewczyk, E. (1988). Effect of various immunosuppressants on heterotopic and orthotopic osteogenesis (in Polish). Doctoral thesis. Medical Academy in Warszawa, Poland.

Wight, P. A. L. and Duff, S. R. I. (1985). Ectopic pulmonary cartilage and bone in domestic fowl. *Res. Vet. Sci.*, **39**: 188–195.

Williams, L. M., Fahrere, W., and Rintoul, J. R. (1970). Electron microscopic observation of transitional epithelium of the urinary bladder of guinea-pig. *J. Anat.*, **106**: 409.

Wlodarski, K. (1984). Induction of heterotopic and orthotopic cartilage and bone formation in mice. *Acta Biol. Hung.*, **35**: 205–218.

Wlodarski, K. (1982). Heterotopic bone marrow formation in xenogeneic implants of insoluble bone matrix gelatin. *Clin. Orthop.*, **171**: 210–212.

Wlodarski, K. (1978). Failure of heterotopic osteogenesis by epithelial mesenchymal cell interactions in xenogeneic transplants in the kidney. *Calcif. Tissue Res.*, **25**: 7–11.

Wlodarski, K. (1969). The inductive properties of epithelial established cell lines. *Exp. Cell Res.*, **57**: 446–448.

Wlodarski, K. (1990). Properties and origin of osteoblasts. *Clin. Orthop.*, **252**: 276–293.

Wlodarski, K. H. (1985). Orthotopic and ectopic chondrogenesis and osteogenesis mediated by neoplastic cells. *Clin. Orthop.*, **200**: 248–265.

Wlodarski, K. and Hancox, N. M. (1972). Antilymphocytic serum as immunosuppressant in experimental bone induction by xenogeneic epithelial cells. *Calcif. Tissue Res.*, **8**: 262–264.

Wlodarski, K., Hancox, N. M., and Brooks, B. (1973). The influence of cortisone and implantation site on bone and cartilage induction in various animals. *J. Bone Jt. Surg.*, **55B**: 595–603.

Wlodarski, K. H., Hinek, A., and Ostrowski, K. (1970). Investigations on cartilage and bone induction in mice grafted with FL and WISH line human amniotic cells. *Calcif. Tissue Res.*, **5**: 70–79.

Wlodarski, K. and Jakóbisiak, M. (1981). Heterotopic induction of osteogenesis in mice lethally irradiated and repopulated with syngeneic bone marrow cells. *Arch. Immunol. Ther. Exp.*, **29**: 509–514.

Wlodarski, K. and Jakóbisiak, M. (1978a). Cytological analysis of bone marrow present in the bone nodules induced by human FL cells in mice. *Folia Biol. (Praha)*, **24**: 215–218.

Wlodarski, K., Jakóbisiak, M., and Janowska-Wieczorek, A. (1980). Heterotopically induced bone marrow formation: morphology and transplantation. *Exp. Hematol.*, **8**: 1016–1023.

Wlodarski, K. H., Jakóbisiak, M., and Kossakowska, A. (1976a). Quantitative and morphological analysis of bone marrow associated with bone induction phenomenon in mice. *Folia Haematol. (Leipzig)*, **103**: 177–182.

Wlodarski, K. H., Jakóbisiak, M., and Zaleska-Rutczynska, Z. (1976b). Colony forming units (CFU) in bone marrow associated with heterotopic bone formation by epithelial cells grafted in mice. *Arch. Immunol. Ther. Exp.*, **24**: 395–400.

Wlodarski, K. H. and Jakóbisiak, M. (1978b). Heterotopically induced bone marrow. I. Cellular composition of bone marrow derived from the heterotopic ossicles induced in mice by xenogenic epithelia of human amnion and dog's transitional epithelium. *Arch. Immunol. Ther. Exp.*, **26**: 1027–1031.

Wlodarski, K., Kobus, M., and Luczak, M. (1979). Orthotopic bone induction at sites of Moloney sarcoma virus inoculation in mice. *Nature*, **281**: 386–387.

Wlodarski, K., Moskalewski, S., Skarzyńska, S., Poltorak, A., and Ostrowski, K. (1971a). Irradiation and the bone inductive properties of epithelial cells. *Bull. Acad. Pol. Sci. Ser. Sci. Biol.*, **19**: 821–825.

Wlodarski, K. and Ostrowski, K. (1979). Further investigations on possible correlation between agglutinability and osteoinductive properties of established cell lines. *Arch. Immunol. Ther. Exp.*, **27**: 113–119.

Wlodarski, K. and Ostrowski, K. (1975). Investigations on the properties of established cell lines of human origin to induce cartilage and bone and properties of human fibroblasts transformed by varicella virus. *Mater. Med. Polona*, **7**: 3–7.

Wlodarski, K., Ostrowski, K., Chlopkiewicz, B., and Koziorowska, J. (1974). Correlation between the agglutinability of living cells by Concanavalin A and their ability to induce cartilage and bone formation. *Calcif. Tissue Res.*, **16**: 251–255.

Wlodarski, K., Poltorak, A., and Koziorowska, J. (1971b). Species specificity of osteogenesis induced by WISH cell line and bone induction by vaccinia virus transformed human fibroblasts. *Calcif. Tissue Res.*, **7**: 345–352.

Wlodarski, K., Poltorak, A., Zaleski, M., and Ostrowski, K. (1971c). Bone induction evoked in mouse by xenogenic grafts of the transitional epithelium. *Experientia*, **27**: 688–689.

Wlodarski, K. H. and Reddi, A. H. (1986a). Alkaline phosphatase as a marker of osteoinductive cells. *Calcif. Tissue Int.*, **39**: 382–385.

Wlodarski, K. H. and Reddi, A. H. (1986b). Heterotopically induced bone does not develop functional periosteal membrane. *Arch. Immunol. Ther. Exp.*, **34**: 583–593.

Wlodarski, K. H. and Reddi, A. H. (1986c). The age-dependence of endochondral bone formation in mice. Biochemical evidence for decreased bone forming capacity. *Bull. Pol. Acad. Sci. Ser. Biol. Sci.*, **34**: 155–159.

Wlodarski, K. H. and Reddi, A. H. (1986d). Importance of skeletal muscle environment for ectopic bone induction in mice. *Folia Biol. (Krakow)*, **34**: 425–434.

Wozney, J. M., Rosen, V., Celeste, A. J., Mitsock, L. M., Whitters, M. J., Kriz, R. W., Hewick, R. M., and Wang, E. A. (1988). Novel regulators of bone formation: molecular clones and activities. *Science*, **242**: 1528–1534.

Yarkony, G. M., Lee, M. Y., Green, D., and Roth, E. (1989). Heterotopic ossification pseudophlebitis. *Am. J. Med.*, **87**: 342–344.

Yoshikawa, H., Hashimoto, J., Masuhara, K., Takaoka, K., and Ono, K. (1989). Inhibition by tumor necrosis factor of induction of ectopic bone formation by osteosarcoma-derived bone-inducing substance. *Bone*, **9**: 391–396.

Zaleski, M. (1960). Obserwacje morfologiczne przeszczepow homogennych sciany pecherza moczowego chomlow syryjskich *(Mesocricetus auratus)*. *Folia Morphol. (Warszawa)*, **12**: 275–266.

Zaleski, M. (1961). Zachowanie sie tkanki kostnej indukowanej przez przeszczepy homogenne sciany pecherza moczowego swinki morskiej. *Folia Morphol. (Warszawa)*, **12**: 267–277.

Zaleski, M. (1962). The structure and development of induced bone tissue. *Bull. Acad. Pol. Sci. Ser. Sci. Biol.*, **10**: 555–558.

Zaleski, M., Krassowski, T., and Wlodarski, K. H. (1963). Attempts of bone induction by heterogeneous grafts of urinary bladder mucosa. *Folia Morphol. (Warszawa)*, **14**: 45–51.

Zaleski, T. and Moskalewski, S. (1963). Investigation on autologus transplants of urinary bladder wall in mouse. *Bull. Acad. Pol. Sci. Ser. Sci. Biol.*, **11**: 403–406.

Zarrin, K. (1977). The bone inducing capacity of syngeneic thyroid tissue in guinea-pig muscle. *J. Pathol.*, **125**: 99–101.

Index

A

abdominal scars, bone formation if postoperative, 323

β-acetylglucosaminidase, increase of in bony callus, 15

achondroplasia, 249

acid phosphatase
demonstration of in ossifying cells, 15
increase of in bony callus, 15
post coupling reactions for, 5
presence of in proliferating cartilage, 14

acidic fibroblast growth factor (aFGF), 211, 145

acidic polysaccharides, presence of in rabbit fracture callus, 97

adenosine triphosphate, in proliferative zone cells, 236

adhesive substances, 129

aerobic glycolysis, 14

aFGF, *see* acidic fibroblast growth factor

Alcian Blue, binding of, 105

alkaline phosphatase, 16, 101
activity of in cartilage, 14
activity of in rat metatarsal, 18, 21, 22
appearance of in early fibrocartilage, 15
association between endochondral calcification and, 16
effect of vitamin B_6 deficiency on activity of, 24
increase in activity of, 14
metabolic activity of in cortical and trabecular bone from human iliac crest biopsies, 10
periosteal activity of, 23
presence of in proliferative stages of fracture healing, 20
simultaneous capture reaction for, 5

allogeneic embryonal chick chondrocytes, 135

allogeneic transplantation, *see* xenogeneic transplantation

aluminium salt, 328

aminopeptidase, activity of, 15

amphibians, limb regeneration in, 263, 297, 306

amputation plane, 295, 298, 303

amputation sites, 308

anaerobic glycolysis, 14

angiogenesis, local inhibition of, 97

arthrograph, assessment of knee contracture using, 37

arthroplasty surface, conversion of to fibrocartilage, 46

arthroscopy, treatment of knee contractures, 51

articular cartilage, 35, 111, 124
cartilaginous adaptation in, 51
changes of, 36
fracture lines in, 47
lack of at extremities, 275
repair of, 140
role of fluid movement in, 40
treatment of by activity protocols, 45

articular defects, 142

articular surface replacement matrix, composition of by fibrocartilage, 46

autogenous bone graft, 224

B

basement membrane
lack of in apical epithelium, 298
proteinous component of, 314

basic fibroblast growth factor (bFGF), 211

BDGF, *see* bone-derived growth factor

bFGF, *see* basic fibroblast growth factor

biochemical studies, fibrous collagen identified by, 90

Bioglass, 170–171

biological resorbable immobilizing vehicles (BRIV), 129

blastema, 293

blood supply, changes in, 234

blood vessels
cartilaginous segment reabsorbed by, 246
fibrous tissue with, 79
lack of, 97
maintenance of, 84

blood-borne cells, 64

BMP, *see* bone morphogenetic protein

bone
biological repair of, 123
expression of mRNA in, 93

position of, 36
immobilized animals, recovery from stress
    deprivation in, 39
immobilized joints, 35, 37
immobilized limbs
  changes in capsular and ligamentous
      structures of, 37
  in fiberglass cast, 48
immobilized rabbit, cross-linking of collagen
      from, 42
immune reaction, 130, 131
immunohistochemical investigations, 90
immunosuppression, 130
immunosuppressive agents, 131
implant, introduction of into body, 153
implantation, site of, 138
implants
  quality tests, 125
  reconstitution, 128
  solid framework, 137
in situ hybridization, 97
inducible osteoprogenitor cells (IOPC), 323
inductive molecules, 145
inductive stimuli, target for, 315
inherited connective tissue, 117
inomethacin, nonsteroidal anti-inflammatory
      therapy with, 323
integrins, 34, 53
intermedullary nail, 104
intermittent passive motion, blocking of
      extrinsic mechanism by, 48
internal callus, 142
internal fixation, 61–63
interrupted motion, philosophy of early
      mobilization, 44
IOPC, *see* inducible osteoprogenitor cells

J

joint transplantation, 261
junctional cartilage, 264, 269–271
  ablation of by reamputation series, 276
  physeal cell architecture in, 280
  total excision of, 275

K

keratan sulfate, 26, 100, 109
  antibodies to, 111, 112
  confirmation of using monoclonal
      antibodies, 105
  presence of in cartilaginous matrix, 106
kidney, transplantation under, 324

knee arthroplasties, 176–177
knee immobilization, 36
knee joint, disuse of, 53
Krebs cycle, enzymes related to, 15

L

Lacroix, perichondrial ring of, 237, 238
lactate
  activity of in callus, 14
  production of under aerobic conditions, 8
lactate dehydrogenase
  activity of in callus of rat metatarsal, 22
  change in activity of, 13
  enzymatic activity of in metatarsal growth
      plate, 10
  metabolic activity of in cortical and
      trabecular bone from human iliac
      crest biopsies, 10
laminin, adhesion of cells to, 53
leg length discrepancy, 249
leucine aminopeptidase
  activity of in resting osteocytes, 15
  appearance of in early fibrocartilage, 15
leucine naphthylamidase, use of to define
      osteoclastic activity, 22
ligament tissue, adhesive protein receptors of,
      53–54
limb development, 80, 82
lipids, 236
long bones, healing of, 61
longitudinal growth, inhibition of, 243
longitudinally directed screws, 171
low oxygen tension, occurrence of differen-
      tiation into chondrocytes, 27
lysosomal enzyme, activity of throughout
      fracture callus, 22
lysosomes, fragility of, 19

M

macrophages, 69, 75, 77, 79
macroporous stem implants, 157
macrorough and microrough surfaces, 167
Madreporique hip prosthesis, 168
malic dehydrogenase, activity of in callus, 14
mammalian limb regeneration, attempted
      induction of, 304
mammalian regeneration, 308
marrow stromal cells, 324
massive segmental defects, 141
matrix coat, immunoprotection, 128
matrix flow phenomenon, in cartilage, 125

transforming growth factor α, 213
transforming growth factor β, 211, 213, 326
transplantation antigens, 133
transversally directed screws, 171–173
trauma, 280
  control of in bone surgery, 192
  inflammatory response to, 9
  at insertion of implants, 191
  regeneration induced by, 275
  repeated surgical, 281
  treatments, 306
  unrelated forms of, 274
two-stage surgical procedure, 194

U

undifferentiated callus, presence of acid
    phosphatase in, 15
uninjured cartilage, interstitial growth of, 282
unstable fractures
  callus of, 93
  presence of type II collagen in, 95
unstable mechanical conditions, healing
    under, 105
urinary bladder mucosa, auto- and allogeneic
    implants of, 317
urinary tract mucosa, autologous grafts of,
    315

V

vaccinia-virus transformed fibroblasts, 318
varicella-virus transformed fibroblasts, 318
vascular supply, in mammalian growth plate,
    235
very late antigens (VLA), 53
viscoelastic properties, importance of fluid
    movement in importing, 40
vitamin B_6, effect of deficiency, 24

vitamin B_6 deficient diet, delay in callus
    maturation in rats fed, 24
vitamin D deficiency, 130
vitamin K cycle
  antagonistic effect against vitamin K_1 in, 23
  inhibition of, 22–23
  use of NADPH in, 27
vitamins, influence of on speed of fracture
    healing, 22
VLA, *see* very late antigens

W

Wagner cup, 160
water content, paralleling of to GAG ranges,
    40
Wolff's Law, 35
wound epidermis, in frogs, 274
wound healing, 50, 124
woven bone, 3
  features of young, 316
  formation of, 302
  generation of new, 296
  ossification with areas of, 11
  osteoblasts of in rat fracture callus, 19
  remodeling, 292
  sealing of marrow by, 300

X

X-linked hypophosphatemic mice, 327
xenogeneic cultured cartilage, 131
xenogeneic embryonal chick chondrocytes,
    132
xenogeneic transplantation, 124, 131, 223

Z

Zweymüller prosthesis, 168